The Echo Manual

The Echo Manual

from the
Mayo Clinic

Jae K. Oh, M.D.
Consultant, Division of Cardiovascular Diseases and Internal Medicine,
Mayo Clinic and Mayo Foundation; Associate Professor of Medicine,
Mayo Medical School, Rochester, Minnesota

James B. Seward, M.D.
Director, Cardiovascular Ultrasound Imaging and Hemodynamic Laboratory,
Mayo Clinic and Mayo Foundation; Professor of Medicine and Pediatrics,
Mayo Medical School, Rochester, Minnesota

A. Jamil Tajik, M.D.
Chair, Division of Cardiovascular·Diseases, and Thomas J. Watson, Jr., Professor,
Mayo Clinic and Mayo Foundation; Professor of Medicine and Pediatrics,
Mayo Medical School, Rochester, Minnesota

Little, Brown and Company
Boston   New York   Toronto   London

Library of Congress Cataloging-in-Publication Data

Oh, Jae K.
    The echo manual / Jae K. Oh, James B. Seward, A. Jamil Tajik.
        p.   cm.
    Includes bibliographical references and index.
    ISBN 0-316-63374-7
    1. Echocardiography—Handbooks, manuals, etc. I. Seward, J.B.
(James B.) II. Tajik, A. Jamil. III. Title.
    [DNLM: 1. Echocardiography—handbooks. WG 39 036e 1994]
RC683.5.U5O37   1994
616.1′2′07543—dc20
DNLM/DLC
for Library of Congress   93-27159
                                                      CIP

Printed in the United States of America

KP

Second   Printing

Editorial: Nancy Chorpenning
Production Editor: Marie A. Salter
Copyeditor: Mary Babcock
Indexer: Dorothy Hoffman
Production Supervisor/Designer:
    Michael A. Granger
Cover Designer: Linda Dana Willis

Contents

Preface   ix

1. Overview   1
Development of Echocardiography   1
Echocardiography at the Mayo Clinic   2
Examination   2
   Operator   2
   Instrumentation   3
   Patient   5

2. Transthoracic Echocardiography   7
M-mode and 2D Echocardiography   7
Doppler Echocardiography   15
Color-Flow Imaging   18

3. Transesophageal Echocardiography   21
Instrumentation   21
Patient Preparation   22
Anatomic Correlations   22
   Horizontal Plane   23
   Longitudinal Plane   24
   Multiplane   31
   Thoracic Aorta   34
Clinical Applications   35
Complications   35
Training and Role of Sonographer   35
Future Development   36

4. Assessment of Ventricular Function   39
Quantitation of the Left Ventricle   39
   Dimensions and Area   41
   Volume   41
   Mass   41
Systolic Function   43
   Global Function   43
   Regional Function   44
Diastolic Filling Profiles   46
   Definition of Diastole   46
   Abnormal Relaxation   47

Restrictive Physiology   47
Pseudonormalization   49
Venous Flow Pattern in Diastolic Filling
   Assessment   49
Automated Edge Detection System   50

5. Hemodynamic Assessment   51
Doppler Echocardiography   52
   Stroke Volume and Cardiac Output   52
   Regurgitant Volume and Regurgitant
      Fraction   55
   Pulmonary-Systemic Flow Ratio
      (Qp/Qs)   55
   Transvalvular Gradients   55
   Valve Area   58
   Intracardiac Pressures   60
   Systolic and Diastolic Function   61
   Time Constant of Left Ventricular
      Relaxation Time (TAU)   64

6. Coronary Artery Disease   67
Regional Wall Motion Analysis   67
   Technical Caveats   69
Digital Echocardiography   69
Stress Echocardiography   70
   Caveats for Technical and
      Interpretation Skills   72
Acute Myocardial Infarction   72
   Evaluation of Chest Pain Syndromes   72
   Role of Echocardiography in the
      Emergency Room   73
   Detection of Complications   73
   Evaluation of Reperfusion Therapy   80
   Evaluation of Stunned and Hibernating
      Myocardium   81
   Post–Myocardial Infarction Risk
      Stratification   82
Diastolic Function   82
Coronary Artery Visualization   82
Intravascular Ultrasound   84
Clinical Impact   84

7. **Valvular Heart Disease**   **87**
   Evaluation of Valvular Stenosis   87
      Aortic Stenosis   88
      Mitral Stenosis   96
   Evaluation of Valvular
      Regurgitation   100
   Aortic Regurgitation   101
   Mitral Regurgitation   104
   Tricuspid Regurgitation   109
   Valvular Regurgitation in Normal
      Subjects   110
   Transesophageal Echocardiography   110
   Clinical Impact   113

8. **Prosthetic Valve Evaluation**   **117**
   Obstruction   120
      Calculation of Effective Prosthetic
         Orifice Area   123
   Regurgitation   123
   Transesophageal Echocardiography   124
   Clinical Impact   124
      Caveat   127

9. **Infective Endocarditis**   **129**
   Diagnosis   129
   Complications   132
   Transesophageal Echocardiography   133
   Echocardiographic-Pathologic
      Correlation   135
   Limitations and Pitfalls   135

10. **Cardiomyopathies**   **137**
   Dilated Cardiomyopathy   137
      2D Echocardiography   137
      Doppler (Pulsed-Wave, Continuous-
         Wave) and Color-Flow Imaging   139
      Familial Dilated Cardiomyopathy
         and Arrhythmogenic Right
         Ventricular Dysplasia   139
   Hypertrophic Cardiomyopathy   140
      2D/M-mode Echocardiography   140
      Doppler (Pulsed-Wave, Continuous-
         Wave) and Color-Flow Imaging   143
      Transesophageal Echocardiography   146
      Limitations and Pitfalls   147
   Restrictive Cardiomyopathy   149

11. **Cardiac Diseases due to Systemic
    Illness**   **153**
   Amyloidosis   154
   Carcinoid   157
   Hemochromatosis   159

   Hypereosinophilic Syndrome   160
   Sarcoidosis   160
   Systemic Lupus Erythematosus   161
   Other Conditions   162

12. **Pericardial Diseases**   **165**
   Pericardial Effusion/Tamponade   165
      Echo-guided Pericardiocentesis   166
   Constrictive Pericarditis   166
   Congenitally Absent Pericardium   172
   Pericardial Cyst   173
   Pericardial Effusion Versus Pleural
      Effusion   173
   Transesophageal Echocardiography   173
   Clinical Impact   175

13. **Pulmonary Hypertension**   **177**
   2D Echocardiography   177
   Doppler Echocardiography   178
      Tricuspid Regurgitation Velocity   178
      Right Ventricular Outflow Tract Flow
         Acceleration Time   180
      Pulmonary Regurgitation Velocity   180
   Cor Pulmonale and Pulmonary
      Embolism   182
      Transthoracic Echocardiography   182
      Transesophageal Echocardiography   183

14. **Tumors and Masses**   **185**
   Primary Tumor   185
   Metastatic Tumor and Other
      Masses   188
   Transesophageal Echocardiography   189
   Role of Echocardiography in
      Nonrheumatic Atrial Fibrillation   191
   Pseudotumor—Pitfalls   191

15. **Diseases of the Aorta**   **195**
   Aortic Dissection   196
      Transthoracic Echocardiography   196
      Transesophageal Echocardiography   198
   Other Pathologies   200
      Aortic Rupture   200
      Aortic Debris   200
      Aortic Aneurysm   200
      Coarctation of the Aorta   203

16. **Congenital Heart Disease**   **205**
   Systematic Tomographic
      Approach   205
      Short-Axis View   206
      Long-Axis View   206
      Four-Chamber View   206

2D Examination 206
Step 1: Short-Axis Image of the
Upper Abdomen 207
Step 2: Long-Axis Image of the
Upper Abdomen 207
Step 3: Four-Chamber Image 207
Step 4: Precordial Examination 207
Overview of Adult Congenital
Heart Disease 207
Atrial Septal Defect 208
Outflow Tract Obstruction 209
Internal Cardiac Crux 210
Ventricular Septal Defect 214
Patent Ductus Arteriosus 216
Coarctation 217
Overriding Aorta 217
Pediatric Congenital Heart
Disease 217
Fetal Congenital Heart Disease 217
Heart Disease in Pregnancy 218
Transesophageal
Echocardiography 218
Wide-Field and 3D Imaging 218
Intraoperative
Echocardiography 220

17. **Intraoperative
Echocardiography** **221**
Mode 222
Implementation 222
Indications and Mitral Valve
Repair 222
Intraoperative Monitoring 227

18. **Echocardiography in
Conjunction with Other
Procedures or Techniques** **229**
Stress Echocardiography 229
Pericardiocentesis 229
Intraoperative Echocardiography 230
Mitral Balloon Valvuloplasty 230
Closure of Atrial Septal Defect or
Patent Foramen Ovale 230
Catheter Placement 231
Contrast Echocardiography for
Detection of Shunt 231

19. **Comprehensive Examination
According to the Referral
Diagnosis** **237**
Evaluation of Ventricular
Function 237
Evaluation of Dyspnea or Heart
Failure 238
Murmur or Mitral Valve Prolapse 238
Nonspecific ECG Abnormalities 238
Chest Pain 239
Cardiac Source of Emboli 239
Hypotension or Cardiogenic
Shock 240
Cardiac Contusion and Donor
Heart Evaluation 240
Systemic Hypertension 241

Index *243*

Preface

With the rapid advances in technology and clinical application of echocardiography, there is a need for a concise but comprehensive manual to assist proper performance, interpretation, and clinical use of this readily available diagnostic modality. Although there are several excellent echocardiography textbooks available, none is designed for quick reference. This manual provides readers with the basic concepts of echocardiographic examination, including the steps required to obtain adequate information, especially for Doppler examination, hemodynamic calculations, and echocardiographic differential diagnoses. The potential limitations of echocardiography are also discussed. The transesophageal approach has become such an integral part of the comprehensive echocardiographic examination that it is discussed throughout the manual to illustrate its characteristic images and clinical impact in various cardiovascular disorders.

In each chapter, the discussion of basic concepts and applications is supplemented by numerous schematic drawings, still-frames of actual echocardiographic images, and M-mode and Doppler-strip chart recordings to enhance the reader's comprehension. These valuable illustrations and examples were gathered from the patient files of the Mayo Clinic Cardiovascular Imaging and Hemodynamic Laboratory (formerly Echocardiography Laboratory), where more than 25,000 examinations are performed annually.

There are many individuals to whom we are indebted for the publication of this manual. We express our thanks to the entire medical and paramedical staff of our laboratory, for their superb echocardiographic skills, meticulous archiving, ability to quickly identify interesting cases (from more than 30,000 file tapes), and

unselfish dedication to patient care; to the cardiology fellows, for challenging existing concepts and making us better teachers; to members of Medical Graphics and Photography, for preparing "the best" figures; to Robert Benassi, for drawing all the schematics with precision and love of medical art; to members of the Section of Publications, for proofreading the manuscript; to the entire staff of Little, Brown, for accommodating the special needs of this manual (especially to Nancy Chorpenning, Editor-in-Chief, and Marie Salter, Production Editor, for their frequent reminders and telephone calls); and to Gail Ludens, Jamie Kramer, and Kristen Albee, for typing the manuscript and arranging the references during multiple revisions.

We are also grateful to Drs. Robert L. Frye and Hugh C. Smith, the Chair of the Department of Internal Medicine and the immediate past-Chair of the Division of Cardiovascular Diseases, respectively, as well as all colleagues in our division, the Department of Cardiovascular-Thoracic Surgery, and the Division of Cardiac Pathology, for their continuous support of research and development of echocardiography at Mayo.

Our parents deserve recognition for providing the guidance and support necessary for us to be where we are. Most of all, we are heavily indebted to our wives (Terry, Judith, and Zeest) and children, whose need for us was frequently sacrificed and whose loving support, understanding, and patience have kept us going all of these years. To them we dedicate this book.

JKO
JBS
AJT

Abbreviations

General

A	Anterior
Asc	Ascending
Dsc	Descending
L	Left, lateral
P	Posterior
R	Right
2D	Two-dimensional
3D	Three-dimensional

Anatomy

AL	Anterolateral papillary muscle
Ao, AO	Aorta
AS	Anteroseptum
AV	Aortic valve
AW	Anterior wall
B	Bronchus
D	Diastole, diastolic
E	Esophagus
FO	Fossa ovalis
IL	Inferolateral
IS	Inferoseptum
IVC	Inferior vena cava
LA	Left atrium
LAA	Left atrial appendage
LLPV	Left lower pulmonary vein
LUPV	Left upper pulmonary vein
LV	Left ventricle
LVOT	Left ventricular outflow tract
MV	Mitral valve
OT	Outflow tract
PM	Posteromedial papillary muscle
PV	Pulmonary vein
PW	Posterior wall
RA	Right atrium

RPA	Right pulmonary artery
RV	Right ventricle
S	Systole, systolic
SVC	Superior vena cava
TV	Tricuspid valve
VS	Ventricular septum

Echo and Diagnosis

A	Late-filling velocity
AFP	Atrial filling phase
AR	Aortic regurgitation
ARVD	Arrhythmogenic right ventricular dysplasia
AS	Aortic stenosis
AVA	Aortic valve area
CHF	Congestive heart failure
CM	Cardiomyopathy
CSA	Cross-sectional area
CW	Continuous-wave
D	Diameter
DT	Deceleration time
E	Early-filling velocity
EDP	End-diastolic pressure
EF	Ejection fraction
ET	Ejection time
IVRF	Isovolumic relaxation flow
IVRT	Isovolumic relaxation time
LAA	Left atrial area
LVED	Left ventricular end-diastole
LVEDP	Left ventricular end-diastolic pressure
LVES	Left ventricular end-systole
LVH	Left ventricular hypertrophy
MIG	Maximum instantaneous gradient
MVA	Mitral valve area
MVP	Mitral valve prolapse

PE	Pericardial effusion	RJA	Regurgitant jet area
PISA	Proximal isovelocity surface area	SAM	Systolic anterior motion
		$t^{1/2}$	Pressure half-time
PHT	Pressure half-time	(*also* PHT)	
(*also* $t^{1/2}$)		TEE	Transesophageal echocardiography
P-P	Peak-to-peak		
PRF	Pulse repetition frequency	TTE	Transthoracic echocardiography
PW	Pulsed-wave		
Qp/Qs	Pulmonary-systemic flow ratio	TVI	Time velocity integral
RES	Regional expansion selection	VSD	Ventricular septal defect
RF	Regurgitant fraction	WMSI	Wall motion score index
RFP	Rapid filling phase		

The Echo Manual

Overview

Development of Echocardiography

Echocardiography is a noninvasive diagnostic technique that utilizes high-frequency ultrasound (2.0–7.0 MHz) to evaluate structural, functional, and hemodynamic status of the cardiovascular system. Edler and Hertz of Sweden were the first to record movements of cardiac structures, in particular, the mitral valve, by ultrasound in 1954 [1]. The reflected ultrasound pattern was so distinctive in patients with mitral stenosis that it became diagnostic, and the severity of mitral stenosis could be semiquantitatively measured by analysis of the M-mode echocardiogram. In the United States, Joyner and Reid at the University of Pennsylvania were the first to use ultrasound to examine the heart [2]. Shortly after, in 1965, Feigenbaum, with his colleagues at Indiana University, reported the first ultrasound detection of pericardial effusion [3] and is responsible for introducing echocardiography into the clinical practice of cardiology. M-mode echocardiography, however, produced only an "ice pick" view of the heart; two-dimensional (2D) sector scanning, developed in the mid-1970s, allowed real-time tomographic images of cardiac morphology and function [4]. Although the development of Doppler echocardiography parallels that of M-mode and 2D echocardiography from the early 1950s, it was not clinically utilized until the late 1970s. Pressure gradients across a fixed orifice could be reliably obtained by blood flow velocities measured by Doppler echocardiography [5]. Numerous validation studies subsequently confirmed the accuracy of Doppler

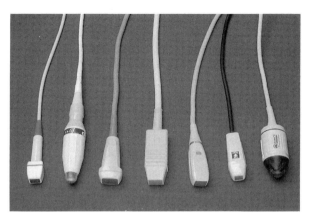

Fig. 1-1. Various transducers for transthoracic echocardiography with different sizes and shapes depending on the transducer ultrasound frequency, number of elements, and manufacturer.

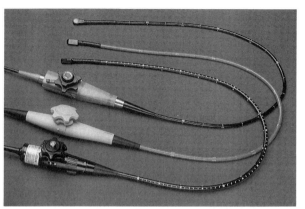

Fig. 1-2. Examples of a TEE probe. Transducers are mounted on the tip of an endoscopy probe. The distal end of the probe is maneuvered to different directions by a control knob at the other end of the probe. Usually there are two controls: one knob to move the tip side to side and another knob for antero-flexion or retroflexion. The position of the probe can also be locked in when it needs to remain at one location for an extended period. When the probe has biplane transducers, either the transverse or the longitudinal plane is selected. With a multiplane probe, the transducer rotates up to 180 degrees by dialing a control button at the operator's end. The distance from the tip of the probe is clearly shown on the shaft. (The length of a probe is usually 100–110 cm.)

ever, up to the individual echocardiographer to optimize the examination utilizing optimal transducer, knob settings, and transducer positions.

Diagnostic ultrasound requires a frequency of at least 2.0 MHz. As the sound frequency increases, there is less penetration of the ultrasound beam into the body tissue; therefore, the usual echocardiography examination in the adult begins with a 2.0- to 2.5-MHz transducer (Fig. 1-1). However, the image resolution improves with a higher-frequency transducer (i.e., shorter wavelength). In a thin individual or a pediatric patient, a 3.0- to 5.0-MHz transducer should provide adequate penetration and also improves the image resolution. In the TEE probe, a modification of an endoscopy probe (Fig. 1-2) with a higher-frequency (3.5–7.5-MHz) transducer is utilized since the distance between the transducer and the cardiac structure is quite short and is not interrupted greatly by other body tissues; therefore, the penetration is not as significant an issue. However, in the Doppler examination, a lower-frequency transducer is required to record high velocities since the measurable velocities are inversely proportional to the transmitted frequency (see Doppler equation in Chap. 5).

Once a proper transducer is selected, all the available ultrasound windows should be utilized. Gray scales and gains are manually con-

trolled to minimize background noise and to maximize the delineation of cardiac structures. The depth of the fields can be controlled to provide the optimal image size and depends on the goal of the study. When a certain structure needs to be carefully examined, a "zoom" or an "RES" (i.e., regional expansion selection) function can enlarge the selected portion of the image. Field depth is important during Doppler and color-flow imaging examinations since the Nyquist limit (i.e., the maximum velocity to be recorded without aliasing) is related to the depth of the examination: The shallower the field depth, the higher the Nyquist limit.

The setting of filters depends on the type of Doppler study being performed. When low-velocity flow is being measured by pulsed-wave Doppler echocardiography, the filter setting should be low, but when high-velocity flow is to be measured by continuous-wave Doppler echocardiography (e.g., aortic flow

Overview

Development of Echocardiography

Echocardiography is a noninvasive diagnostic technique that utilizes high-frequency ultrasound (2.0–7.0 MHz) to evaluate structural, functional, and hemodynamic status of the cardiovascular system. Edler and Hertz of Sweden were the first to record movements of cardiac structures, in particular, the mitral valve, by ultrasound in 1954 [1]. The reflected ultrasound pattern was so distinctive in patients with mitral stenosis that it became diagnostic, and the severity of mitral stenosis could be semiquantitatively measured by analysis of the M-mode echocardiogram. In the United States, Joyner and Reid at the University of Pennsylvania were the first to use ultrasound to examine the heart [2]. Shortly after, in 1965, Feigenbaum, with his colleagues at Indiana University, reported the first ultrasound detection of pericardial effusion [3] and is responsible for introducing echocardiography into the clinical practice of cardiology. M-mode echocardiography, however, produced only an "ice pick" view of the heart; two-dimensional (2D) sector scanning, developed in the mid-1970s, allowed real-time tomographic images of cardiac morphology and function [4]. Although the development of Doppler echocardiography parallels that of M-mode and 2D echocardiography from the early 1950s, it was not clinically utilized until the late 1970s. Pressure gradients across a fixed orifice could be reliably obtained by blood flow velocities measured by Doppler echocardiography [5]. Numerous validation studies subsequently confirmed the accuracy of Doppler in the assessment of cardiac pressures. The Doppler technique, therefore, made echocardiography not only an imaging but also a hemodynamic technique. Based on the Doppler concept, color-flow imaging was developed in the mid-1980s so that blood flow could also be noninvasively visualized.

With M-mode, 2D, Doppler, and color-flow imaging as the basic armamentarium, echocardiography has branched into numerous areas including transesophageal echocardiography (TEE), stress, contrast, fetal, intravascular, and intracardiac imaging. Tissue characterization and three-dimensional (3D) reconstruction remain active areas of clinical investigation.

Echocardiography at the Mayo Clinic

The first Mayo Clinic publication on echocardiography, titled "Echocardiography diagnosis of left atrial myxoma," was by Dr. T. T. Schattenberg and was published in the *Mayo Clinic Proceedings* in 1968 [6]. From the very beginning, the Mayo Clinic echocardiography laboratory was interested in validation of the echocardiographic technique. We published the feasibility and the anatomic correlation of transthoracic 2D echocardiography in the late 1970s [7]. Soon after the clinical introduction of Doppler echocardiography in the early 1980s, Doppler-derived pressure gradients were correlated with simultaneous catheter-derived pressure measurements [8], and excellent correlation was demonstrated in various clinical conditions. TEE was introduced in 1976, and clinical outpatient TEE became established by 1987 in the United States. Comprehensive monographs on TEE anatomic correlations (monoplane, biplane, and multiplane) and clinical applications were published, based on the experience of our group at the Mayo Clinic [9–11].

Examination

Echocardiography is an interactive procedure involving the echocardiographer, the cardiac ultrasound unit, and the patient. To produce the most optimal echocardiographic images and signals, these three components of the examination should meet the following requirements.

Operator

The person who performs echocardiographic examinations should have satisfactory cognitive and technical skills. Guidelines for clinical competence in performing adult echocardiography were developed by the American College of Cardiology, American College of Physicians, and the American Heart Association [12] and are listed in Tables 1-1 and 1-2.

To obtain the necessary cognitive and technical competence for adult echocardiography, a guideline for minimum physician training was established [12]. There are three levels of echocardiography training. The *first level* (level 1) is designed to provide an understanding of the basic principles, indications and applications, and limitations of echocardiography. All cardiovascular specialty trainees are expected to achieve this level of echocardiography training. The first level of training usually requires 3 months solely dedicated to echocardiography, including performance of at least 120 2D/M-mode and 60 Doppler examinations. The *second level* (level 2) of training allows independent echocardiographic examination and interpretation and requires 3 additional months with performance of at least 120 2D/M-mode and 120 Doppler examinations beyond those conducted at the first level. Training for an additional 6 months is needed to qualify the physician to direct an echocardiography laboratory. This *third-level* (level 3) training requires an additional 350 2D/M-mode and 350 Doppler examinations. Further training is necessary for transesophageal, stress, contrast, and any other special areas of echocardiography. At the Mayo Clinic, a cardiology trainee spends 3 months in the echocardiography laboratory during the first year of the fellowship program to achieve the level 1 training. During the 3 months, the training is entirely dedicated to echocardiography. If the individual wants to perform echocardiography independently or to direct an echocardiography laboratory, training for an additional 6 to 12 months is required.

Table 1-1. Cognitive skills needed to perform adult echocardiography competently

1. Knowledge of the appropriate indications for echocardiography and its elements.
2. Knowledge of the differential diagnostic problem in each patient and echocardiographic techniques needed to investigate these possibilities.
3. Knowledge of the alternatives to echocardiography.
4. Knowledge of the physical principles of echocardiographic image formation and blood flow velocity measurement.
5. Knowledge of the normal cardiac anatomy.
6. Knowledge of the pathologic changes in cardiac anatomy due to acquired and congenital heart disease.
7. Knowledge of the fluid dynamics of normal blood flow.
8. Knowledge of the pathologic changes in cardiac blood flow due to acquired and congenital heart disease.
9. Knowledge of cardiac auscultation and electrocardiography for correlation with results of the echocardiogram.
10. Ability to distinguish an adequate from an inadequate echocardiographic examination.
11. Ability to communicate results of the examination to the patient, medical record, and other physicians.

Source: From RL Popp, WL Winters. Clinical competence in adult echocardiography: a statement for physicians from the ACP/ACC/AHA Task Force on Clinical Privileges in Cardiology. *J Am Coll Cardiol* 1990;15:1466.

Table 1-2. Technical skills needed to perform adult echocardiography competently

1. Technical proficiency with operation of ultrasonography equipment and all controls affecting the quality of the received signals.
2. Ability to position and direct the ultrasound transducer to obtain the desired tomographic images and Doppler flow velocity signals.
3. Ability to perform a complete standard examination including all locally available elements of an echocardiographic study.
4. Ability to record and recognize the electrocardiogram for correlation with the echocardiographic data.
5. Ability to recognize abnormalities of anatomy and flow to modify the standard examination to accommodate perceived diagnostic needs.
6. Ability to perform quantitative analysis of the echocardiographic study and to produce a written report.

Source: From RL Popp, WL Winters. Clinical competence in adult echocardiography: a statement for physicians from the ACP/ACC/AHA Task Force on Clinical Privileges in Cardiology. *J Am Coll Cardiol* 1990;15:1467.

Because echocardiographic data acquisition is usually performed by a sonographer, the importance of sonographer training in echocardiography should also be recognized. Sonographer training depends on the individual's background and should be done under the supervision of a physician echocardiographer who has completed level 3 training. Technical skills similar to those outlined for physicians should be obtained by sonographers. The ultimate responsibility for interpretation of echocardiographic findings, however, should rest with the physician with appropriate training (level 2 or 3). The role of the sonographer during transesophageal and stress echocardiography varies depending on his or her qualifications and experience. This is discussed separately in subsequent chapters.

Instrumentation

All ultrasound units should be equipped with the basic requirements—M-mode, 2D sector scanning, Doppler, and color-flow imaging capabilities, although some portable units only provide M-mode and 2D imaging. It is, how-

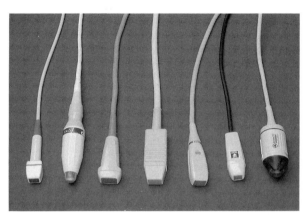

Fig. 1-1. Various transducers for transthoracic echocardiography with different sizes and shapes depending on the transducer ultrasound frequency, number of elements, and manufacturer.

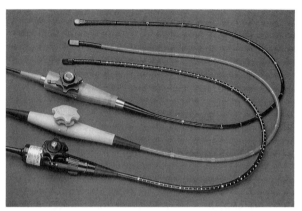

Fig. 1-2. Examples of a TEE probe. Transducers are mounted on the tip of an endoscopy probe. The distal end of the probe is maneuvered to different directions by a control knob at the other end of the probe. Usually there are two controls: one knob to move the tip side to side and another knob for antero-flexion or retroflexion. The position of the probe can also be locked in when it needs to remain at one location for an extended period. When the probe has biplane transducers, either the transverse or the longitudinal plane is selected. With a multiplane probe, the transducer rotates up to 180 degrees by dialing a control button at the operator's end. The distance from the tip of the probe is clearly shown on the shaft. (The length of a probe is usually 100–110 cm.)

ever, up to the individual echocardiographer to optimize the examination utilizing optimal transducer, knob settings, and transducer positions.

Diagnostic ultrasound requires a frequency of at least 2.0 MHz. As the sound frequency increases, there is less penetration of the ultrasound beam into the body tissue; therefore, the usual echocardiography examination in the adult begins with a 2.0- to 2.5-MHz transducer (Fig. 1-1). However, the image resolution improves with a higher-frequency transducer (i.e., shorter wavelength). In a thin individual or a pediatric patient, a 3.0- to 5.0-MHz transducer should provide adequate penetration and also improves the image resolution. In the TEE probe, a modification of an endoscopy probe (Fig. 1-2) with a higher-frequency (3.5–7.5-MHz) transducer is utilized since the distance between the transducer and the cardiac structure is quite short and is not interrupted greatly by other body tissues; therefore, the penetration is not as significant an issue. However, in the Doppler examination, a lower-frequency transducer is required to record high velocities since the measurable velocities are inversely proportional to the transmitted frequency (see Doppler equation in Chap. 5).

Once a proper transducer is selected, all the available ultrasound windows should be utilized. Gray scales and gains are manually con-

trolled to minimize background noise and to maximize the delineation of cardiac structures. The depth of the fields can be controlled to provide the optimal image size and depends on the goal of the study. When a certain structure needs to be carefully examined, a "zoom" or an "RES" (i.e., regional expansion selection) function can enlarge the selected portion of the image. Field depth is important during Doppler and color-flow imaging examinations since the Nyquist limit (i.e., the maximum velocity to be recorded without aliasing) is related to the depth of the examination: The shallower the field depth, the higher the Nyquist limit.

The setting of filters depends on the type of Doppler study being performed. When low-velocity flow is being measured by pulsed-wave Doppler echocardiography, the filter setting should be low, but when high-velocity flow is to be measured by continuous-wave Doppler echocardiography (e.g., aortic flow velocity in aortic stenosis), the filter setting should be high to eliminate the low-velocity flow signals. In color-flow imaging, the filter setting should be high to eliminate the noise artifacts near the cardiac walls. Theoretically, to obtain the highest available velocity by Doppler echocardiography, the Doppler beam should be parallel with the direction of the blood flow jet (angle of θ should be 0). However, the error introduced by the angle of θ is quite acceptable as long as the angle remains less than 20 degrees. Sometimes, an angle correction can overestimate the velocity of a Doppler on examination, and is therefore rarely used in daily practice.

Color-flow imaging also depends on the gain setting. It is very important to make certain that the area of abnormal blood flow is not underestimated by a low gain setting since the severity of valvular regurgitation or shunt flow depends on the area of abnormal blood flow detected by color-flow imaging. The optimal setting should be where the entire flow jet is displayed with minimal background noise. It is usually best to start with maximum color gain to identify the largest area of abnormal blood flow and then decrease the gain gradually to minimize the background noise without compromising the visualization of abnormal flow. It should also be noted that the gain settings for 2D tissue imaging may affect color gains in flow imaging in some instruments.

Patient

Occasionally, the patient is a limiting factor in the echocardiography examination, due to emphysema, obesity, or a unique body habitus. These features may preclude meaningful transthoracic echocardiography examination. However, completely uninterpretable echo images are rare even with these limiting factors, and clinical questions can be answered by transthoracic echocardiography in most of the patients. When a better image is required, the transesophageal approach provides an alternative ultrasound window. Even in the most ideal patient, visualization of certain structures such as the left atrial appendage, left main coronary artery, and descending thoracic aorta requires the TEE view.

References

1. Edler I, Hertz CH. The use of ultrasonic reflectoscope for the continuous recording of the movements of heart walls. *Kungliga Fysiografiska Sallskapets i Lund förhandlingar* 1954; Bd 24, No. 5:1–19.

2. Joyner CR, Reid JM. Application of ultrasound in cardiology and cardiovascular physiology. *Prog Cardiovasc Dis* 1963;5:482–497.

3. Feigenbaum H, Waldhaussen JA, Hyde LP. Ultrasound diagnosis of pericardial effusion. *JAMA* 1965;191:711–714.

4. Feigenbaum H. *Echocardiography* (3rd ed). Philadelphia: Lea & Febiger, 1981.

5. Holen J, et al. Determination of pressure gradient in mitral stenosis with a non-invasive ultrasound Doppler technique. *Acta Med Scand* 1976;199:455–460.

6. Schattenberg TT. Echocardiographic diagnosis of left atrial myxoma. *Mayo Clin Proc* 1968;43:620–627.

7. Tajik AJ, et al. Two-dimensional real-time ultrasonic imaging of the heart and great vessels: technique, image orientation, structure identification, and validation. *Mayo Clin Proc* 1978;53:271–303.

8. Currie PJ, et al. Instantaneous pressure gradient: a simultaneous Doppler and dual catheter correlative study. *J Am Coll Cardiol* 1986; 7:800–806.

9. Seward JB, et al. Transesophageal echocardiography: technique, anatomic correlations, implementation, and clinical applications. *Mayo Clin Proc* 1988;63:649–680.

10. Seward JB, et al. Biplanar transesophageal echocardiography: anatomic correlations, image orientation, and clinical applications. *Mayo Clin Proc* 1990;65:1193–1213.

11. Seward JB, et al. Multiplane transesophageal echocardiography: examination technique, anatomic correlations, image orientation, and clinical applications. *Mayo Clin Proc* 1993;68:523-551.

12. Popp RL, Winters WL. Clinical competence in adult echocardiography: a statement for physicians from the ACP/ACC/AHA Task Force on Clinical Privileges in Cardiology. *J Am Coll Cardiol* 1990;15:1465–1468.

2

Transthoracic Echocardiography

M-mode and 2D Echocardiography

The typical patient examination begins with transthoracic 2D echocardiography utilizing four standard transducer positions: the parasternal, apical, subcostal, and suprasternal windows. The first two views are usually obtained with the patient in the left lateral decubitus position (Fig. 2-1A) and the latter two views with the patient in the supine position (Fig. 2-1B). From each transducer position, multiple tomographic images of the heart relative to its long and short axes are obtained by manually rotating and angulating the transducer, hence, performing a multiplane examination [1–4] (Fig. 2-2). The long-axis view represents a sagittal or coronal section of the heart, bisecting the heart from the base to the apex. The short-axis view is perpendicular to the long-axis view and is equivalent to sectioning the heart like a loaf of bread ("bread-loafing"). The standard long and short tomographic imaging planes and the corresponding anatomic structures of the heart are shown in Figures 2-3 through 2-7. Real-time 2D echocardiography provides high-resolution images of cardiac structures and their movements so that detailed anatomic and functional information of the heart can be obtained. Therefore, 2D echocardiography is the basis (cornerstone) of morphologic and functional assessment of the heart. Quantitative measurements of cardiac dimensions, area, and volume are derived from 2D images. 2D echocardiography also provides the framework for Doppler and color-flow imaging.

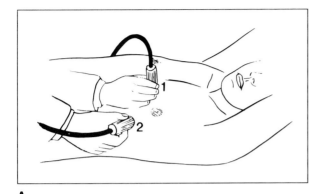

A

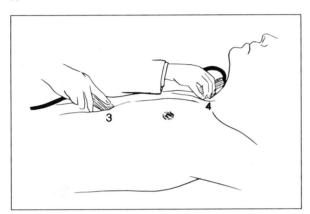

B

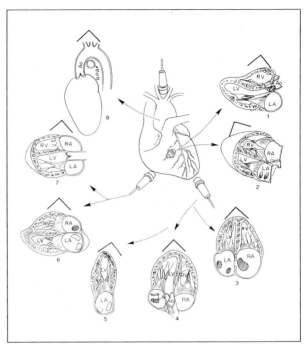

A

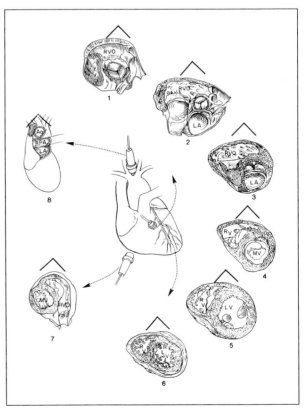

B

▲ **Fig. 2-1.** Four standard transthoracic transducer positions. **A.** Parasternal (1) and apical (2) views are usually obtained with the patient in the left lateral decubitus position. The parasternal view is usually obtained by placing the transducer at the left parasternal area in the second or third intercostal space. The apical view is obtained with the transducer at the maximal apical impulse (usually slightly lateral and inferior to the nipple, but it may be significantly displaced further due to cardiac enlargement or rotation or both). These views may be best imaged during held expiration, especially in patients with chronic obstructive lung disease. The apical view can be difficult to obtain in a thin young individual and the transducer may require superior tilting. **B.** Subcostal (3) and suprasternal notch (4) views are obtained with the patient in the supine position. For subcostal imaging, the flexion of the patient's knees softens the abdominal muscles, and forced inspiration frequently improves the views. For suprasternal notch imaging, the patient's head needs to be extended and turned leftward so the transducer can be placed comfortably in the notch without rubbing the patient's neck.

Fig. 2-2. **A.** Schematic drawing of longitudinal views from four standard transthoracic transducer positions. Shown are the parasternal long-axis view (1), parasternal right ventricular inflow view (2), apical four-chamber view (3), apical five-chamber view (4), apical two-chamber view (5), subcostal four-chamber view (6), subcostal long-axis (five-chamber) view (7), and the suprasternal notch view (8). **B.** Schematic drawing of short-axis views. These views are obtained by rotating the transducer 90 degrees clockwise from the longitudinal position. Drawings 1–6 show parasternal short-axis views at different levels obtained by angulating the transducer from a superior medial position (for imaging of the aortic and pulmonary valves) to an inferolateral position, tilting toward the apex (from level 1 to level 6 short-axis views). Shown are short-axis views of the right ventricular outflow tract (RVO) and pulmonary valve (1), aortic valve and left atrium (2), left ventricular outflow tract (3), and short-axis views at the left ventricular basal (mitral valve [MV]) level (4), the left ventricular mid level (papillary muscle) (5), and the left ventricular apical level (6). A good view to visualize the right ventricular outflow tract is the subcostal short-axis view (7). Also shown is the suprasternal notch short-axis view of the aorta (8).

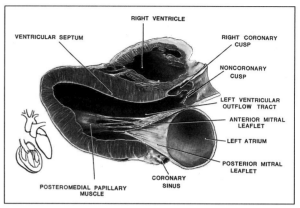

A

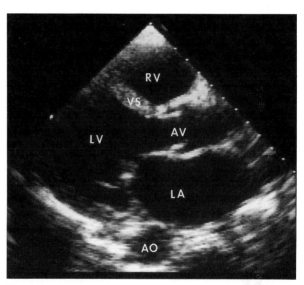

B

Fig. 2-3. Schematic anatomic section **(A)** and corresponding still-frame **(B)** of 2D echo image of the parasternal long-axis view. The parasternal long-axis view allows the visualization of the right ventricle (RV), ventricular septum (VS), aortic valve (AV) cusps, left ventricle (LV), mitral valve, left atrium (LA), and descending thoracic aorta (AO). The coronary sinus may be seen as a small circular echo-free structure in the LV atrioventricular groove. In this view, the true LV apex is not well seen.

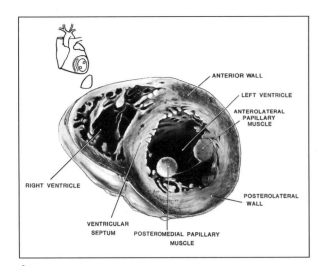

A

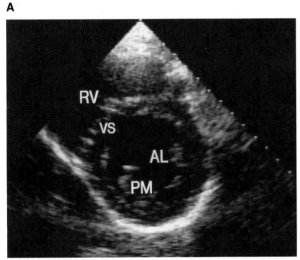

B

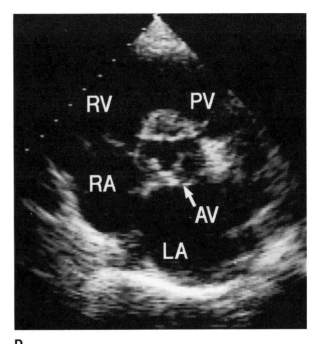

D

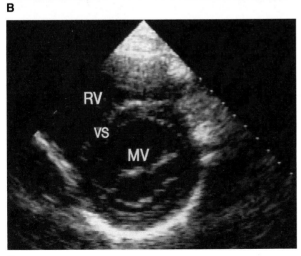

C

Fig. 2-4.   A. Schematic anatomic section of a parasternal short-axis view at the papillary muscle level. **B.** A corresponding still-frame of a 2D image in the parasternal short-axis view at the papillary muscle level. This view is particularly useful in measuring the LV cavity dimension and wall thickness, and in assessing wall motion. **C.** The superior and rightward tilting of the transducer obtains a parasternal short-axis view at the basal level showing the mitral valve (MV). **D.** With even further tilting, the short-axis view of the aortic valve is obtained. In this view, a right ventricular (RV) outflow tract and pulmonary valve (PV) are visualized. Below the aortic valve (AV) lies the left atrium (LA), and the connections of all four pulmonary veins to the left atrium are usually seen. If the transducer is angulated inferiorly and laterally, the apical short-axis view, which is essential in assessing the apical regional wall motion abnormalities, is obtained. (Modified from AJ Tajik et al. Two-dimensional real-time ultrasonic imaging of the heart and great vessels: technique, image orientation, structure identification, and validation. *Mayo Clin Proc* 1978;53:271–303.)

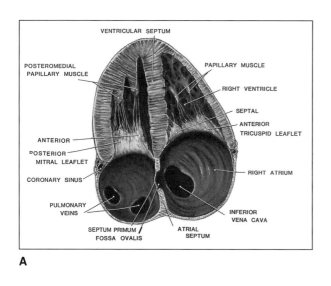

A

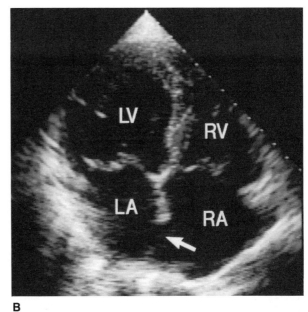

B

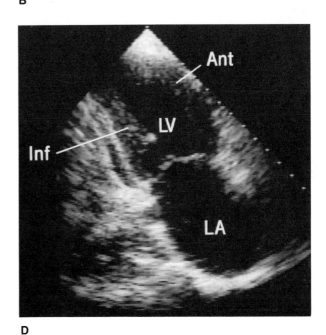

C

D

Fig. 2-5. Schematic anatomic section **(A)** and corresponding 2D echo image **(B)** of the apical four-chamber view. The apical view is obtained by placing the transducer in the immediate vicinity of, or at the point of, maximum apical impulse. The four-chamber view displays all four cardiac chambers, the ventricular and atrial septa, and the crux of the heart. However, it is not uncommon to see a drop-out area in the region of the atrial septum (*arrow* in **B**). It is due to the parallel orientation of the atrial septum to the ultrasound beam rather than an actual atrial septal defect. It should also be noted that the insertion of the septal leaflet of the tricuspid valve is somewhat inferior to the insertion of the anterior mitral leaflet, and this is an important anatomic distinction in the evaluation of congenital heart disease. **C.** By angulating the transducer in a clockwise rotation, the five-chamber or long-axis apical view allows us to see the LV outflow tract and the aortic valve. In this view, inferolateral wall (IL) and anteroseptum (AS) are visualized. **D.** Further clockwise rotation produces the two-chamber view, which is useful to visualize the entire posterior or inferior (Inf) wall and to analyze anterior (Ant) wall motion. (Modified from AJ Tajik et al. Two-dimensional real-time ultrasonic imaging of the heart and great vessels: technique, image orientation, structure identification, and validation. *Mayo Clin Proc* 1978;53:271–303.)

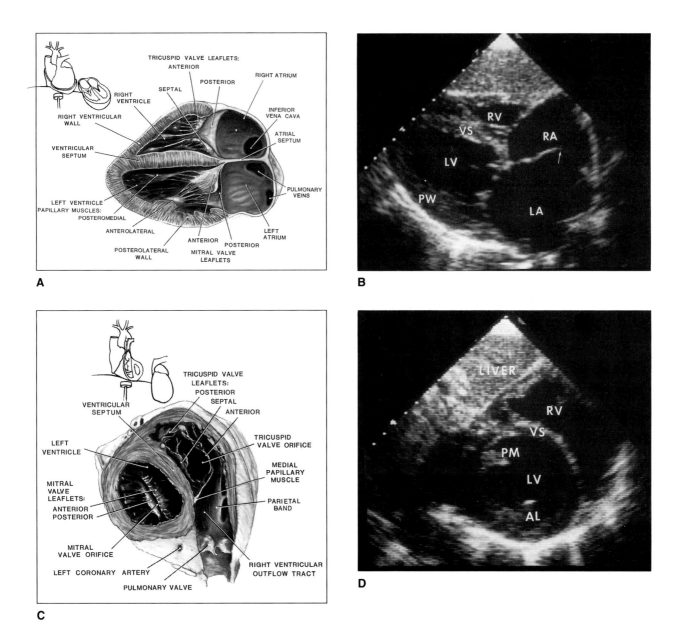

Fig. 2-6. Schematic anatomic section and corresponding 2D echo image in the subcostal view. **A, B.** Long-axis view. **C, D.** Short-axis view. The subcostal view allows better definition of certain cardiac structures such as the atrial septum, right and left atria, right ventricular free wall, and right ventricular outflow tract and pulmonary valve, entrance of the inferior vena cava to the right atrium, hepatic vein, and abdominal aorta. This view may be the only satisfactory echocardiographic window for patients with chronic obstructive lung disease and emphysema. In **B** the arrow indicates the atrial septum bulged to the right atrium. (Modified from AJ Tajik et al. Two-dimensional real-time ultrasonic imaging of the heart and great vessels: technique, image orientation, structure identification, and validation. *Mayo Clin Proc* 1978;53:271–303.)

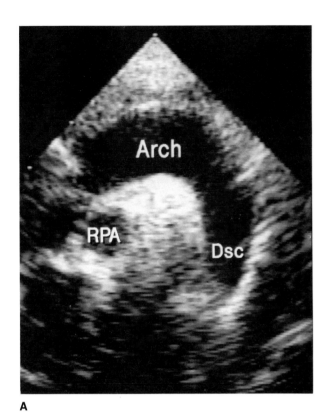

A

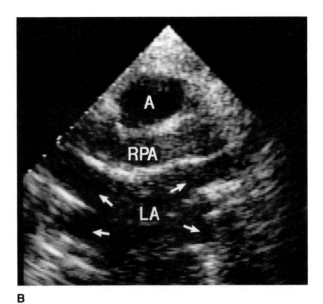

B

Fig. 2-7. Suprasternal notch long-axis **(A)**, and short-axis **(B, C)** views. This transducer position allows the visualization of the ascending aorta, aortic arch (A), origin of the brachiocephalic vessels, and descending thoracic aorta. The short-axis view of the aortic arch is obtained by rotating the transducer clockwise, along with the visualization of the right pulmonary artery (RPA) in its long-axis format, located inferiorly. Inferior to the pulmonary artery, the left atrial (LA) cavity is seen with connections of four pulmonary veins *(arrows)*. The superior vena cava (SVC) is visualized by further clockwise rotation, appearing along the right side of the aorta **(C)**.

C

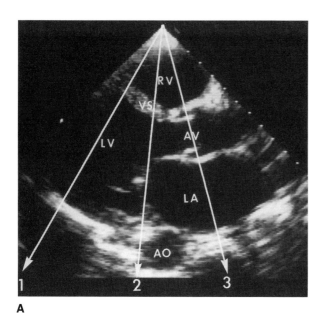

A

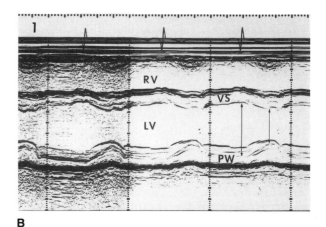

B

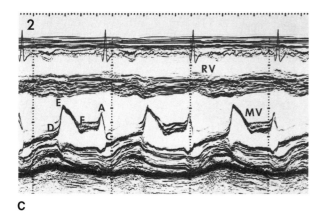

C

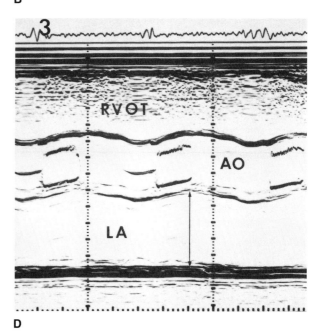

D

Fig. 2-8.   A. An M-mode cursor is placed along different levels (1 = ventricular; 2 = mitral valve; 3 = aortic valve level, in **A–D**) of the heart with parasternal long-axis 2D echo guidance. **B–D.** Representative normal M-mode echocardiograms at the midventricular, mitral valve, and aortic valve levels, respectively. The arrows in **B** indicate end-diastolic (at QRS) and end-systolic dimensions of LV. The M-mode echocardiogram **(C)** of the anterior mitral leaflet has the following alphabetical labeling: D = end-systole prior to mitral valve opening; E = peak of early opening; F = middiastolic closure; A = peak of late opening with atrial systole; C = closure of the mitral valve. The arrow in **D** indicates the dimension of the left atrium at end-systole.

M-mode echocardiography complements the 2D echocardiographic examination by recording detailed motions of cardiac structures and is best derived with guidance from a 2D echocardiographic image by placing a cursor through the desired structure (Fig. 2-8). M-mode is utilized for the measurement of dimension and is essential for the display of subtle motion abnormalities of specific cardiac structures. Methods for measuring cardiac dimensions from M-mode are shown in Figure

Table 2-1. Normal values for cardiac dimensions (mm) in adult population (20–97 years old)

	≤ 30 yr	> 70 yr
LV diastolic dimension	48.1 ± 5.6	45.3 ± 5.6
LV systolic dimension	30.0 ± 5.8	28.4 ± 5.8
Septum	9.8 ± 1.7	11.8 ± 1.7
Posterior wall thickness	10.1 ± 1.4	11.8 ± 1.4
Aortic root	27.4 ± 5.7	33.5 ± 5.7
Left atrium	34.3 ± 7.0	39.7 ± 7.0

LV = left ventricle
Source: Modified from JM Gardin et al. Echocardiographic measurements in normal subjects: evaluation of an adult population without clinically apparent heart disease. *J Clin Ultrasound* 1979;7:439–447.

2-9. Normal values for cardiac dimensions in the adult population have been well established [5, 6] (Table 2-1).

Doppler Echocardiography

Doppler measures blood flow velocities in the heart and the great vessels, based on the *Doppler effect,* which was described by the Austrian physicist Christian Doppler in 1842 [7]. The Doppler effect states that sound frequency increases as a sound source moves toward the observer, and it decreases as the source moves away. One example of the Doppler effect is the sound of an ambulance siren. When an ambulance is coming toward us, the siren becomes louder (i.e., sound frequency increases) and it becomes softer (i.e., sound frequency decreases) when the ambulance drives away. In the circulatory system, the moving target is the red blood cell. When an ultrasound beam with known frequency (fo) is transmitted to the heart or the great vessels, it is reflected by red blood cells. The frequency of the reflected ultrasound waves (fr) increases when red blood cells are moving toward the source of ultrasound. Conversely, the frequency of reflected ultrasound waves decreases when red blood cells are moving away. The change in frequency between the transmitted sound and the reflected sound is termed the *frequency shift* (Δf) or *Doppler shift* (= fr − fo). The Doppler

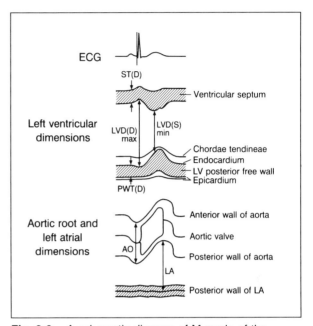

Fig. 2-9. A schematic diagram of M-mode of the LV, aortic root, and the left atrium. The LV internal dimension at end-diastole (D) was measured at onset of the QRS complex, and systolic (S) measurement was done at the maximal excursion of the ventricular septum, which occurs normally before the maximal excursion of the posterior wall. These measurements corresponded, respectively, to the maximum and minimum internal dimensions between the interventricular septum and the posterobasal LV free wall endocardium. Septal thickness (ST) and posterior wall thickness (PWT) were measured at end-diastole at onset of the QRS complex. The aortic root dimension (AO) was measured at onset of the QRS complex from leading edge to leading edge of aortic walls. The left atrial dimension was measured at end-systole as the largest distance between the posterior aortic wall and the center of the line denoting the posterior left atrial wall. (From JM Gardin et al. Echocardiographic measurements in normal subjects: evaluation of an adult population without clinically apparent heart disease. *J Clin Ultrasound* 1979;7:439–447.)

shift depends on the transmitted frequency (fo), velocity of the moving target (v), and the angle (θ) between the ultrasound beam and the direction of the moving target as expressed in the *Doppler equation* (Fig. 2-10):

$$\Delta f = \frac{2 \, fo \times v \times \cos \theta}{c}$$

where c is the speed of sound in blood (1,560 m/sec).

If the angle θ is 0 degrees (i.e., the ultrasound beam is parallel with the direction of blood flow), then the maximum frequency shift is measured since the cosine of 0 is 1. Note that as the angle θ increases, the corresponding cosine becomes progressively less than 1 (Table 2-2) and this will result in underestimation of the Doppler shift (Δf), and hence peak velocity, since peak flow velocity is derived from Δf by rearranging the Doppler equation:

$$v = \frac{c}{2} \times \frac{\Delta f}{fo}$$

Blood flow velocities determined by Doppler echocardiography are in turn used to derive various hemodynamic data (see Chap. 5).

The most common uses of Doppler echocardiography are in the *pulsed-* and *continuous-wave* forms (Fig. 2-11). Both modalities are necessary parts of the Doppler examination and provide complementary information. In the pulsed-wave mode, a single ultrasound crystal sends and receives sound beams. The crystal emits a short burst of ultrasound at a certain frequency (*pulse repetition frequency* [PRF]). The ultrasound is reflected from moving red blood cells and is received by the same crystal. Therefore, the maximal frequency shift that can be determined by pulsed-wave Doppler is half of the PRF, called the *Nyquist frequency*. If frequency shift is higher than the Nyquist frequency, *aliasing* occurs; that is, the Doppler spectrum is cut off at the Nyquist frequency and the remaining frequency shift is recorded on the opposite side of baseline. Pulsed-wave Doppler measures flow velocities at a specific location within a "sample volume" of a cardiac chamber. The PRF varies inversely with the depth of sample volume: the shallower the sample volume location, the higher the PRF and the Nyquist frequency. In other words, higher velocities can be recorded without aliasing by pulsed-wave Doppler as the sample volume location becomes closer to the transducer.

In the continuous-wave mode, the transducer has two crystals—one to send and the other to receive the reflected ultrasound waves continuously. Therefore, the maximal frequency shift that can be recorded by continu-

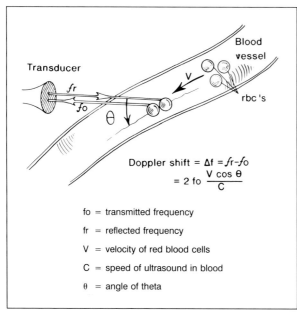

Fig. 2-10. Schematic drawing to demonstrate the Doppler effect (see text).

Table 2-2. Cosine value of angle θ

Angle θ (degrees)	Cosine
0	1.00
10	0.98
20	0.94
30	0.87
40	0.77
50	0.64
60	0.50
70	0.34
80	0.17
90	0.00

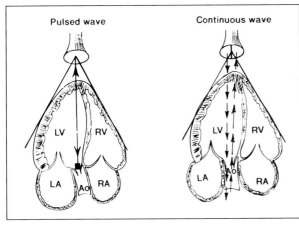

A

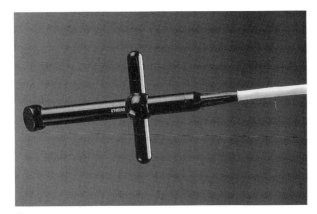

B

ous-wave Doppler is not limited by the PRF or the Nyquist phenomenon. Unlike pulsed-wave Doppler, continuous-wave Doppler measures all the frequency shifts (i.e., velocities) present along its beam path; hence, it is useful for recording high velocities. Continuous-wave Doppler is usually performed with a nonimaging transducer (see Fig. 2-11B). This small transducer is better fit for interrogation of high-velocity jet from multiple windows. Image-guided continuous-wave examination may be necessary when the direction of blood flow is eccentric or the amount of desired blood flow is trivial. Table 2-3 shows a summary of the characteristics and clinical applications of each Doppler modality. Their representative recordings are demonstrated in Figure 2-12. Table 2-4 shows the mean and the range of maximal velocities recorded from normal subjects by Doppler echocardiography.

Fig. 2-11. Schematic drawing of pulsed- and continuous-wave Doppler echocardiography from the apical view **(A)**, and nonimaging continuous-wave Doppler transducer **(B)** (see text).

Table 2-3. Pulsed- versus continuous-wave Doppler

Pulsed-wave	Continuous-wave
Measures specific blood flow velocity by placing the "sample volume" at a precise region of interest.	Measures blood flow velocities along the axis of the entire ultrasound beam (range ambiguous).
Maximum measurable velocity without aliasing is usually less than 2 m/sec.	Able to measure high velocities up to 9 m/sec.
Performed by duplex transducer (2D and Doppler).	Performed by duplex as well as by nonimaging transducer.
Suited for measuring low velocity at a particular intracardiac location.	Suited for measuring peak velocities (i.e., gradients) across the intracardiac orifices.

Clinical applications utilized for determining
    a. LVOT velocity and TVI.
    b. Volume measurements.
    c. Diastolic filling parameters.
    d. Mitral inflow velocity.
    e. Pulmonary and hepatic vein velocity.
    f. Location of flow disturbance.
	Clinical applications utilized for determining
	    a. Peak flow velocity and TVI.
	    b. Valvular pressure gradient.
	    c. Pressure half-time.
	    d. Dynamic LVOT gradient.
	    e. Pulmonary pressure.
	    f. dP/dt.

LVOT = left ventricular outflow tract; TVI = time velocity integral; dP/dt = the rate of ventricular pressure rise obtained from mitral or tricuspid regurgitation Doppler signal.

Color-Flow Imaging

Color-flow imaging, based on the pulsed-wave Doppler principles, displays intracavitary blood flow in three colors (red, blue, and green) or their combinations, depending on velocity, direction, and extent of turbulence [8, 9]. It utilizes multiple sampling sites along multiple ultrasound beams ("multigated"). At each sampling site (or gate), frequency shift is meas-

ured, converted to a digital format, automatically correlated (autocorrelation) to preset color schemes, and displayed as color flow on the monitor (Fig. 2-13). Blood flow directed toward the transducer does have a positive frequency shift (i.e., reflected ultrasound frequency is higher than the transmitted frequency) and is color-encoded in shades of red. Blood flow directed away from the transducer has a negative frequency shift and is color-

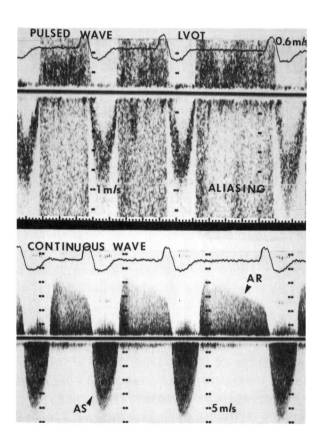

Fig. 2-12. Representative pulsed-wave and continuous-wave Doppler spectra from the apex in a patient with aortic stenosis and regurgitation. The patient is in atrial fibrillation. The pulsed-wave Doppler sample volume is placed at the LV outflow tract (LVOT) and the Doppler spectrum shows systolic LVOT velocity of 1.0 m/sec and turbulent diastolic signal of aortic regurgitation (AR) recorded at both sides of the baseline. Although AR flow is toward the transducer, "aliasing" (velocity wraparound) occurs due to its high velocity (4–6 m/sec). Continuous-wave Doppler detects flow velocities all along its beam and is able to record high velocity. Systolic flow away from the transducer (spectrum below the baseline) represents flow across the stenotic aortic valve (AS) and diastolic flow is from AR, with a peak velocity of 4 m/sec. Peak AS velocity across the stenotic valve varies beat to beat from 5.0 to 5.5 m/sec due to atrial fibrillation.

Table 2-4.   Normal maximal velocities: Doppler measurements

	Children		Adults	
	Mean	**Range**	**Mean**	**Range**
Mitral flow	1.00 m/sec	0.8–1.3 m/sec	0.90 m/sec	0.6–1.3 m/sec
Tricuspid flow	0.60 m/sec	0.5–0.8 m/sec	0.50 m/sec	0.3–0.7 m/sec
Pulmonary artery	0.90 m/sec	0.7–1.1 m/sec	0.75 m/sec	0.6–0.9 m/sec
Left ventricle	1.00 m/sec	0.7–1.2 m/sec	0.90 m/sec	0.7–1.1 m/sec
Aorta	1.50 m/sec	1.2–1.8 m/sec	1.35 m/sec	1.0–1.7 m/sec

Source: From L Hatle, B Angelsen. *Doppler Ultrasound in Cardiology* (2nd ed). Philadelphia: Lea & Febiger, 1985. P 93.

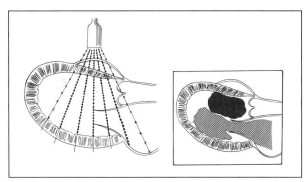

Fig. 2-13. Schematic diagram to illustrate how color-flow imaging is performed and displayed. The small dots indicate the multiple sampling sites (gates). Frequency shift measured at each gate is automatically correlated and converted to preset color schemes (*inset:* dark area = blue; shaded area = red).

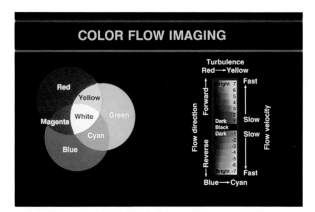

Fig. 2-14. Color-flow imaging is displayed using three primary colors (red, blue, and green) and their combinations based on the velocity, direction, and turbulence of flow. (From R Omoto, C Kasai. Physics and instrumentation of Doppler color flow mapping. *Echocardiography* 1987;4:467–483.)

encoded in shades of blue. Each color has multiple shades and the lighter shades within each primary color are assigned to higher velocities within the Nyquist limit. When flow velocity is higher than the Nyquist frequency limit, color aliasing occurs and is depicted as a color reversal. For example, flow toward the transducer at 1.2 m/sec is displayed blue instead of red if the Nyquist limit allows the maximum velocity of blood flow of only 1.0 m/sec. With each multiple of the Nyquist limit, the color repeatedly reverts to the opposite color. Turbulence, blood moving in multiple directions with multiple velocities, is characterized by the presence of *variance*. The degree of the variance from the mean velocity can be encoded as a variance color, which usually is shades of green. Therefore, abnormal blood flow is easily recognized by combinations of multiple colors according to the directions, velocities, and the degree of turbulence (Fig. 2-14). The width and the size of abnormal intracavitary flows are utilized to semiquantitate the degree of valvular regurgitation or cardiac shunt.

References

1. Tajik AJ, et al. Two-dimensional real-time ultrasonic imaging of the heart and great vessels: technique, image orientation, structure identification, and validation. *Mayo Clin Proc* 1978;53:271–303.

2. Bansal RC, et al. Feasibility of detailed two-dimensional echocardiographic examinations in adults: prospective study of 200 patients. *Mayo Clin Proc* 1980;55:291–308.

3. Edwards WD, Tajik AJ, Seward JB. Standardized normal and anatomic basis for regional tomographic analysis of the heart. *Mayo Clin Proc* 1981;56:479–497.

4. Henry WL, et al. Report of the American Society of Echocardiography Committee on Nomenclature and Standards in Two-dimensional Echocardiography. *Circulation* 1980;62:212–217.

5. Henry WL, et al. Echocardiographic measurements in normal subjects: growth-related changes that occur between infancy and early adulthood. *Circulation* 1978;57:278–285.

6. Gardin JM, et al. Echocardiographic measurements in normal subjects: evaluation of an adult population without clinically apparent heart disease. *J Clin Ultrasound* 1979;7:439–447.

7. Hatle L, Angelsen B. *Doppler Ultrasound in Cardiology: Physical Principles and Clinical Applications* (2nd ed). Philadelphia: Lea & Febiger, 1985.

8. Omoto R, Kasai C. Physics and instrumentation of Doppler color flow mapping. *Echocardiography* 1987;4:467–483.

9. Kisslo J, Adams DB, Belkin RN. *Doppler Color Flow Imaging.* New York: Churchill-Livingstone, 1988.

3

Transesophageal Echocardiography

Transthoracic echocardiographic examination may be suboptimal in patients with morbid obesity, emphysema, chest wall deformity, recent surgical wounds, or trauma. Moreover, certain cardiovascular structures such as the left atrial appendage and the descending thoracic aorta are not readily accessible to transthoracic imaging. Furthermore, a prosthetic valve, because of a high degree of echo reflectance, may prevent adequate imaging of posterior cardiac structures. Since the esophagus is located between the heart and the descending thoracic aorta, transesophageal echocardiography (TEE) provides high-resolution images of cardiac structures and the thoracic aorta in essentially all patients [1–3]. In this chapter, general aspects of TEE are discussed, based on more than 5,000 examinations performed so far at the Mayo Clinic. Specific clinical applications of TEE are presented in detail throughout the manual.

Instrumentation

Usually 5.0-MHz transducers are mounted on the tip of an endoscope and can be maneuvered to various positions in the esophagus and the stomach. The width of the transducer tip varies from 10 to 14 mm for the adult scope but has been miniaturized to 4 mm for pediatric use. The echocardiographer who performs the TEE should be familiar with the intubation technique of the transesophageal probe and transesophageal tomographic image orientation as well as the strengths and the limitations of transthoracic echocardiography. The TEE examination is usually performed with the patient in the left lateral decubitus position (Fig. 3-1A) in a special procedure room equipped

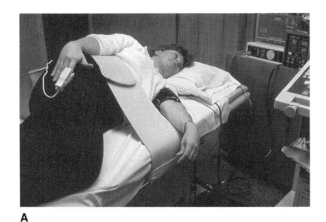

A

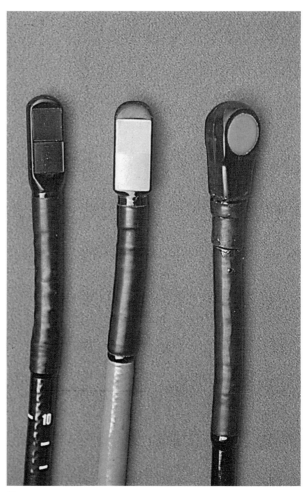

B

Fig. 3-1. **A.** TEE is usually performed with the patient in the left lateral decubitus position. The patient is securely maintained by a belt and is monitored continuously for oxygen saturation and blood pressure. **B.** Biplane (left and center) and multiplane (right) TEE transducers. With the biplane probe, two separate crystals provide orthogonal imaging arrays. The multiplane transducer rotates 180 degrees to provide continuous tomographic images.

with oral suction devices, oxygen supply, pulse oximeter, and cardiopulmonary resuscitation (CPR) capabilities. When the patient is critically ill or difficult to transfer, the examination is performed at the patient's bedside. Intraoperative TEE examination is separately discussed (see Chap. 17).

Patient Preparation

The patient should fast for at least 4 hours prior to TEE and history of dysphagia or esophageal pathology should be excluded (Table 3-1). Lidocaine spray (10%) is used to anesthetize the posterior pharynx and a drying agent (usually glycopyrrolate [Robinul], 0.2 mg) minimizes oral secretion and the possibility of aspiration during the examination. A short-acting sedative (midazolam [Versed], 1.0–5.0 mg) may be necessary to make the TEE examination more pleasant, but should be used cautiously, especially in the elderly patient because of more pronounced respiratory suppression. Additional medication such as me-

peridine hydrochloride (Demerol, 25–50 mg) helps alleviate the gag reflex, especially for young patients. Subacute bacterial endocarditis prophylaxis is recommended in high-risk patients, for example, those with a prosthetic valve, previous endocarditis, or intracardiac conduits [4, 5] (Table 3-2). Every patient should have an intravenous access for administration of a contrast agent (e.g., agitated saline solution) or medications.

Anatomic Correlations

The first generation of ultrasound transducers for TEE had only a horizontal plane. The second generation of transesophageal probes incorporated a second set of ultrasound crystals to provide an orthogonal longitudinal plane (Fig. 3-1B). This additional imaging improved visualization of the cardiac apex, atrial septum, thoracic aorta, venae cavae, pulmonary veins, left and right ventricular outflow tracts, and aortic valve. More recently, a multiplane probe has been developed so that a rotating trans-ducer (see Fig. 3-1B) allows a circular continuum of tomographic images within a 180-degree arc without moving the probe. Using multiplane TEE, one can more easily visualize intermediate, transitional, and off-axis images between the primary planes. Al-though additional tomographic information is obtained by the multiplane probe compared to the biplane probe, the primary advantage of multiplane TEE is the ability to obtain an unin-terrupted series of adjacent images simply by rotation of the transducer array.

Horizontal Plane

There are three primary horizontal trans-esophageal views of the heart: basal short-axis, four-chamber, and transgastric views de-pending on the location of the transesophageal transducer in the esophagus [3]. Serial tomo-graphic images are obtained from each view by angulating or rotating the transducer (Fig. 3-2). Anatomic sections and corresponding

Table 3-1. Transesophageal echocardiography (TEE)

Preparation
    No history of dysphagia or esophageal pathology
    NPO (fasting) for ≥ 4 hr
    Local anesthesia; lidocaine sprays
    IV access with three-way stopcock
Medications
    Drying agent 2–3 min prior to TEE (optional);
      glycopyrrolate (Robinul, 0.2 mg IV)
    Sedation as necessary (midazolam hydrochloride
      [Versed] and/or meperidine hydrochloride
      [Demerol])
    Flumazenil (Mazicon), if needed for reversal of
      midazolam hydrochloride
    Subacute bacterial endocarditis prophylaxis for
      high-risk patients
    High-risk patients include those with:
      a. Prosthetic valve without suspicion of
         endocarditis
      b. Previous endocarditis
      c. Conduits

Table 3-2. Prophylaxis for subacute bacterial endocarditis

For patients with no allergy to penicillin
    30 min before the procedure
      1. Ampicillin, 2 g IV or IM
      2. Gentamicin, 1.5 mg/kg IV or IM (not to
         exceed 80 mg)
For patients allergic to penicillin
    1 hr before the procedure
      1. Vancomycin, 1 g IV over 1 hr
      2. Gentamicin, 1.5 mg/kg IV or IM (not to
         exceed 80 mg)

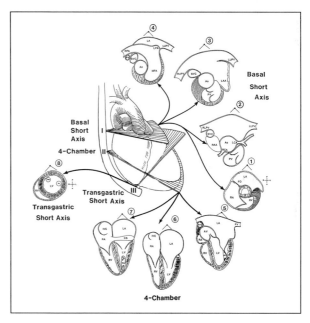

Fig. 3-2. Three primary horizontal (or cross-sectional) tomographic views of the heart by TEE. Multiple tomographic planes are obtained by various transducer positions and angulations. Basal short-axis planes (I) are initially obtained, usually with the transducer tip 25 to 30 cm from the incisors. Four-chamber planes (II) are obtained by retroflexion or slight advancement of the endoscope tip from position 1 (about 30–35 cm from the incisors). Transgastric short-axis planes (III) are obtained from the fundus of the stomach, 35 to 40 cm from the incisors. (From JB Seward et al. Transesophageal echocardiography: technique, anatomic correlations, implementation, and clinical applications. *Mayo Clin Proc* 1988;63:649–680.)

TEE images of these primary scan planes are shown in Figures 3-3 through 3-6.

Longitudinal Plane

With the tip of the transducer lying in the neutral long-axis orientation within the esophagus, a series of four primary views is obtained by rotation of the scope from the left cardiac structures toward the right side (clockwise rotation of the transducer; Fig. 3-7): (1) left ventricular (LV)–left atrial two-chamber view, (2) right ventricular outflow long-axis view, (3) ascending aorta–atrial septal view, and (4) caval–right atrial–atrial septal view [6]. Leftward and rightward flexion of the scope results in additional secondary long- and short-axis tomographic views (Fig. 3-8). The transgastric longitudinal plane provides a long-axis view of the heart (Fig. 3-9). Anatomic sections and corresponding transesophageal primary and secondary longitudinal views are shown in Figures 3-10 through 3-14.

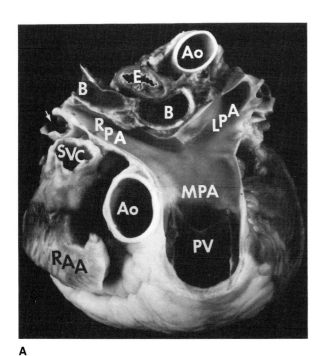

A

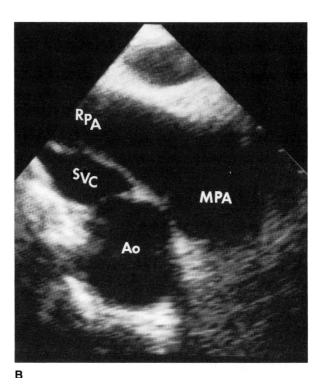

B

Fig. 3-3.   Anatomic specimen **(A)** and corresponding TEE image **(B)** of basal short-axis view at the level of main pulmonary artery (MPA). This is the uppermost tomographic plane from the basal short-axis view. The main pulmonary artery and right pulmonary artery (RPA) are well seen. However, the left pulmonary artery (LPA) is obscured by the bronchus (B). The ascending aorta (Ao) and superior vena cava (SVC) are well seen. (From JB Seward et al.: Transesophageal echocardiography: technique, anatomic correlations, implementation, and clinical applications. *Mayo Clin Proc* 1988;63:649–680.)

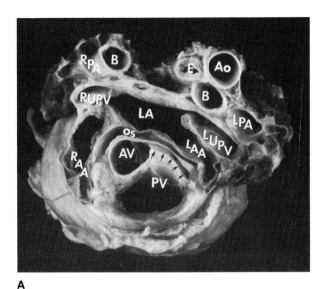

A

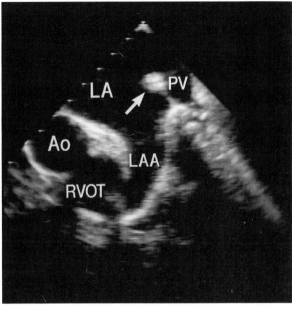

B

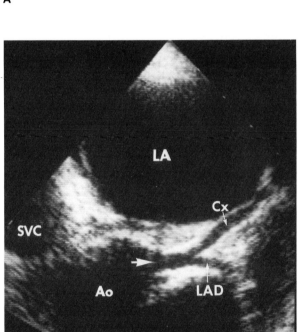

C

Fig. 3-4. Anatomic specimen **(A)** and corresponding TEE images **(B, C)** of basal short-axis scan at the level of the aortic valve. This view is obtained by advancing the transducer slightly further into the esophagus from the previous view or by retroflexing the transducer. The left atrium (LA) and the left atrial appendage (LAA) are well seen as well as the entrance of the left upper pulmonary vein (LUPV) into the LA. A bulbous structure (*arrow* in **B**) separates the left upper pulmonary vein from the left atrial appendage. The membranous structure looks like a Q-tip and should not be mistaken for a left atrial mass. In this view, the aortic valve (AV) is well seen as well as the origin of the left coronary artery (*black arrows* in **A**). There is a potential space or sinus (OS) between the aortic valve and the left atrium, which may be confused with a coronary artery. This space may become larger when pericardial effusion is present. Coronary arteries are located immediately below the left atrial appendage. From the short-axis view of the aortic valve, the left main artery (large arrow in **C**) and its bifurcation to the left anterior descending (LAD) and circumflex (Cx) coronary arteries can be visualized. (From JB Seward et al. Transesophageal echocardiography: technique, anatomic correlations, implementation, and clinical applications. *Mayo Clin Proc* 1988;63:649–680.)

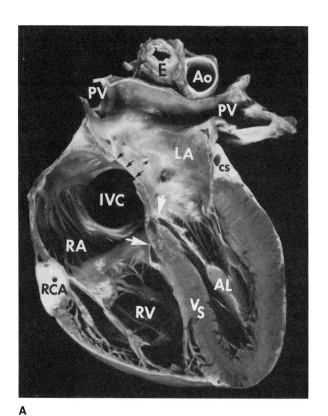

A

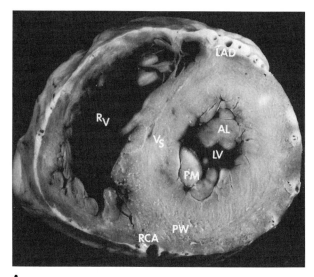

A

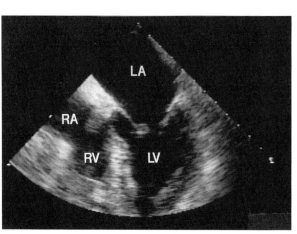

B

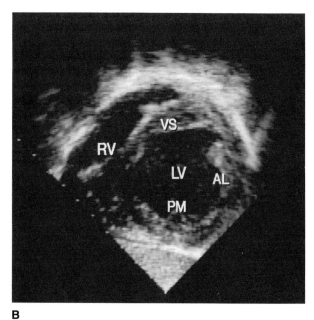

B

▲ **Fig. 3-5.** Anatomic specimen **(A)** and corresponding TEE image **(B).** With further retroflexion of the transducer, a conventional four-chamber view is obtained by TEE. This four-chamber view is best for delineating the morphologic characteristics of the cardiac crux (*large arrow* in **A**). (From JB Seward et al. Transesophageal echocardiography: technique, anatomic correlations, implementation, and clinical applications. *Mayo Clin Proc* 1988;63:649–680.)

◀ **Fig. 3-6.** Anatomic specimen **(A)** and corresponding 2D echo image **(B)** of transgastric short-axis view (40 cm from the incisors). With the transducer control in a neutral position, the instrument is advanced further into the stomach and anteflexed to image the short axis of the heart from the fundus of the stomach. This position is most frequently used to provide a cross-sectional view of the left ventrical (LV) as seen in the anatomic section dissected according to this particular tomographic plane. 2D echo image presentation is electronically inverted so that the posterior wall (PW) or inferior wall (IW) is displayed at the bottom of the screen, and the anterior wall (AW) is displayed at the top of the screen, similar to the transthoracic presentation of the parasternal short-axis view of the LV. This orientation projects the heart as if viewed from the apex toward the base. At the papillary muscle level, anterolateral (AL) and posteromedial (PM) papillary muscles are also seen. The right ventricle (RV) is displayed on the left side of the screen. (From JB Seward et al. Transesophageal echocardiography: technique, anatomic correlations, implementation, and clinical applications. *Mayo Clin Proc* 1988;63:649–680.)

Fig. 3-7. Schematic drawing of primary longitudinal TEE views of the heart. With the TEE transducer in the neutral position in the middle of the esophagus, a sequence of tomographic cardiac sections is obtained by clockwise rotation of the scope from the left side of the heart toward the right side of the heart. These images are in the sagittal plane of the thorax but are oblique to the body of the heart. The scope is advanced or withdrawn to image more inferior and superior structures lying in the same sagittal plane. The left atrial and LV inflow, right ventricular outflow tract, midportion of the ascending aorta, and superior and inferior venae cavae views are in the sagittal plane of the thorax. (From JB Seward et al. Biplanar transesophageal echocardiography: anatomic correlations, image orientation, and clinical applications. *Mayo Clin Proc* 1990;65:1193–1213.)

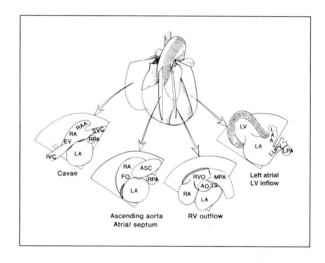

Fig. 3-8. Schematic drawing of secondary long- and short-axis tomographic views by longitudinal plane. The longitudinal array can be reoriented from the sagittal plane of the thorax planes that are in the long axis or short axis of the heart. This manipulation necessitates leftward and rightward flexion of the tip of the endoscope from the neutral position. The leftward flexion results in the long-axis view of the heart, whereas a rightward flexion orients the longitudinal plane into the short-axis view of the heart. (From JB Seward et al. Biplanar transesophageal echocardiography: anatomic correlations, image orientation, and clinical applications. *Mayo Clin Proc* 1990;65:1193–1213.)

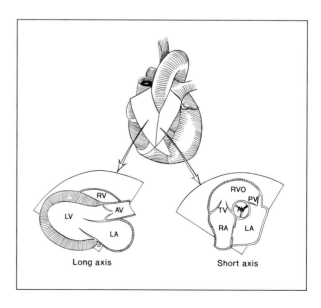

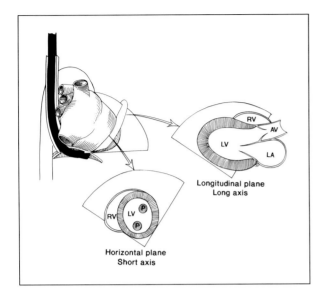

Fig. 3-9. Schematic drawing of horizontal and longitudinal transgastric views. The transducer is usually advanced into the transgastric position with the use of the horizontal plane of image (approximately 35–40 cm from the incisors). The transgastric short-axis view, obtained with the use of a horizontal array, is displayed with a transducer artifact at the bottom of the video screen. The result is a view compatible to a parasternal short-axis view of the LV. From this orientation, switching to a longitudinal array results in a long-axis view of the LV. The LV apex is often best appreciated by transgastric longitudinal plane imaging. For optimal long-axis orientation of the scanning array, slight leftward or rightward flexion and rotation of the tip of the transducer may be necessary. Rotation of the scope medially images the right ventricular inflow. Anteflexion of the scope produces an apical long-axis equivalent view of the LV and aortic and mitral valves.

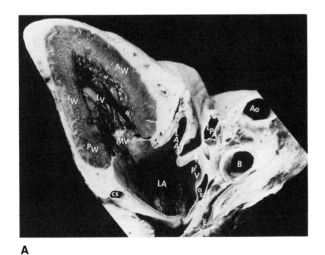

A

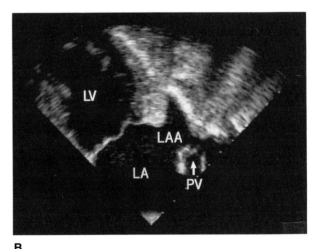

B

Fig. 3-10. Anatomic section **(A)** and corresponding 2D echo image **(B)** of the LV–left atrial two-chamber view. With the longitudinal array directed leftward within the esophagus, the body of the left atrial cavity is adjacent to the transducer. This section transects the left atrium, mitral valve orifice, and portions of the LV inflow tract. The left atrial appendage (LAA) and the left upper pulmonary vein are visualized anteriorly. (From JB Seward et al. Biplanar transesophageal echocardiography: anatomic correlations, image orientation, and clinical applications. *Mayo Clin Proc* 1990;65:1193–1213.)

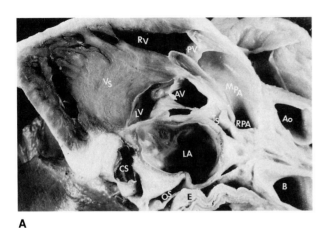

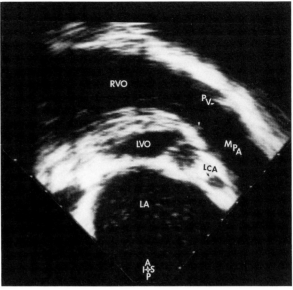

A　　　　　　　　　　　　　　　　　　　　　**B**

Fig. 3-11. Anatomic section **(A)** and corresponding 2D echo image **(B)** of the right ventricular outflow long-axis view. Slight rightward rotation of the longitudinal array results in imaging of the right ventricular outflow (RVO) tract, pulmonary valve (PV), main pulmonary artery (MPA), and proximal portion of the left pulmonary artery in the long axis. Posteriorly, the transducer is adjacent to the left atrial cavity. (From JB Seward et al. Biplanar transesophageal echocardiography: anatomic correlations, image orientation, and clinical applications. *Mayo Clin Proc* 1990;65:1193–1213.)

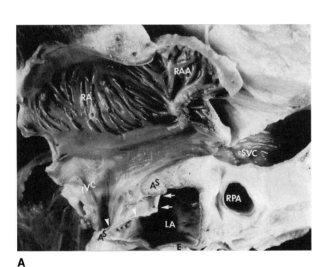

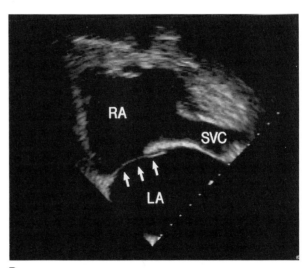

A　　　　　　　　　　　　　　　　　　　　　**B**

Fig. 3-12. Anatomic section **(A)** and corresponding 2D echo image **(B)** of caval–right atrial–atrial septal view. Still further rightward rotation of the longitudinal array allows for visualization of the superior vena cava (SVC) in the long axis, which lies to the right of and adjacent to the ascending aorta. Posterior or superior to the superior vena cava is the right pulmonary artery (RPA) transected in the short axis. The left atrium (LA) is adjacent to the transducer. The limbus of the atrial septum (AS) separates the right and the left atrial cavities. Anteriorly, the right atrium and the right atrial appendage (RAA) are seen in sagittal cross section. Advancement of the scope allows imaging of the eustachian valve and proximal portion of the inferior vena cava (IVC) in the long axis. The arrows indicate the atrial septum (AS). (From JB Seward et al. Biplanar transesophageal echocardiography: anatomic correlations, image orientation, and clinical applications. *Mayo Clin Proc* 1990;65:1193–1213.)

29

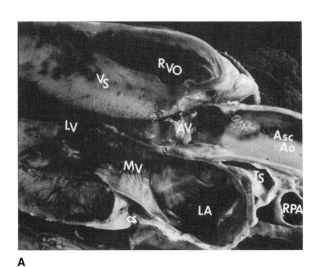

A

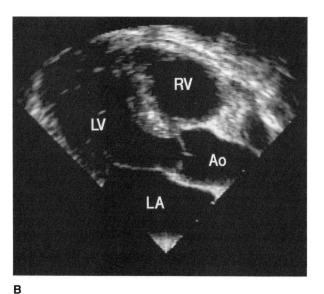

B

Fig. 3-13. Anatomic section **(A)** and corresponding 2D echo image **(B)** of the secondary long-axis view, which is good for visualization of the aortic valve, the LV outflow tract (LVOT), and the ascending aorta (Asc Ao). In order to image LVOT in the long axis, the tip of the scope is flexed leftward (laterally). This maneuver is achieved by fine manipulation and adjustment of an outer or a smaller control on the handle of the scope. Concomitant medial rotation of the tip of the scope is usually necessary to optimize this long-axis view of the LVOT, aortic valve, and the aortic root. This maneuver also best images the sagittal plane of the mitral valve (MV) orifice. Medial and lateral rotation of the scope allows sequential long-axis views comparable to a precordial parasternal long-axis image. (From JB Seward et al. Biplanar transesophageal echocardiography: anatomic correlations, image orientation, and clinical applications. *Mayo Clin Proc* 1990;65:1193–1213.)

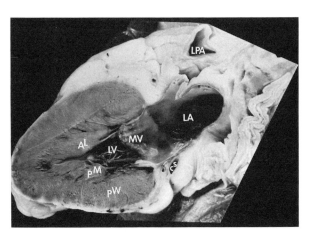

A

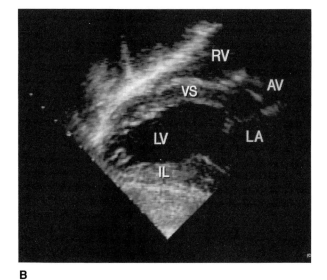

B

Fig. 3-14. Anatomic section **(A)** and corresponding 2D echo image **(B)** of the transgastric longitudinal view, which is similar to the transthoracic parasternal long-axis view. (From JB Seward et al. Biplanar transesophageal echocardiography: anatomic correlations, image orientation, and clinical applications. *Mayo Clin Proc* 1990;65:1193–1213.)

Multiplane

The multiplane probe has a rotating transducer along an axis perpendicular to the axis of the probe shaft (Fig. 3-15A). At 0-degree orientation, the acquired tomographic plane is equivalent to the horizontal plane, and at approximately 90-degree orientation, longitudinal plane images are obtained with the transducer about 30 cm from the patient's teeth [7]. The transducer can be rotated up to 180 degrees, which provides a mirror image of the 0-degree orientation (Fig. 3-15B). Therefore, multiple tomographic image planes are continuously developed by rotating the transducer without significant manipulation of the probe (Figs. 3-16 and 3-17).

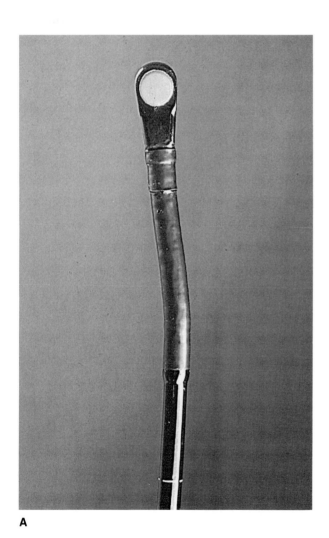

A

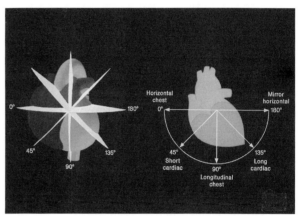

B

Fig. 3-15. **A.** A circular rotating multiplane TEE transducer. **B.** Array rotations at selected degrees (0, 45, 90, 135, and 180 degrees) permits a logical sequence of standard transducer orientations and resultant images. Such a display assists the examiner in the acquisition of desired views (i.e., 0-degree transverse orientation, which is horizontal to the chest at the midesophageal level; 45-degree short-axis orientation to the base of the heart from the midesophagus; 90-degree longitudinal orientation, which is in the sagittal plane of the body; 135-degree long-axis orientation to the heart from the midesophagus; and 180-degree rotation, which produces a mirror-image transverse plane). (From JB Seward et al. Multiplane transesophageal echocardiography: image orientation, examination technique, anatomic correlations, and clinical applications. *Mayo Clin Proc* 1993;68:523–551.)

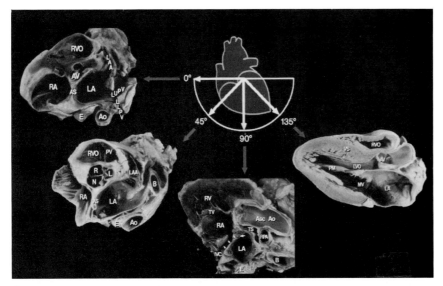

A

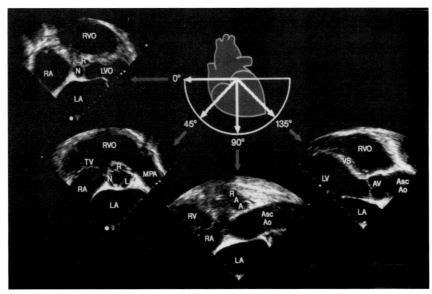

B

Fig. 3-16.   A. Tomographic anatomic sections of primary multiplane views at 0, 45, 90, and 135 degrees. The oblique short-axis cut of the base of the heart corresponds to the section at 0 degrees. The esophagus (E) is posterior and adjacent to the left atrium (LA). The tomographic cut is along the short axis of the body and not the short axis of the heart; consequently, the aortic valve (AV) cusps are cut obliquely. Often the left atrial appendage (LAA) and left upper (LUPV) and left lower (LLPV) pulmonary veins are best visualized in this short-axis view. The right atrium (RA) is to the viewer's left. The right ventricular outflow (RVO) is anterior. At 45 degrees, a short-axis view of the basal structure (i.e., aortic valve) is obtained. At 90 degrees, this tomographic section is equivalent to the longitudinal plane seen on biplane examination. A long-axis view of the ascending aorta (Asc Ao) and the atrial septum *(arrows)* is visualized. At 135 degrees, the tomographic section is similar to the transthoracic parasternal long-axis view demonstrating the LV outflow tract (LVO). **B.** Corresponding primary multiplane TEE images obtained by placing the probe at 30 cm from the patient's teeth. (From JB Seward et al. Multiplane transesophageal echocardiography: image orientation, examination technique, anatomic correlations, and clinical applications. *Mayo Clin Proc* 1993;68:523–551.)

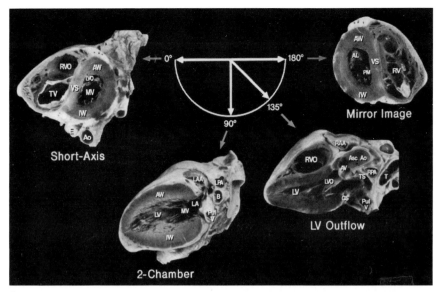

A

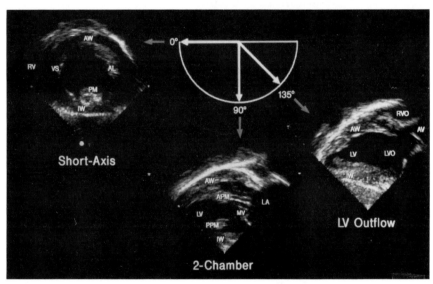

B

Fig. 3-17. **A.** Tomographic anatomic section of multiplane transgastric views.

Short-axis midventricle, 0-degree view: Short-axis cut of the left (LV) and right (RV) ventricles with the specimen viewed from the apex toward the base. The esophagus (E) is posterior and adjacent to the inferior wall (IW) of the LV. The LV is to the viewer's right and RV to the viewer's left. The right ventricular outflow (RVO) and LV anterior wall (AW) are viewed anteriorly. The thoracic aorta (Ao) is posterior and to the left of the esophagus (E).

Two-chamber, 90-degree view: The LV and left atrium (LA) are in the same long-axis tomographic cut. This is an excellent view for assessing mitral support apparatus and LV wall motion.

LV outflow, 135-degree view: The aortic valve (AV) and LV outflow are cut in long axis. The esophagus is posterior to the LV inferior wall.

Transgastric mirror-image short-axis, 180-degree view: Anatomic specimen viewed from the base toward the apex.
B. Multiplane transgastric views. With the transducer tip in a stable position, the array can be rotated to obtain a sequence of short- and long-axis views:

Short-axis view of LV—array at 0 degrees (transverse plane).

Two-chamber view of the LV—array at 90 degrees (longitudinal plane) with slight leftward rotation of the scope.

Long-axis view of the LV outflow—array at 110 to 135 degrees, which best visualizes the LV outflow (LVO) and aortic valve (AV) from the gastric transducer position.

A multitude of intermediate and oblique sections are provided (obtained) and are complementary for a thorough spatial anatomic diagnosis. (From JB Seward et al. Multiplane transesophageal echocardiography: image orientation, examination technique, anatomic correlations, and clinical applications. *Mayo Clin Proc* 1993;68:523–551.)

33

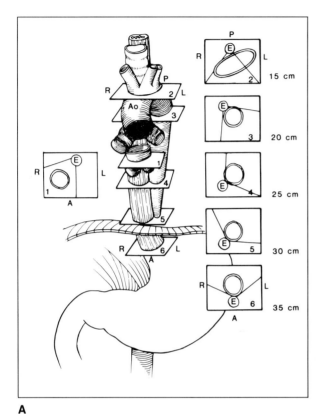

A

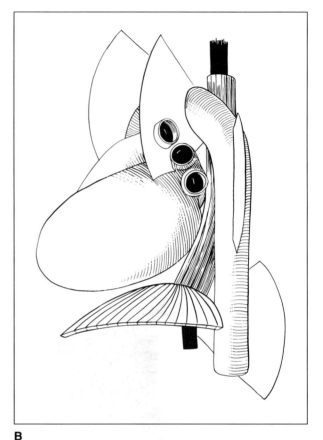

B

Fig. 3-18. **A.** The anatomic relationships of the aorta (Ao), trachea, and esophagus (E). Also shown are various levels of horizontal planes of the thoracic aorta: aortic root (1), transverse aortic arch (2), upper descending aorta (3), midthoracic aorta (4 and 5), and upper abdominal aorta (6). Note that the esophagus lies anterior to the aorta at the diaphragm and posterior at the level of the transverse arch. A portion of the ascending aorta directly anterior to the trachea is a blind area for TEE. A few internal landmarks allow the examiner to accurately designate anterior-posterior and right-left orientation of the midthoracic aorta. The examiner *must* record, in centimeters, the depth of the tip of the transducer and must relate orientation to an anatomic depiction, such as that shown in this diagram. A = anterior; L = left; P = posterior; R = right. **B.** The longitudinal imaging technique for the aortic arch, brachiocephalic vessels, and descending thoracic aorta. (From JB Seward et al. Transesophageal echocardiography: technique, anatomic correlations, image orientation, and clinical applications. *Mayo Clin Proc* 1988;63:649–680.)

Thoracic Aorta

By rotating the transducer laterally and posteriorly from cardiac views, the entire descending thoracic aorta and transverse arch can be visualized. Although the proximal part of the arch and the distal portion of the descending aorta may not be accessible to the horizontal plane of transesophageal imaging due to the interposed trachea [8], the longitudinal view allows visualization of the mid to upper portion of the ascending aorta, as well as the proximal part of the aortic arch. Schematic biplane imaging views of the aorta are shown in Figure 3-18. The short- and long-axis views of the normal descending thoracic aorta are shown in Figure 3-19.

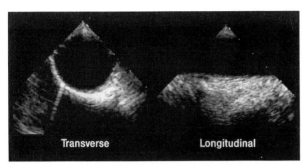

Fig. 3-19. Transverse (horizontal) and longitudinal TEE view of a normal descending thoracic aorta. The intimal surface is smooth and the luminal diameter is about 2 cm.

Table 3-3. Indications for TEE: 5,441 procedures

Indication	Frequency (%)
Source of embolism	36
Endocarditis	13
Native valvular disease	11
Prosthetic valvular disease	7
Congenital heart disease	7
Aortic pathology	7
Tumor/mass	6
Critically ill patients	3
Others	10

Data analyzed by Dr. BK Khandheria.

Clinical Applications

Table 3-3 shows the indications for 5,441 TEE procedures at the Mayo Clinic; this does not include intraoperative TEE. Although indications may vary from institution to institution depending on the patient populations, TEE has been shown to be essential in the evaluation of mitral valve pathology (both native and prosthetic), thrombus in the left atrium or left atrial appendage, atrial septal defect, valvular vegetation, ring abscess, aortic dissection, and critically ill patients. Clinical applications of TEE are discussed in detail individually in the appropriate chapters.

Complications

During the 5,441 procedures, most of the complications were benign (transient hypotension, supraventricular tachycardia, hypertension, parotid swelling). However, there were significant complications in 28 patients (0.5%): 1 died, 2 had ventricular tachycardia requiring electric cardioversion, 11 patients had laryngospasm, and 14 patients had hypoxia or worsening of heart failure. The European multicenter survey of 10,419 TEE examinations carried out by 54 physicians reported a similarly low rate of complications, including one death [9]. Since TEE is a semiinvasive procedure with potentially serious complications, it should be performed only by echocardiologists who are well trained in echocardiography and in the management of critical situations. The patient's vital signs, including oxygen saturation (pulse oximeter), cardiac rhythm, and blood pressure, should be monitored throughout the procedure.

Training and Role of Sonographer

TEE complements the transthoracic examination. Therefore, it is mandatory that the physician who performs TEE have prior training in transthoracic echocardiography including 2D, Doppler, and color-flow imaging. Since the endoscopy procedure is not routinely a part of the internal medicine training program, echocardiographers need to learn esophageal intubation under the supervision of an endoscopist. A minimum of 30 to 50 esophageal intubations is necessary to provide adequate exposure to the inexperienced individual [10].

The sonographer plays an essential role in the preparation of patients for TEE and in assisting the physician during the examination

[11]. The sonographer's role in TEE is summarized in Table 3-4. In our laboratory, a registered nurse sonographer coordinates and assists TEE. Because of the semiinvasive nature of TEE, the skills of a registered nurse are preferred for monitoring the patient closely; obtaining vital signs; administering medications; inserting intravenous lines; and using suction, oxygen, or other emergency equipment. A properly trained non-nurse sonographer can perform all of these functions except the administration of medications.

Future Development

Within a few years of clinical use, TEE has made a significant impact on the practice of

Table 3-4. A summary of the sonographer's role in TEE

Before procedure
  Preparation of equipment and supplies
    Assemble supplies
      Medications, normal saline flushes, and contrast medium
      Intravenous supplies (angiocatheter, three-way stopcock)
      Lidocaine spray and tongue blade
      Scope lubricant: lubricating jelly or viscous lidocaine
      Gloves, safety glasses, TEE probe, and bite block
    Maintain and check suction, oxygen, and basic life-support equipment
  Patient preparation
    Confirm that patient has had no oral intake for 4–6 hr before TEE
    Obtain brief history of drug allergies and current medications
    Explain procedure to patient
    Obtain baseline vital signs and monitor rhythm
    Remove patient's dentures, oral prostheses, and eyeglasses
    Establish intravenous line for administration of medications
    Place patient in the left lateral decubitus position with wedge support and safety restraints
    Assist patient during esophageal intubation, such as head position, breathing, and reassurance
  Drugs
    Endocarditis prophylaxis: American Heart Association recommendations
    Pharyngeal anesthesia: lidocaine 10% spray
    Drying agent: glycopyrrolate (Robinul)
    Sedative: midazolam hydrochloride (Versed), meperidine hydrochloride (Demerol)
During procedure
  Position and maintain bite block
  Monitor vital signs: rhythm, respiration, blood pressure, and oxygen saturation
  Use oral suction if necessary
  Have basic life-support equipment available
After procedure
  Assist patient during recovery period
  Remove intravenous line
  Instruct patient not to drive for 12 hr if sedation was used
  Record vital signs and patient's condition on dismissal
  Arrange for escort if patient is not completely recovered
  Clean scope with enzyme solution and glutaraldehyde disinfectant

Source: Modified from JM Mays et al. Transesophageal echocardiography: a sonographer's perspective. *J Am Soc Echocardiogr* 1991;4:513–518.

cardiovascular medicine. However, this technology is in its infancy and further progress in the following areas will be seen: multiplane probe, miniaturization of probe, wide-field imaging (Fig. 3-20), tissue characterization using TEE, and 3D reconstruction [12, 13].

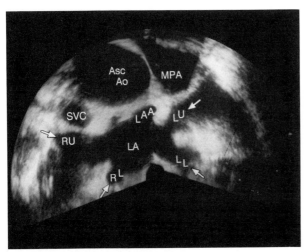

Fig. 3-20. Wide-field tomographic transesophageal image of four pulmonary vein connections—left upper (LU), left lower (LL), right upper (RU), and right lower (RL)—to the left atrium (LA). This was obtained by manual rotation of the transducer in the esophagus. Several images were positioned side by side to produce a circular composite photograph.

References

1. Frazin L, et al. Esophageal echocardiography. *Circulation* 1976;54:102–108.

2. Schluter M, et al. Transesophageal cross-sectional echocardiography with a phased array transducer system: technique and initial clinical results. *Br Heart J* 1982;48:67–72.

3. Seward JB, et al. Transesophageal echocardiography: technique, anatomic correlations, implementation, and clinical applications. *Mayo Clin Proc* 1988;63:649–680.

4. Gorge G, et al. Positive blood cultures during transesophageal echocardiography. *Am J Cardiol* 1990;65:1404–1405.

5. Steckelberg JM, et al. Prospective evaluation of the risks of bacteremia associated with transesophageal echocardiography. *Circulation* 1991;84:177–180.

6. Seward JB, et al. Biplanar transesophageal echocardiography: anatomic correlations, image orientation, and clinical applications. *Mayo Clin Proc* 1990;65:1193–1213.

7. Seward JB, et al. Multiplane transesophageal echocardiography: image orientation, examination technique, anatomic correlations, and clinical applications. *Mayo Clin Proc* 1993;68:523–551.

8. Erbel R, et al. Echocardiography in diagnosis of aortic dissection. *Lancet* 1989;1:457–461.

9. Daniel W, et al. Safety of transesophageal echocardiography: a multicenter survey of 10,419 examinations. *Circulation* 1991;83:817–821.

10. Khandheria BK. Transesophageal echocardiography: technique and training (letter to the editor). *J Am Soc Echocardiogr* 1990;3:177–178.

11. Mays JM, et al. Transesophageal echocardiography: a sonographer's perspective. *J Am Soc Echocardiogr* 1991;4:513–518.

12. Khandheria BK, Oh JK. Transesophageal echocardiography: state-of-the-art and future directions. *Am J Cardiol* 1992;16:9–20.

13. Seward JB, Khandheria BK, Tajik AJ. Wide-field transesophageal echocardiographic tomography: feasibility study. *Mayo Clin Proc* 1990;65:31–37.

4

Assessment of Ventricular Function

"Assess left ventricular (LV) function" is one of the most common referral reasons for echocardiography since clinical management decisions rely heavily on the status of LV function. 2D echocardiography visualizes in real time directly the entire myopericardial layers at any point in the cardiac cycle, and hence is best suited for the evaluation of regional as well as global myocardial contraction and relaxation. Doppler echocardiography determines the diastolic filling pattern of the ventricles by measuring ventricular relaxation, compliance, and filling velocities during various diastolic phases. Therefore, systolic and diastolic ventricular function and filling characteristics can be readily, reliably, and serially measured by the comprehensive echocardiography examination.

Quantitation of the Left Ventricle

The American Society of Echocardiography has recommended the quantitation method of 2D echocardiography for determining the linear dimensions, area, and volume of the LV cavity [1]. Once the most satisfactory 2D echocardiographic images are obtained to optimize endocardial definitions, measurements of the dimensions, area, volume, and mass are derived as described in the following discussion. Their normal values are listed in Tables 4-1 through 4-4.

Table 4-1.   Heart chamber measurements by 2D echocardiography

View	Normal range (cm) (mean ± 2 SD)	Mean (cm)	Index range (cm/m²)	Absolute range (cm)
Apical four-chamber				
LVED major	6.9–10.3	8.6	4.1–5.7	7.2–10.3
LVED minor	3.3–6.1	4.7	2.2–3.1	3.8–6.2
LVES minor	1.9–3.7	2.8	1.3–2.0	2.1–3.9
LVFS	0.27–0.50	38.0	—	0.26–0.47
RV major	6.5–9.5	8.0	3.8–5.3	6.3–9.3
RV minor	2.2–4.4	3.3	1.0–2.8	2.2–4.5
Parasternal long-axis				
LVED	3.5–6.0	4.8	2.3–3.1	3.8–5.8
LVES	2.1–4.0	3.1	1.4–2.1	2.3–3.9
FS	0.25–0.46	36.0	—	0.26–0.45
RV	1.9–3.8	2.8	1.2–2.0	1.9–3.9
Parasternal short-axis				
Chordal level				
LVED	3.5–6.2	4.8	2.3–3.2	3.8–6.1
LVES	2.3–4.0	3.2	1.5–2.2	2.6–4.2
LVFS	0.27–0.42	34.0	—	0.27–0.41
Papillary muscle level				
LVED	3.5–5.8	4.7	2.2–3.1	3.9–5.8
LVES	2.2–4.0	3.1	1.4–2.2	2.5–4.1
LVFS	0.25–0.43	34.0	—	0.25–0.43

LVED = left ventricle, end-diastole; LVES = left ventricle, end-systole; LVFS = left ventricular fractional shortening; RV = right ventricle; FS = fractional shortening.
Note: Although it is a common and useful practice in adult cardiology to correct values for body surface area, for pediatric applications or for smaller or larger than average subjects, charts based on subjects of a wide range of body sizes should be consulted.
Source: Data from I Schnittger et al. Standardized intracardiac measurements of two-dimensional echocardiography. *J Am Coll Cardiol* 1983;2:934–938.)

Table 4-2.   Linear dimensions and areas from the LV base (normal values)*

	Range	Range corrected for BSA	No.
LV diameter, diastole	3.6–5.2 cm	2.0–2.8 cm/m²	49
LV diameter, systole	2.3–3.9 cm	1.3–2.1 cm/m²	49
Fractional shortening	0.18–0.42	—	49
LV short-axis area, diastole	9.5–22.3 cm²	5.5–11.9 cm/m²	44
LV short-axis area, systole	4.0–11.6 cm²	2.4–6.4 cm/m²	44
Fractional area change	0.36–0.64	—	—

BSA = body surface area.
*Values are derived from 50 subjects; age range, 19–63 yr; mean age, 31.2 ± 10.0 yr; BSA range, 1.44–2.48 m²; mean BSA, 1.84 ± 0.18 m².
Source: Data from H Feigenbaum. *Echocardiography* (4th ed). Philadelphia: Lea & Febiger, 1986.

Table 4-3. LV volumes (normal values)

Methods	End-diastole mean ± SD (ml) (range)	End-systole mean ± SD (ml) (range)
Four-chamber area length		
Male patients	112 ± 27 (65–193)	35 ± 16 (13–86)
Female patients	89 ± 20 (59–136)	33 ± 12 (13–59)
Two-chamber area length		
Male patients	130 ± 27 (73–201)	40 ± 14 (17–74)
Female patients	92 ± 19 (53–146)	31 ± 11 (11–53)
Biplane disk summation (modified Simpson's rule)		
Male patients	111 ± 22 (62–170)	34 ± 12 (14–76)
Female patients	80 ± 12 (55–101)	29 ± 10 (13–60)

Source: Data from DW Wahr, YS Wang, NB Schiller. Left ventricular volumes determined by two-dimensional echocardiography in a normal adult population. *J Am Coll Cardiol* 1983;1:863–868.

Table 4-4. Left ventricular mass (normal values, means ± SD) determined by the truncated ellipsoid method

	Males (n = 44)	Females (n = 40)
Mass (g)	148 ± 26	108 ± 21
Mass index (g/m²)	76 ± 13	66 ± 11

Source: Data from JW Helak, N Reichek. Quantitation of human left ventricular mass and volume by two-dimensional echocardiography in vitro anatomic validation. *Circulation* 1981;63:1398–1407.

Dimensions and Area

The LV cavity size is determined from multiple linear dimensions taken directly from the parasternal long-axis and short-axis views at the papillary muscle level, and apical views (Fig. 4-1). These dimensions can be obtained either by separate manual measurements or by an automatic endocardial tracing for area and volume determinations. To obtain the basal LV contractile function, another linear dimension can be obtained at the mitral valve level using the parasternal long-axis view. Dimensions are aligned perpendicular to the major axis of the LV cavity at the level of the mitral valve and chordal junction in systole and diastole (Fig. 4-2). Representative LV cavity areas are deter-mined from the short-axis papillary muscle view from which fractional area changes are calculated. However, it does not accurately reflect changes in the apical segment.

Volume

LV cavity volume is measured from the dimensions and area obtained from orthogonal apical views (four-chamber and two-chamber views). Quantitative programs digitize the endocardial surface of the LV in the two apical views, and utilize the *modified Simpson's rule* (or disk summation method) to calculate volume (Fig. 4-3). If only one apical view is available, a single-plane area length method is used.

Mass

There are two methods of calculating LV mass from 2D echocardiography—the *area length method* and the *truncated ellipsoid method* [1]. For both methods, the short-axis view of the LV at the papillary muscle level and the apical four- and two-chamber views at end-diastole are required. Myocardial mass is equal to the product of volume and the specific gravity of the myocardium, 1.04 g/ml. Built-in software in the ultrasound unit can make both

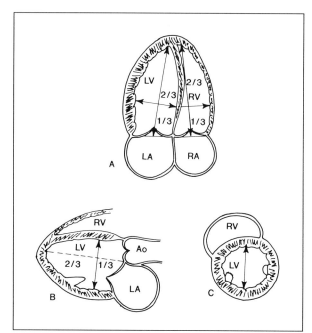

Fig. 4-1. Measurement of ventricular dimensions. **A.** The major long-axis measurement is obtained from the apical four-chamber view from the apical endocardium to middle mitral valve plane. The minor short axis is measured from one-third of the length of the long axis from the base and orthogonal to it. **B.** The long and short axes can be measured similarly from the parasternal long-axis view, but this view rarely shows the true LV apex. **C.** The short axis is measured from the parasternal short-axis view at the level of the papillary muscle tip. (Modified from N Schiller et al. Recommendations for quantitation of the left ventricle by two-dimensional echocardiography. *J Am Soc Echocardiogr* 1989;2:358.)

Fig. 4-3. Calculation of LV volume from two orthogonal apical views obtained by 2D echocardiography (modified Simpson's rule). **A.** The two-chamber view. **B.** The four-chamber view. The modified Simpson's rule is based on the summation of areas from diameters ai and bi of the number (n) of cylinders or disks of equal height. The number (n) of cylinders varies from 4 to 256. L = length; Σ = summation. (Modified from N Schiller et al. Recommendations for quantitation of the left ventricle by two-dimensional echocardiography. *J Am Soc Echocardiogr* 1989;2:358.)

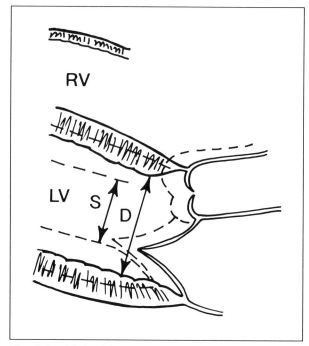

Fig. 4-2. Method for measurement of basal LV contractile function. Dimensions are aligned perpendicular to the major axis of the ventricular cavity at the level of the chordal-mitral junction. This can be utilized to predict the outcome of LV apical aneurysmectomy. (From N Schiller et al. Recommendations for quantitation of the left ventricle by two-dimensional echocardiography. *J Am Soc Echocardiogr* 1989;2:358.)

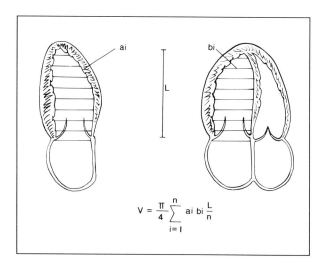

$$V = \frac{\pi}{4} \sum_{i=1}^{n} ai \; bi \; \frac{L}{n}$$

methods available so that the mass is automatically calculated once all the variables are entered. LV mass can also be estimated from 2D-guided M-mode measurements of LV dimension and wall thicknesses at the papillary muscle level. Without measuring the LV major axis, LV mass is reliably obtained from the LV short-axis dimension and a simple geometric cube formula. The following equation provides an accurate determination of LV mass according to Devereux and associates [2]:

LV mass (g) =
1.04 ([LVID + PWT + IVST]³ − LVID³) × 0.8 + 0.6

where LVID = LV internal dimension,
    PWT = posterior wall thickness,
    IVST = interventricular septal thickness
       measured at end-diastole,
    1.04 = specific gravity of the
       myocardium, and
    0.8 = correction factor.

Values for the upper LV mass index (LV mass in g/m² body surface area) determined by the above formula at the Mayo Clinic are shown in Figure 4-4.

Systolic Function

Global Function

Two parameters are most frequently used to express LV global systolic function: (1) fractional shortening or ejection fraction, and (2) cardiac output. *Fractional shortening* is a percent change in LV cavity dimension with systolic contraction and can be calculated from the following equation:

$$\text{Fractional shortening} = \frac{\text{LVED} - \text{LVES}}{\text{LVED}} \times 100\%$$

where LVED = LV end-diastolic dimension, and
    LVES = LV end-systolic dimension.

Ejection fraction represents stroke volume as a percent of end-diastolic LV volume; hence, its determination requires LV volume measurement.

$$\text{Ejection fraction} = \frac{\text{EDV} - \text{ESV}}{\text{EDV}} \times 100\%$$

where EDV = end-diastolic volume, and
    ESV = end-systolic volume.

Most current echocardiographic units do have volume measurement capability by digitizing the LV endocardial surface. The American Society of Echocardiography recommends the simplified Simpson's method to estimate ventricular volume from two orthogonal apical views (see Fig. 4-3). Quinones and coauthors [3] proposed a simplified method for determining ejection fraction by measuring LV internal dimensions.

Ejection fraction = (%ΔD²) + ([1 − %ΔD²][%ΔL])

where %ΔD² = $\dfrac{\text{LVED}^2 - \text{LVES}^2}{\text{LVED}^2} \times 100\%$
       fractional shortening of the square
       of the minor axis, and
    %ΔL = fractional shortening of the long
       axis, mainly related to apical
       contraction, where 15% is normal;
       5%, hypokinetic apex; 0%, akinetic
       apex; −5%, mildly dyskinetic apex;
       and −10%, apical aneurysm.

The equation has two components: fractional shortening of the square of the minor axis and fractional shortening of the long axis. LVED and LVES can be measured as an average of three short-axis dimensions at the basal, mid

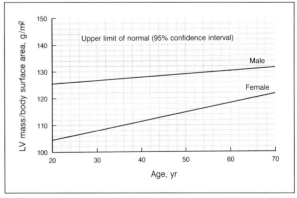

Fig. 4-4. Upper normal LV mass index values according to age and sex. (Courtesy of C Shub, M.D.)

(papillary muscle), and apical levels using a pair of calipers on the video screen, or from a midlevel short-axis dimension assuming a uniform contraction of minor axes. Since it is difficult to measure the fractional shortening of the long axis, empirical values are assigned according to apical wall motion. An example of estimating LV ejection fraction from the midlevel short-axis view is shown in Figure 4-5.

Cardiac output is the product of stroke volume and heart rate. Stroke volume is determined either by 2D volumetric measurement, as in calculation of ejection fraction, or by Doppler method using LV outflow tract diameter and time velocity integral (see Chap. 5).

Regional Function

LV regional wall motion analysis is usually based on grading of contractility of individual segments [4]. There are various LV segmental models depending on how the LV is subdivided. For the purpose of standardized analysis, the LV is divided into three levels (basal, mid, and apical) and 16 segments (Fig. 4-6)[1]. The basal and mid (papillary muscle) levels

are each subdivided into 6 segments, and the apical level is subdivided into 4 segments. All 16 segments can be visualized from multiple tomographic planes of surface echocardiography. With transesophageal echocardiography (TEE), regional wall motion analysis is best done using the biplane transgastric view (Fig. 4-7). Transesophageal views analogous to transthoracic apical four- and two-chamber views are obtained by horizontal and longitudinal views (see Fig. 4-7) with the transesophageal transducer in the midesophagus area (about 30 cm from the teeth). When the multiplane probe is available, rotation of the transducer crystal to 120 to 135 degrees from the horizontal plane (at 0 degrees) produces an imaging plane similar to the parasternal long-axis view (Fig. 4-8). Based on the contractility of the individual segments, a numerical scoring system has been adopted in which higher scores indicate more severe wall motion abnormality (1 = normal; 2 = hypokinesis;

Fig. 4-6. Sixteen-segment model for regional wall motion analysis proposed by the American Society of Echocardiography. The LV is divided into three levels (basal, mid or papillary muscle, and apical). The basal and mid levels are each subdivided into 6 segments and the apical level is subdivided into 4 segments. All 16 segments can be visualized from multiple tomographic planes. According to contractility, each segment is given a wall motion score. Segment 13 (apical septum) should be used only once, depending on the coronary anatomy. Also, it should be noted that there is no apical segment of the posterolateral wall.

Fig. 4-5. An M-mode echocardiogram of the LV at the papillary muscle level. The LV end-diastolic internal dimension *(long arrow)* measured at the onset of QRS is 48 mm and LV end-systolic internal dimension *(short arrow)* is 32 mm. Therefore,

$$\text{LV ejection fraction} = \frac{48^2 - 32^2}{48^2} \times 100 = 56\%$$

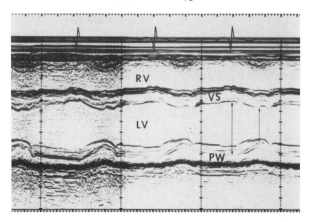

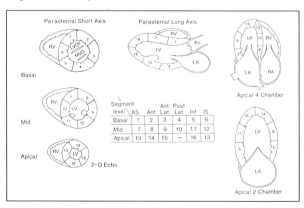

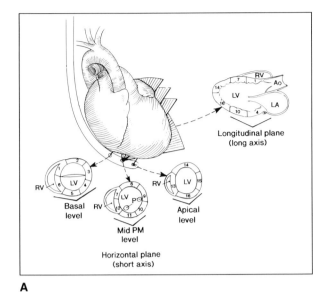

A

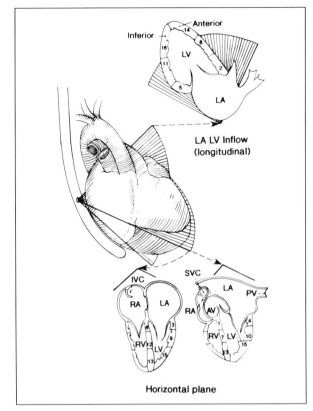

B

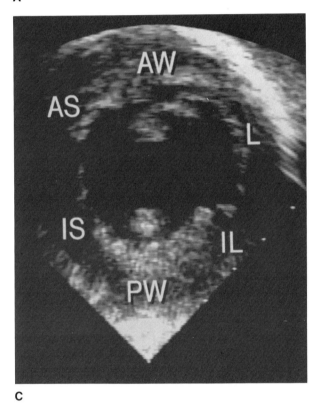

C

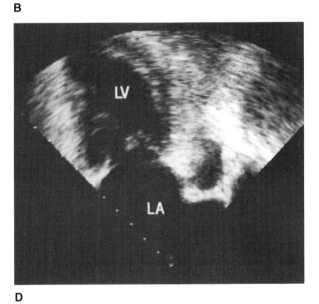

D

Fig. 4-7. Schematic diagram of LV regional wall motion analysis by transesophageal echocardiography (TEE). This is done primarily by placing the transducer at the transgastric **(A)** and midesophagus **(B)** positions, about 30 cm from teeth. Transgastric imaging in the horizontal plane provides a series of short-axis views similar to parasternal short-axis views. The transducer tip needs to be maneuvered in the fundus to obtain the short-axis views at different levels. The transgastric longitudinal plane provides a long-axis view of the LV similar to the parasternal long-axis view. The LV apex may not be visualized in all patients. The LV walls are segmented according to the American Society of Echocardiography recommendation, and the numbering of each segment is identical to that for transthoracic echocardiography (see Fig. 4-6). With the transducer at the midesophagus position **(B)**, the horizontal plane provides views similar to the apical four-chamber and long-axis views and the longitudinal plane provides views similar to the apical two-chamber view. **C, D.** Corresponding TEE images of the LV from the transgastric horizontal view at the papillary muscle level **(C)** and the midesophagus longitudinal view **(D).** The images were electronically inverted so that the position of the transducer and the posterior structures are located at the bottom.

3 = akinesis; 4 = dyskinesis; 5 = aneurysmal). A *wall motion score index* (WMSI) is derived by dividing the sum of wall motion scores by the number of visualized segments, and represents the extent of regional wall motion abnormalities.

$$WMSI = \frac{\text{sum of wall motion scores}}{\text{number of visualized segments}}$$

Diastolic Filling Profiles

It is now well recognized that congestive heart failure (CHF) syndrome can be seen in the presence of an entirely normal LV systolic function. In these patients (an estimated 30% of patients with CHF), the CHF is secondary to LV diastolic dysfunction. It is, therefore, mandatory that not only systolic but also diastolic LV function be assessed in all patients with CHF.

Definition of Diastole

Diastole begins with myocardial relaxation at the end of systolic contraction (A_2, aortic valve closure) and ventricular pressure starts to decline (isovolumic relaxation). When the left atrial pressure exceeds the LV pressure, the mitral valve opens to allow an early (E) rapid filling phase of the LV. The LV pressure continues to decline after the onset of E, but soon increases again with continuous ventricular filling equalizing with left atrial pressure, resulting in a period of diastasis. Another bolus of ventricular filling occurs with left atrial contraction (A) whose contribution to the total cardiac output depends on LV filling pressure and atrial contractility. Therefore, diastole is divided into four phases:

1. Isovolumic relaxation time (IVRT): A_2 to mitral valve opening
2. Rapid filling phase (RFP)
3. Diastasis
4. Atrial filling phase (AFP)

The transmitral pressure changes during diastole are reflected by pulsed-wave Doppler mi-

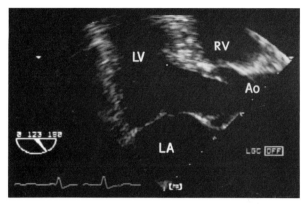

Fig. 4-8. Multiplane 2D TEE image with the transducer rotated 123 degrees from the horizontal plane (0 degrees). This provides an excellent view of the aortic valve, LV outflow tract, anteroseptum, and the mitral valve, similar to the parasternal long-axis view.

tral flow velocities [5, 6] (Fig. 4-9). Mitral flow velocities are measured by pulsed-wave Doppler, with the sample volume placed between the leaflet tips, and the following diastolic filling parameters are derived: IVRT, early filling velocity (E), late filling velocity (A), and deceleration time (DT) of E. When the ventricular filling pattern is evaluated, it is important to keep the sample volume between the leaflet tips since Doppler parameters are dependent on the sample volume location. Both E and A velocities are smaller with the sample volume at the mitral annulus compared to the leaflet tip position [7]. The DT is also shorter at the annulus position (Fig. 4-10).

Based on the Doppler velocity patterns, the diastolic filling abnormalities can be classified into three broad categories [8, 9]: *relaxation abnormality, restrictive physiology,* and *pseudonormalization* (Fig. 4-11).

Abnormal Relaxation

When myocardial relaxation is the predominant diastolic abnormality, IVRT is prolonged and the initial decline in LV pressure is slow. Hence, early filling is reduced, and there is a

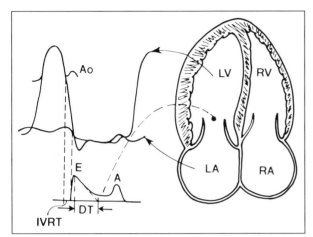

Fig. 4-9. Schematic drawing of pressure tracings from the LV, left atrium (LA), and aorta (Ao) and the corresponding transmitral Doppler flow velocities. Mitral velocities reflect transmitral pressure gradients and are used to derive diastolic parameters as shown.

large compensatory filling with atrial contraction. The ventricle continues to relax even after the opening of the mitral valve, and it takes longer to equalize ventricular pressure with atrial pressure, resulting in a longer DT. Therefore, abnormal myocardial relaxation is characterized by a constellation of abnormalities consisting of

1. Prolonged IVRT (≥ 110 msec)
2. Low E velocity and high A velocity
3. Reversed E/A ratio (< 1.0)
4. Prolonged DT (≥ 240 msec)

Restrictive Physiology

When ventricular compliance is decreased, the rise in ventricular diastolic pressure is very rapid during the early filling phase (short DT) and the elevated LV end-diastolic pressure minimizes ventricular filling due to atrial contraction (decreased A). With the resultant high left atrial pressure, the IVRT becomes shortened and the E velocity is high. This particular diastolic filling pattern is indicative of "restric-

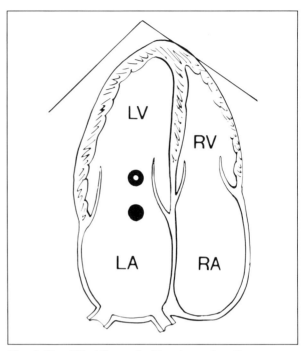

Fig. 4-10. Mitral flow velocities depend on the sample volume locations. The early filling wave (E) and late filling wave (A) peak velocities are significantly higher at the tips. The E velocity increase is greater than the A velocity increase, producing a higher E/A ratio at the tips than at the annulus *(closed circle)*. Therefore, the sample volume should be located between the leaflet tip to assess ventricular filling pattern, to determine the deceleration or pressure half-time, and to evaluate constrictive hemodynamics with respiration. The sample volume location should be at the level of the mitral annulus when the velocities are utilized for calculation of stroke volume. (From ZP Ding et al. Effect of sample volume location on Doppler-derived transmitral inflow velocity values. *J Am Soc Echocardiogr* 1991;4:451–456.)

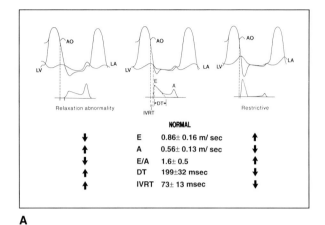

A

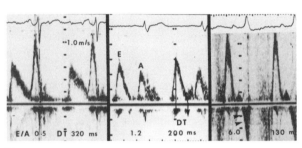

B

Fig. 4-11.   A. Schematic LV, aortic, and left atrial (LA) pressure tracings in three different filling conditions, along with corresponding mitral inflow Doppler spectrum. The mitral inflow velocity tracing represents the LA-LV diastolic pressure gradient. Normally, early rapid filling (E) has a velocity higher than that of filling due to atrial contraction (A). Deceleration time (DT) measures the interval between peak E velocity and the time it reaches the baseline (i.e., time to equilibrate LA and LV diastolic pressure). Isovolumic relaxation time (IVRT) is the interval from aortic valve closure to mitral valve opening. It is prolonged in patients with relaxation abnormalities and shortened in restrictive conditions. **B.** Examples of normal (center), relaxation abnormality (left), and restrictive diastolic filling (right) in mitral inflow. The arrowheads indicate diastolic mitral regurgitation, which is common in restrictive filling. It should also be noted that atrial flow duration is short in restrictive filling (right).

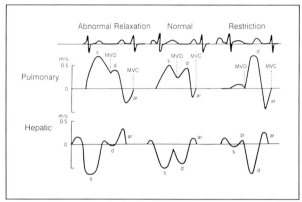

Fig. 4-12.   Schematic drawing of pulmonary and hepatic venous flow velocities in different diastolic filling patterns. Pulmonary venous flow velocity is recorded by placing a sample volume in a pulmonary vein using the transthoracic apical view or the transesophageal basal short-axis view. Normal pulmonary venous flow has systolic (s) and diastolic (d) components. Systolic velocity is usually higher than diastolic velocity with sinus rhythm. A small amount of atrial flow reversal (ar) is normal. In restrictive filling, systolic flow is limited due to increased atrial pressure, and predominant forward flow is during diastole after the opening of the mitral valve (MVO). The velocity and flow duration of pulmonary vein atrial flow reversal are increased and lengthened in restrictive physiology. In relaxation abnormality, systolic flow is the predominant antegrade flow.

Hepatic venous flow is recorded by placing a sample volume in the hepatic vein at least 1 cm away from its junction with the inferior vena cava, from the subcostal window. Normal hepatic venous flow (in sinus rhythm) has larger systolic (s) and smaller diastolic (d) components than does pulmonary venous flow. In restriction, systolic flow is diminished, whereas it is increased in relaxation abnormality. Normal hepatic venous Doppler velocities are usually higher with inspiration. Normally, there are small systolic (sr) and diastolic atrial reversal (ar) velocities that get accentuated slightly with expiration.

In patients with atrial fibrillation, systolic forward flow velocity is lower than that of diastolic forward flow both in the pulmonary and the hepatic veins.

tive" physiology characterized by the following diastolic parameters:

1. Shortened IVRT (< 60 msec)
2. High E velocity and low A velocity
3. Increased E/A ratio (≥ 2.0)
4. Shortened DT (≤ 150 msec)

Restrictive physiology pattern is seen whenever LV diastolic pressure rises rapidly and end-diastolic pressure is high, as in LV failure, restrictive cardiomyopathy, volume overload, and severe acute aortic regurgitation.

Pseudonormalization

When relaxation abnormality and restrictive hemodynamics coexist, Doppler features of the latter predominate. However, there is a transitional period when they become "pseudonormalized." The pseudonormalization pattern is present when the left atrial pressure rises moderately in the setting of abnormal myocardial relaxation, producing a diastolic filling pattern similar to the normal pattern. Pulmonary venous flow velocity is helpful in separating pseudonormal from true normal diastolic filling. Pulmonary venous systolic forward flow velocity is decreased in pseudonormalization, whereas it is higher than diastolic forward flow in the true normal filling pattern. Furthermore, the elevated left atrial pressure in the patient with pseudonormal mitral inflow produces a longer duration and higher velocity of pulmonary vein atrial flow reversal.

Venous Flow Pattern in Diastolic Filling Assessment

Venous flow (pulmonary and hepatic vein) velocity patterns are also useful in the evaluation of diastolic filling of a respective ventricle [10, 11] (Fig. 4-12). These Doppler parameters need to be recorded simultaneously with respirometer recording during the evaluation of pericardial effusion, tamponade, or constriction. Right-side flow velocities normally do vary with respiration, but left-side flow veloci-

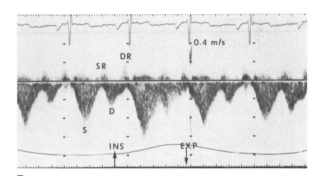

Fig. 4-13. **A.** Pulsed-wave Doppler recording from the left upper pulmonary vein (PV) using TEE. Systolic (S) forward flow velocity is increased and atrial reversal (R) is also increased, consistent with relaxation abnormality. **B.** Normal pulsed-wave Doppler recording from the hepatic vein. Systolic (S) forward flow is greater than diastolic (D) forward flow. Both components are higher during inspiration (INS) than expiration (EXP). Short systolic (SR) and diastolic (DR) reversals are normally present.

ties do not change significantly unless the patient has cardiac tamponade, constrictive pericarditis, right ventricular infarct, or chronic obstructive lung disease [12–14]. Representative pulmonary and hepatic venous Doppler patterns are shown in Figure 4-13. See Chapter 5 for hemodynamic assessment by diastolic filling parameters.

Automated Edge Detection System

The accuracy of quantitating LV dimensions, area, volume, and mass depends on how well the endocardial border is defined. Current commercially available ultrasound units permit manual border tracing, but it is time-consuming and subject to significant interobserver variability, which make routine quantitative measurements difficult. Most recently, an on-line, automated, endocardial border edge detection system has been developed [15]. This system allows instantaneous determination of LV cavity areas, displayed as a continuous waveform throughout the cardiac cycle. The area changes derived from the automated edge detection system correlate well with LV volume changes. Therefore, relative volume changes, ejection fraction, and diastolic filling fractions can be readily determined on a beat-to-beat basis. Once a more refined automated edge detection system is commercially available, quantitation of LV function will be easier and will become a routine part of the comprehensive echocardiographic examination.

References

1. American Society of Echocardiography Committee on Standards. Recommendations for quantification of the left ventricle by two-dimensional echocardiography. *J Am Soc Echocardiogr* 1989;2:358–367.
2. Devereux RB, et al. Echocardiographic assessment of left ventricular hypertrophy: comparison to necropsy findings. *Am J Cardiol* 1986;57:450–458.
3. Quinones MA, et al. A new simplified and accurate method for determining ejection fraction with two-dimensional echocardiography. *Circulation* 1981;64:744–753.
4. Shiina A, et al: Prognostic significance of regional wall motion abnormality in patients with prior myocardial infarction: a prospective correlative study of two-dimensional echocardiography and angiography. *Mayo Clin Proc* 1986;61:254–262.
5. Nishimura RA, et al. Assessment of diastolic function of the heart: background and current applications of Doppler echocardiography. Part I: physiologic and pathophysiologic features. *Mayo Clin Proc* 1989;64:71–81.
6. Nishimura RA, et al. Assessment of diastolic function of the heart: background and current applications of Doppler echocardiography. Part II: Clinical Studies *Mayo Clin Proc* 1989;64:181–204.
7. Ding ZP, et al. Effect of sample volume location on Doppler-derived transmitral inflow velocity values. *J Am Soc Echocardiogr* 1991;4:451–456.
8. Appleton CP, Hatle LK, Popp RL. Relation of transmitral flow velocity patterns to left ventricular diastolic function: new insights from a combined hemodynamic and Doppler echocardiographic study. *J Am Coll Cardiol* 1988;12:426–440.
9. Appleton CP, Hatle LK, Popp RL. Demonstration of restrictive ventricular physiology by Doppler echocardiography. *J Am Coll Cardiol* 1988;11:757–768.
10. Appleton CP, Hatle LK, Popp RL. Superior vena cava and hepatic vein Doppler echocardiography in healthy adults. *J Am Coll Cardiol* 1987;10:1032–1039.
11. Klein AL, Tajik AJ. Doppler assessment of pulmonary venous flow in healthy subjects and in patients with heart disease. *J Am Soc Echocardiogr* 1991;4:379–392.
12. Appleton C, Hatle LK, Popp RL. Cardiac tamponade and pericardial effusion: respiratory variation in transvalvular flow velocities studied by Doppler echocardiography. *J Am Coll Cardiol* 1988;11:1020–1030.
13. Burstow DJ, et al. Cardiac tamponade: characteristic Doppler observations. *Mayo Clin Proc* 1989;64:312–324.
14. Hatle LK, Appleton CP, Popp RL. Differentiation of constrictive pericarditis and restrictive cardiomyopathy by Doppler echocardiography. *Circulation* 1989;79:357–370.
15. Vandenberg BF, et al. Estimation of left ventricular cavity area with an on-line, semiautomated echocardiographic edge detection system. *Circulation* 1992;86:159–166.

5

Hemodynamic Assessment

Conventionally, cardiac hemodynamics have been obtained by invasive catheterization techniques. Now it is possible to determine various hemodynamic parameters (Table 5-1) noninvasively using echocardiography.

M-mode and 2D echocardiography provide only indirect evidence of hemodynamic abnormalities, but this evidence may be the initial clue to suggest such problems [1]. Table 5-2 and Figures 5-1 to 5-4 demonstrate various M-mode and 2D echocardiographic signs of hemodynamic derangements. However, it should be noted that these signs are not highly sensitive or specific. Intracardiac hemodynamic assessment is best performed by Doppler

Table 5-1. Echocardiographic determination of intracardiac flows and pressures

1. Stroke volume and cardiac output
   a. Stroke volume calculation
   b. Regurgitant volume and fraction
   c. Pulmonary-systemic circulation ratio (Qp/Qs)
2. Pressure gradients
   a. Maximum instantaneous gradient
   b. Mean gradient
   c. Comparison with peak-to-peak gradient
3. Valve area
   a. Continuity equation
   b. Pressure half-time
4. Intracardiac pressures
   a. Pulmonary artery pressures
   b. Left atrial pressure
   c. Left ventricular end-diastolic pressure
5. Systolic and diastolic function
   a. dP/dt
   b. Diastolic filling parameters

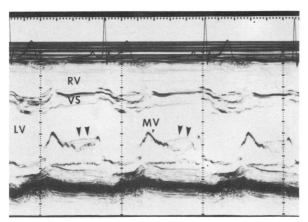

Fig. 5-1. M-mode echocardiogram of the mitral valve (MV) with fluttering *(double arrowhead)* from aortic regurgitation. However, this M-mode sign may not be present if the aortic regurgitation jet is eccentric toward the ventricular septum rather than toward the mitral valve.

echocardiography. The accuracy of Doppler-derived hemodynamic measurements has been confirmed by simultaneously derived catheterization data.

Doppler Echocardiography

Based on the Doppler shift (see Chap. 2), Doppler measures blood flow velocities in the cardiac chambers as well as in the great vessels [2, 3]. Blood flow velocities can then be con-

verted to pressure gradients (in millimeters of mercury) according to the *Bernoulli equation* (Fig. 5-5).

In most clinical situations, flow acceleration and viscous friction terms can be ignored. Furthermore, flow velocity proximal to a fixed orifice (V_1) is much lower than the peak flow velocity (V_2); hence, V_1 can also be frequently ignored. Therefore, pressure gradient (or pressure drop) across a fixed orifice can be calculated by the *simplified Bernoulli equation:*

$$\text{Pressure gradient } (\Delta P) = 4 \times (V_2)^2$$

Stroke Volume and Cardiac Output

Flow across an orifice is equal to the product of the cross-sectional area (CSA) of the orifice and flow velocity (Fig. 5-6). Since flow velocity varies during a flow ejection period, individual velocities of Doppler spectrum need to be summed (i.e., integrated) to measure total flow during a given ejection period. The sum of velocities is called *time velocity integral* (TVI) and is equal to the area enclosed by the baseline and Doppler spectrum. TVI can be readily measured by the built-in calculation package in the ultrasound unit. Once TVI is determined, *stroke volume* (SV) is calculated by multiplying TVI by CSA. Cardiac output is obtained by multiplying stroke volume by heart rate. The most frequently utilized location for stroke volume determination is the left ventricular outflow tract (LVOT) [4]. Figure 5-7 demonstrates how to

Table 5-2.   Signs of hemodynamic derangements

M-mode/2D findings	Hemodynamic abnormality
Fluttering of the mitral valve	Aortic regurgitation
Midsystolic aortic valve closure	Dynamic obstruction of LV outflow tract
Midsystolic pulmonary valve closure	Pulmonary hypertension
Dilated RV + D-shape LV	Increased RV systolic pressure
Dilated inferior vena cava with lack of inspiratory collapse	Increased RA pressure
Persistent bowing of atrial septum	
To RA	Increased LA pressure
To LA	Increased RA pressure
Diastolic RA and RV wall inversion or collapse	Cardiac tamponade

RV = right ventricle; RA = right atrium; LV = left ventricle; LA = left atrium.

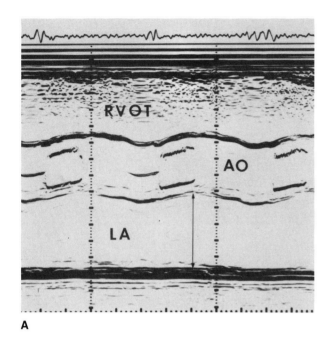

A

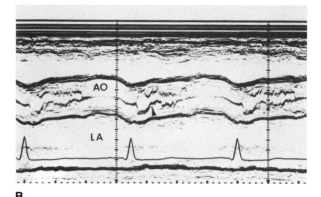

B

Fig. 5-2. M-mode echocardiograms of the aortic valve and the aorta (AO). **A.** Normal aortic valve with the same amount of opening throughout systole. **B.** Midsystolic closure *(arrowhead)* due to dynamic obstruction of the left ventricular outflow tract.

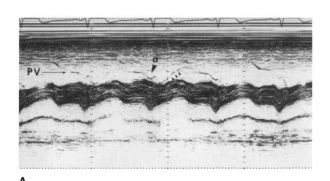

A

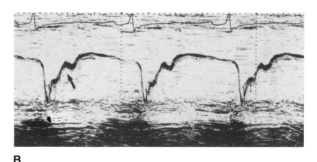

B

Fig. 5-3. M-mode echocardiograms of the pulmonary valve (PV). **A.** Normal pulmonary valve with prominent a wave (a). The valve closure is smooth *(small arrowheads)*. **B.** Midsystolic closure *(arrow)* of the pulmonary valve producing a W shape. There is no a wave.

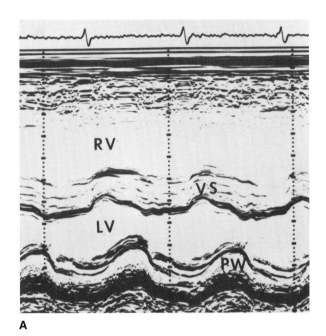

A

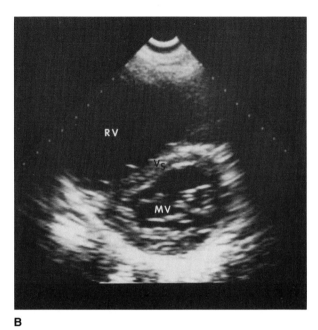

B

Fig. 5-4. **A.** M-mode echocardiogram of the dilated right ventricle (RV), flattened ventricular septum (VS) with abnormal motion, and small LV cavity (LV). This is typical of right ventricular systolic pressure overload. **B.** 2D echocardiogram of the dilated right ventricle, flattened ventricular septum, and D-shaped LV typically seen in patients with pulmonary hypertension.

Fig. 5-5. Schematic drawing of blood flow through a narrowed orifice to illustrate the Bernoulli equation, which measures pressure gradient across the orifice using blood flow velocities. The Bernoulli equation has three components: convective acceleration, flow acceleration, and viscous friction. Since the velocity profile in the center of the lumen is usually flat, the viscous friction factor can be ignored in the clinical setting. The flow acceleration term causes a delay between the pressure drop curve and the velocity curve but provides a reasonably accurate estimation of pressure gradient, and this flow acceleration factor is ignored. Therefore, in a clinical situation, the flow gradient across a narrowed orifice can be derived from the convective acceleration term alone. (From L Hatle, B Angelsen. *Doppler Ultrasound in Cardiology. Physical Principles and Clinical Applications* (2nd ed). Philadelphia: Lea & Febiger, 1985 P. 23.)

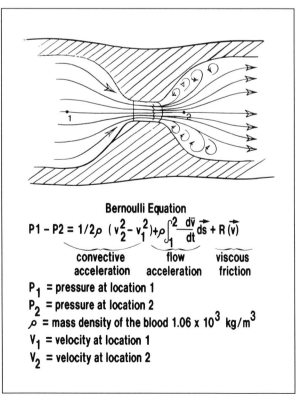

Bernoulli Equation

$$P1 - P2 = 1/2\rho\ (\underbrace{v_2^2 - v_1^2}_{\text{convective acceleration}}) + \underbrace{\rho\int_1^2 \frac{d\vec{v}}{dt}\,\vec{ds}}_{\text{flow acceleration}} + \underbrace{R\,(\vec{v})}_{\text{viscous friction}}$$

P_1 = pressure at location 1

P_2 = pressure at location 2

ρ = mass density of the blood 1.06×10^3 kg/m^3

V_1 = velocity at location 1

V_2 = velocity at location 2

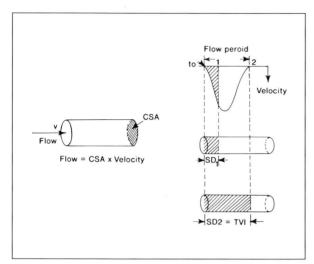

Fig. 5-6. **A.** Schematics to illustrate the basic hydraulic orifice formula. The amount of blood flow going through a fixed orifice is directly proportional to the orifice cross-sectional area (CSA) and flow velocity (flow = CSA × velocity). Therefore, for a given orifice size, blood flow velocity is determined by the flow volume. Flow velocities vary during the ejection or filling period and provide a distinct Doppler profile for a given orifice in the pulsatile cardiovascular system. **B.** A schematic example of a Doppler spectrum of the LV outflow tract. The area enclosed by the velocity curve is equivalent to stroke distance (SD); that is, the shaded area is equal to the distance blood travels from the time of valve opening (to) to time 1 (1). The entire area under the velocity curve represents the total distance the blood traveled with each stroke and is the same as integration of the entire velocity spectrum (time velocity integral [TVI]).

calculate stroke volume from the LVOT. Flow across the other cardiac orifices can be calculated using the same formula. Table 5-3 lists orifice areas according to measured diameters.

Regurgitant Volume and Regurgitant Fraction

Total forward flow across a regurgitant valve (Q valve) is the sum of systemic flow (Qs) and regurgitant volume (Reg Vol). Hence, regurgitant volume (Fig. 5-8) can be obtained by sub-

tracting systemic flow volume from forward flow through the regurgitant valve.

Reg Vol = Q valve − Qs

Systemic flow (Qs) can be calculated from another valve with no or little regurgitation. For example, to calculate regurgitant volume of the mitral valve, stroke volume across the mitral valve represents Q valve, and stroke volume across the aortic valve (or LVOT) represents Qs. Their difference is mitral regurgitant volume [5].

Regurgitant fraction is simply the percentage of regurgitant volume compared to flow across the regurgitant valve.

$$\text{Regurgitant fraction} = \frac{\text{Reg Vol}}{\text{Q valve}} \times 100 \ (\%)$$
$$= \frac{\text{Q valve} - \text{Qs}}{\text{Q valve}} \times 100 \ (\%)$$

Pulmonary-Systemic Flow Ratio (Qp/Qs)

In the presence of intracardiac shunt, the flow ratio between the pulmonary and systemic circulation usually indicates the magnitude of shunt. Pulmonary flow (Qp) is calculated from the right ventricular outflow tract (RVOT) and systemic flow (Qs), from the LVOT.

Qp = RVOT TVI × RVOT CSA
Qs = LVOT TVI × LVOT CSA

Hence,

$$\frac{\text{Qp}}{\text{Qs}} = \frac{\text{RVOT TVI} \times \text{RVOT CSA}}{\text{LVOT TVI} \times \text{LVOT CSA}}$$

Figure 5-9 demonstrates the calculation of right ventricular outflow tract flow from the parasternal or subcostal short-axis view.

Transvalvular Gradients

Blood flow velocity measured by Doppler echocardiography is an *instantaneous* event and the pressure gradients derived from Doppler velocities are *instantaneous gradients*. When maximum Doppler velocity is converted to pressure gradient using the simplified Bernoulli equation, it represents *maximum instantaneous gradient* (MIG). It should be noted that

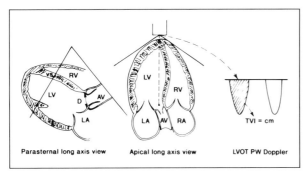

A

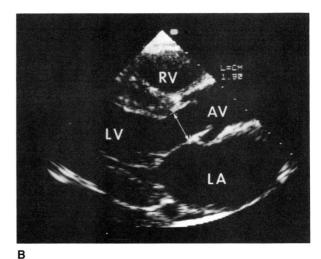

B

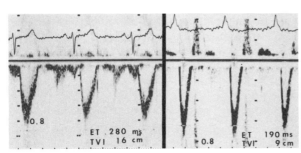

C

Fig. 5-7.   A. Schematics of calculation of stroke volume (SV) from the LVOT.

Step 1: Measurement of LVOT diameter (D) from the parasternal long-axis view. The diameter is measured at the level of the aortic annulus during systole. The line is drawn from where the anterior aortic cusp meets the ventricular septum (VS) to where the posterior aortic cusp meets the anterior mitral leaflet, and perpendicular to the anterior aortic wall.

Step 2: Calculation of LVOT area. Assuming a circular shape of LVOT,

$$\text{LVOT area (cm}^2) = (D/2)^2 \times \pi$$
$$= D^2 \times 0.785$$

Table 5-3 lists area in square centimeters according to the measured diameters.

Step 3: Measurement of LVOT velocity and time velocity integral (TVI), from the apical long-axis view. Pulsed-wave (PW) sample volume is placed at the center of the aortic annulus or 0.5 cm proximal to it (in a patient with aortic stenosis). TVI (cm) is the area under the velocity curve and is equal to the sum of velocities (cm/sec) during the ejection time (sec).

Step 4: Calculation of stroke volume (SV) across the LVOT.

$$\text{SV (ml)} = \text{Area (cm}^2) \times \text{TVI}$$
$$= D^2 \times 0.785 \times \text{TVI}$$

B. Parasternal long-axis view, systolic frame. LVOT diameter is measured to be 1.8 cm. LVOT area $= 1.8^2 \times 0.785 = 2.5 \text{ cm}^2$. **C.** Two different LVOT velocity patterns. Despite similar peak velocities, the TVI is different due to a difference in ejection time (ET). Stroke volume is calculated as follows:

$$\text{(Left) SV} = 2.5 \times 16 = 41 \text{ ml}$$
$$\text{(Right) SV} = 2.5 \times 9 = 23 \text{ ml}$$

Table 5-3. Area calculation from diameter (D): Area $=$ D² $\times$ 0.785

Diameter (cm)	Area (cm²)	Diameter (cm)	Area (cm²)
1.5	1.77	3.3	8.55
1.6	2.01	3.4	9.07
1.7	2.27	3.5	9.62
1.8	2.54	3.6	10.17
1.9[a]	2.83	3.7	10.75
2.0	3.14	3.8	11.34
2.1[b]	3.46	3.9	11.94
2.2	3.80	4.0	12.56
2.3	4.15	4.1	13.20
2.4	4.52	4.2	13.85
2.5	4.90	4.3	14.51
2.6	5.31	4.4	15.20
2.7	5.72	4.5	15.90
2.8	6.15	4.6	16.61
2.9	6.60	4.7	17.34
3.0	7.06	4.8	18.09
3.1	7.54	4.9	18.73
3.2	8.04	5.0	19.63

[a]Mean diameter of LV outflow tract for adult female.
[b]Mean diameter of LV outflow tract for adult male.

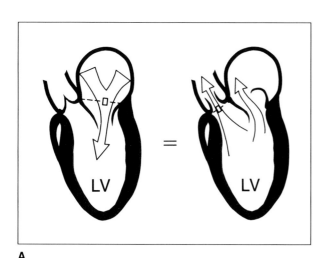

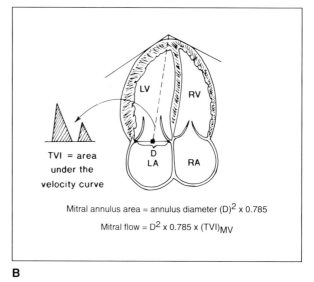

A   B

Fig. 5-8. Estimation of regurgitant volume and regurgitant fraction using mitral regurgitation as an example. **A.** Let's assume that regurgitation is present only in the mitral valve. Therefore, forward flow across the mitral valve (MV) (left) is the sum of systemic flow across the LVOT and mitral regurgitant volume; what goes in (mitral inflow) must come out (LVOT flow + mitral regurgitant flow). **B.** Mitral inflow volume is the product of mitral flow TVI and mitral annulus area (flow = TVI $\times$ area). For this volumetric calculation, the sample volume must be placed at the level of the mitral annulus. Systemic flow is calculated from another orifice without regurgitation, e.g., LVOT (see Fig. 5-7). Then,

$$\text{Mitral regurgitant volume} = \text{mitral inflow} - \text{LVOT flow}$$

$$\text{Regurgitant fraction} = \frac{\text{mitral regurgitant volume}}{\text{mitral inflow volume}} \times 100(\%)$$

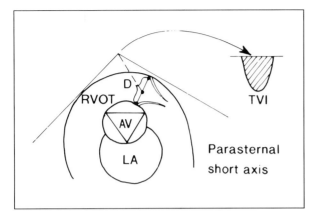

Fig. 5-9. Calculation of blood flow through the pulmonary circulation (Qp), and the pulmonary-systemic flow ratio (Qp/Qs). Pulmonary flow is estimated from the right ventricular outflow tract (RVOT). The right ventricular outflow tract is well visualized from the parasternal short axis or the subcostal short-axis view. The sample volume is located at the level of the pulmonary valve annulus; then,

$$Qp = RVOT \ diameter^2 \times 0.785 \times TVI$$

Systemic flow is estimated from the LVOT as in Figure 5-7 unless there is significant aortic regurgitation. Therefore,

$$\frac{Qp}{Qs} = \frac{RVOT \ D^2 \times 0.785 \times RVOT \ TVI}{LVOT \ D^2 \times 0.785 \times LVOT \ TVI}$$

$$= \frac{RVOT \ D^2 \times RVOT \ TVI}{LVOT \ D^2 \times LVOT \ TVI}$$

the MIG by Doppler will always be higher than the customary peak-to-peak (p-p) gradient measured in the catheterization laboratory (Fig. 5-10). *Peak-to-peak gradient* in the case of aortic stenosis is the pressure difference between the peak LV and peak aortic pressures, which do not occur simultaneously, and hence is a nonphysiologic measurement. *Mean gradient* is an average of pressure gradients during the entire flow period, and mean gradient by Doppler has been shown to correlate well with cardiac catheterization. From the Doppler tracing, mean gradient can be derived by the built-in calculation package. Several studies have validated that Doppler-derived pressure gradients are highly accurate, with an excellent correlation with catheter-derived pressure gradients across left or right ventricular outflow

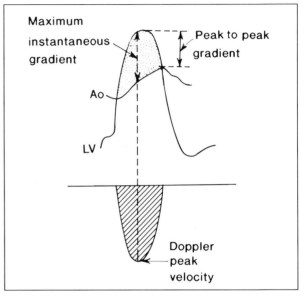

Fig. 5-10. Schematic drawing of pressure tracings of the LV and the aorta (Ao) in aortic stenosis along with the corresponding Doppler velocity spectrum. It is important to understand how different pressure gradients are derived. The average of pressure differences between the LV and the aorta *(dotted area)* represents the *mean gradient* (see text).

obstruction, mitral stenosis, pulmonary artery band, and various prosthetic valves [6–12] (Fig. 5-11).

Valve Area

Continuity Equation

Continuity equation (Fig. 5-12) is the Gorlin formula of echocardiography and is used to calculate valve area (A)[13]. It utilizes the concept that flow is the same upstream and downstream to a stenotic orifice ($F_1 = F_2$): "What comes in must go out."

Since flow is the product of area and TVI,

$$A_1 \times TVI_1 = A_2 \times TVI_2$$

where TVI is measured by pulsed- or continuous-wave Doppler. If A_1 is known, then A_2 can be calculated from the following equation:

$$A_2 = A_1 \times \frac{TVI_1}{TVI_2}$$

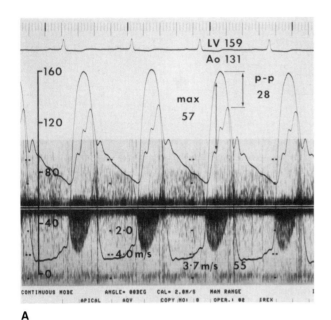

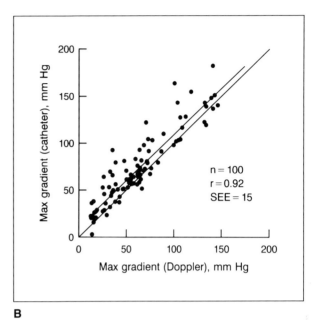

Fig. 5-11. Simultaneous Doppler and cardiac pressure recordings show an excellent correlation between Doppler-derived and catheter-derived pressure gradients in aortic stenosis. **A.** Peak Doppler velocity (3.7 m/sec) from the third cardiac cycle is converted to a maximum instantaneous gradient (max) of 55 mm Hg, which corresponds well to the maximum gradient determined by catheter (57 mm Hg) but not to the peak-to-peak (p-p) gradient of 28 mm Hg. **B.** Plot of maximum instantaneous gradients by Doppler and catheterization with a good correlation in 100 patients with aortic stenosis. r = correlation coefficient; SEE = standard error of estimate.

It should be noted that the ratio of the areas is inversely proportional to their TVI ratio.

$$\frac{A_2}{A_1} = \frac{TVI_1}{TVI_2}$$

The TVI ratio is another measure of severity of aortic stenosis.

Pressure Half-time

Pressure half-time (PHT) (Fig. 5-13) is the time interval for the peak pressure gradient to reach its half level [14] and is the same as the interval for the peak velocity to decline to the peak velocity divided by the square root of 2 (= 1.4) [15, 16]. It is always proportionally related to the deceleration time (DT).

PHT = 0.29 × DT

PHT is utilized to estimate mitral valve area (MVA) using an empiric formula:

MVA = 220/PHT

Fig. 5-12. Schematic drawing to illustrate the derivation of the continuity equation. Area 1 is known cross-sectional area at site 1. Area 2 is unknown cross-sectional area to be calculated at site 2.

(Flow)1 = Flow thru Area$_1$ (known) = Area$_1$ × (TVI)$_1$

(Flow)$_2$ = Flow thru Area$_2$ (unkown) = Area$_2$ × (TVI)$_2$

(Flow)$_2$ = (Flow)$_1$

Area$_2$ × (TVI)$_2$ = Area$_1$ × (TVI)$_1$

Area$_2$ = Area$_1$ × $\frac{(TVI)_1}{(TVI)_2}$

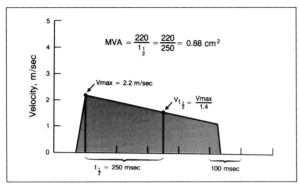

Fig. 5-13. Schematic drawing to illustrate the calculation of pressure half-time. Pressure half-time (t½, or PHT) is the time interval required for maximal pressure gradient (Pmax) to reach its half level (P½). Hence,

$$P½ = ½ \, Pmax$$
$$4 \times (Vt½)^2 = ½ \, (4 \times Vmax^2)$$
$$Vt½ = Vmax/\sqrt{2} = Vmax/1.4$$

In this example, Vmax = 2.2 m/sec; hence, Vt½ = 2.2/1.4 = 1.6 m/sec. The time interval from the Vmax (2.2 m/sec) to Vt½ (1.6 m/sec) is the pressure half-time (t½ = 250 msec). In patients with native mitral valvular stenosis, mitral valve area (MVA) is estimated by dividing the constant, 220, by t½.

Another important clinical application of PHT is to assess the severity of aortic regurgitation (AR). PHT of AR Doppler velocity becomes significantly shorter (≤ 250 msec) with severe AR, due to a rapid rise in LV diastolic pressure and decrease in aortic pressure [17, 18].

Intracardiac Pressures

The velocity of a regurgitant valve is a direct representation of pressure drop across that valve and therefore is utilized for the determination of intracardiac pressure (Table 5-4).

Tricuspid regurgitation (TR) velocity reflects the systolic pressure difference between the right ventricle and atrium (see also Chap. 13). Therefore, right ventricular systolic pressure can be obtained by adding the estimated right atrial pressure to TR velocity² × 4. For example

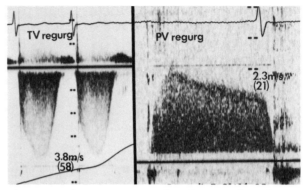

Fig. 5-14. Continuous-wave Doppler recording of tricuspid regurgitation (left) and pulmonary regurgitation (right) in a patient with pulmonary hypertension. Systolic and end-diastolic pulmonary artery pressures are derived from peak tricuspid regurgitation velocity and end-diastolic pulmonary regurgitation velocity, respectively.

Table 5-4. Doppler estimation of intracardiac pressures

1. Peak TR velocity→RV systolic pressure
                              PA systolic pressure
2. Peak PR velocity→mean PA pressure
3. End-diastolic PR velocity→PA end-diastolic
                              pressure
4. Peak MR velocity→LA pressure
5. End-diastolic AR velocity→LV end-diastolic
                              pressure

TR = tricuspid regurgitation; RV = right ventricle; PA = pulmonary artery; PR = pulmonary regurgitation; MR = mitral regurgitation; LA = left atrium; AR = aortic regurgitation; LV = left ventricle.

(Fig. 5-14), if TR velocity is 3.8 m/sec, the pressure drop across the tricuspid valve during systole is 58 mm Hg (= 3.8² × 4). If the right atrial (RA) pressure is 10 mm Hg, the right ventricular systolic pressure is 58 + 10 = 68 mm Hg.

In the absence of right ventricular outflow tract obstruction, the pulmonary artery systolic pressure will be the same as the calculated right ventricular systolic pressure.

Pulmonary regurgitation (PR) velocity represents the diastolic pressure difference between the pulmonary artery and the right ventricle. Hence, pulmonary artery end-diastolic pressure (PAEDP) can be obtained by adding the right ventricular end-diastolic pressure (RVEDP) (which is equal to RA pressure) to $(PR\ end\text{-}diastolic\ velocity)^2 \times 4$. The pulmonary artery mean pressure correlates well with the early diastolic pressure difference between the pulmonary artery and right ventricle, hence, $(PR\ peak\ velocity)^2 \times 4$. For example, PR end-diastolic velocity is around 1.0 m/sec when the pulmonary artery pressure is normal; PAEDP − RVEDP = $1.0^2 \times 4$ = 4 mm Hg. PAEDP = RA pressure + 4 = 14 mm Hg since right atrial pressure is assumed to be 10 mm Hg. When pulmonary artery pressure is elevated, PR end-diastolic velocity is increased. If PR end-diastolic velocity is 2.3 m/sec (see Fig. 5-14), PAEDP − RVEDP = $2.3^2 \times 4$ = 21 mm Hg. Pulmonary artery end-diastolic pressure is, therefore, equal to 21 + RA pressure. Right atrial pressure is roughly estimated by inspecting jugular venous pressure at bedside, or an empiric value of 10 or 14 mm Hg can be used; PAEDP = 21 + 14 = 35.

Mitral regurgitation (MR) velocity represents the systolic pressure difference between the LV and the left atrium. In patients without LV outflow obstruction, systolic blood pressure is practically the same as LV systolic pressure; hence,

Left atrial pressure = SBP − 4 × MRV²

where SBP = systolic blood pressure, and
    MRV = MR velocity.

Aortic regurgitation (AR) velocity reflects the diastolic pressure difference between the aorta and the LV. LV end-diastolic pressure (LVEDP) can be estimated by the following:

DBP − (AR EDV)² × 4

where DBP = diastolic blood pressure, and
    EDV = end-diastolic velocity.

Figure 5-15 shows a continuous-wave Doppler recording of AR velocity with an end-diastolic

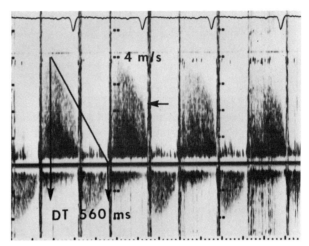

Fig. 5-15. Continuous-wave Doppler recording from the apex of severe aortic regurgitation with elevated LV end-diastolic pressure (LVEDP). The deceleration time (DT) is only 560 msec; hence, the PHT is 160 msec (PHT < 250 msec indicates severe aortic regurgitation). End-diastolic aortic regurgitation velocity is only 2.2 m/sec *(arrow)* due to elevated LV end-diastolic pressure (see text).

velocity of 2.2 m/sec. If the diastolic blood pressure is 40 mm Hg, LVEDP = 40 − $(2.2)^2 \times 4$ = 21 mm Hg. LV end-diastolic pressure can also be estimated by various diastolic filling parameters from mitral inflow and pulmonary venous flow velocities (see next section).

Systolic and Diastolic Function

dP/dt

dP/dt represents the isovolumic phase index of LV contractility. From a continuous-wave Doppler MR jet, rate of LV pressure rise (dP/dt) can be estimated. During the isovolumic contraction period, there is no significant change in the left atrial pressure. Therefore, MR velocity changes during this period reflect dP/dt. Usually, the time interval between 1 and 3 m/sec on MR velocity spectrum is measured (Fig. 5-16A). Using the Bernoulli equation, the pressure change from 1 to 3 m/sec is 32 mm Hg ($4 \times 3^2 − 4 \times 1^2$). The dP/dt (in mm Hg/sec) is calculated from the following formula: 32 mm Hg/time (sec). Several studies demonstrated good correlations between the noninvasive Doppler-derived and the catheter-derived dP/dt [19–21] (Fig. 5-16B). Case examples of determining dP/dt are illustrated in Figure 5-16C–E. Normal dP/dt is more than 1200 mm Hg/sec.

The rate of pressure rise in the right ventricle is derived similarly from the TR jet as in the LV using the MR jet except that the time interval beween 1 and 2 m/sec is used for the right side. Therefore, for the right ventricle,

$$dP/dt = (4 \times 2^2 - 4 \times 1^2)/time$$
$$= 12 \text{ mm Hg/time (sec)}$$

Diastolic Filling
Doppler evaluation of diastolic filling is also discussed in Chapter 4.

Mitral or Tricuspid Flow
Diastolic filling is assessed primarily by analysis of the pulsed-wave Doppler flow velocities of mitral inflow (for the LV) and tricuspid inflow (for the right ventricle). The sample volume is placed between the leaflet tips during diastole. The following variables are obtained: isovolumic relaxation time (IVRT), E velocity, A velocity, E to A ratio (E/A), and deceleration time (DT) of E velocity. Depending on their values, diastolic filling is categorized into three patterns:

1. Relaxation abnormality
2. (Pseudo)normal
3. Restrictive physiology

Variables	Abnormal relaxation	Normal	Restrictive
IVRT (msec)	≥ 110	73 ± 13	≤ 60
E (m/sec)	≤ 0.5	0.86 ± 0.16	≥ 1.2
A (m/sec)	≥ 0.8	0.56 ± 0.13	≤ 0.3
E/A	< 1.0	1.6 ± 0.5	≥ 2.0
DT (msec)	≥ 240	199 ± 32	≤ 150

Diastolic filling pattern is *not disease-specific*, but rather it is dynamic depending on volume status, compliance, atrial pressure, and stage of disease process.

With aging, myocardial relaxation becomes abnormally prolonged and is expected to have

Fig. 5-16. Calculation of dP/dt. **A.** Schematics of LV and left atrial (LA) pressure tracings along with continuous-wave Doppler velocity spectrum of mitral regurgitation (MR). The rate of pressure rise in the LV is estimated from the time interval (dt) required to achieve MR velocity from 1 to 3 m/sec assuming no significant change in left atrial pressure during that period.

$$dP/dt = (4 \times 3^2 - 4 \times 1^2) \text{ mm Hg} \times 1,000/dt$$
$$\text{(in msec)}$$
$$= 32,000/dt \text{ (mm Hg/sec)}$$

Normal LV dP/dt is greater than 1,000 mm Hg/sec. **B.** Transmitral pressure gradients measured by continuous-wave Doppler of an MR jet and by the Millar catheter. Both correlate well with each other. (From C Chen et al. Noninvasive estimation of the instantaneous first derivative of left ventricular pressure using continuous-wave Doppler echocardiography. *Circulation* 1991;83:2101–2110.) **C.** Plot of dP/dt measured by the continuous-wave Doppler method and by the Millar catheter. The noninvasive Doppler determination correlates well with the invasive determination. (From C Chen et al. Noninvasive estimation of the instantaneous first derivative of left ventricular pressure using continuous-wave Doppler echocardiography. *Circulation* 1991;83:2101–2110.) **D.** Continuous-wave Doppler spectrum of MR in a patient with severe LV systolic dysfunction. The Doppler velocities were recorded at two different speeds. In order to measure dt accurately, it is better to record the signal at 50 mm/sec than at 25 mm/sec. The velocity scale is expanded so that only a jet up to 3 m/sec is recorded. It should also be noted that the peak velocity of MR in this patient is 3.5 m/sec, corresponding to only a 49 mm Hg gradient across the mitral valve during systole. Pulmonary capillary wedge pressure in this patient was 50 mm Hg and the systolic blood pressure was 96 mm Hg. The depressed systolic function is also reflected in a decreased dP/dt to 533 mm Hg/sec. **E.** Continuous-wave Doppler spectrum of MR in atrial fibrillation demonstrating changes in dt; therefore, contractility of the LV varies depending on the preceding cardiac cycle length. The time to reach from 1 to 3 m/sec is much shorter after a longer RR cycle (second MR jet) compared to that of MR after a shorter RR cycle (third MR jet).

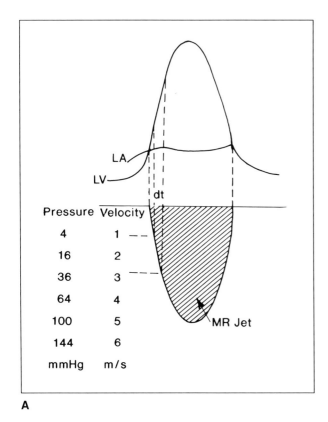

A

Pressure	Velocity
4	1
16	2
36	3
64	4
100	5
144	6
mmHg	m/s

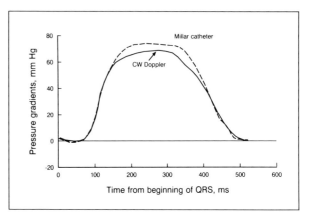

B

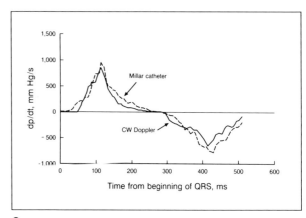

C

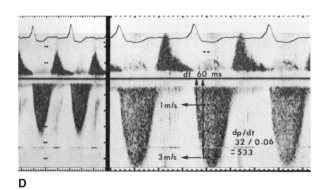

D

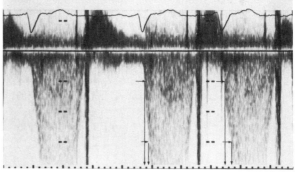

E

an abnormal pattern in subjects 60 years and older. An abnormal relaxation pattern is also seen in patients with a hypertrophied ventricle (hypertension, hypertrophic cardiomyopathy, chronic renal failure), myocardial ischemia, or infiltrative cardiomyopathy without significant elevation of atrial pressure. As compliance decreases or atrial pressure increases, the diastolic filling becomes pseudonormalized and subsequently, restrictive.

Generally, a restrictive diastolic filling pattern indicates a poor prognosis irrespective of the underlying pathophysiology mechanisms. The ultimate prognosis depends on whether the underlying disease entity can be successfully treated, for example, relief of ischemia by revascularization, or fluid overload by diuresis. When the underlying pathology is not reversible, as in cardiac amyloidosis, the patient's prognosis is extremely poor.

Pulmonary or Hepatic Vein Flow

Pulmonary and hepatic vein Doppler flow velocities provide complementary information regarding diastolic filling (see Fig. 4-12). In normal subjects with sinus rhythm, there is a biphasic (systole and diastole) forward flow and a reversal flow during atrial contraction. In older subjects or patients with mainly a relaxation abnormality, the pulmonary or hepatic venous forward flow is greater during systole than during diastole and atrial flow reversals increase. As the atrial pressure increases (i.e., volume overload or restrictive hemodynamics), systolic forward flow is decreased and diastolic forward flow is increased along with increased flow reversals with atrial contraction. In patients with atrial fibrillation, the predominant forward flow occurs during diastole. When there is severe mitral or tricuspid regurgitation, regurgitant flow produces systolic flow reversals in the pulmonary or hepatic vein, respectively.

Determination of Left Atrial Pressure

Since left atrial pressure is one of the most important determinants of diastolic filling profile, it can be estimated from various diastolic filling velocity variables. The following Doppler values indicate elevated LV end-diastolic pressure or left atrial pressure (in middle-aged and older patients):

1. IVRT $\leq$ 60 msec
2. Atrial filling fraction (AFF)* $\leq$20%
3. E/A $\geq$ 2.0
4. DT $\leq$ 130 msec

When all the variables are combined, the following multilinear regression equation provides a more accurate estimate of LV end-diastolic pressure (LVEDP) [22].

$$LVEDP = 46 - 0.22\ IVRT - 0.10\ AFF - 0.03\ DT - (2 \div E/A) + 0.05\ MAR$$

where MAR = the interval from the end of the A wave to the R wave on the electrocardiogram.

However, the equation is too complex for routine daily use. The pulmonary venous flow velocity pattern can also be used to estimate the left atrial pressure. When the left atrial pressure is elevated, systolic forward flow is decreased and atrial reversal is increased [23, 24]. Peak velocity and duration of pulmonary venous atrial flow reversal increase with elevated pulmonary capillary wedge pressure, whereas duration of mitral flow during atrial systole decreases. The difference in duration between pulmonary venous atrial flow reversal and forward mitral flow during atrial systole was found to be the best indicator of elevated LV end-diastolic pressure [25]. A longer duration of the pulmonary venous atrial flow reversal than that of the mitral A wave predicts an end-diastolic pressure of more than 15 mm Hg.

Time Constant of Left Ventricular Relaxation (TAU)

TAU (T) is the most reliable measurement of the rate of LV isovolumic relaxation and is obtained with high-fidelity catheter, invasively. Recently, the Doppler mitral regurgitation velocity profile has been used to provide

---

*AFF is the percentage of LV filling due to atrial contraction and is calculated as the fraction of TVI of A velocity compared to the entire mitral inflow TVI.

noninvasive determination of T in animals and humans [26, 27]. Because the left ventriculoatrial pressure gradient can be reliably calculated from continuous-wave mitral regurgitation velocity profile using the simplified Bernoulli equation, the descending limb of the mitral regurgitation Doppler velocity can be used to measure T from the time of maximal negative dP/dt to LV-LA pressure crossover. Although this method requires knowledge of LA pressure, an empirical LA pressure of 10 mmHg [26] or 20 mmHg [27] yields reliable estimates of T. Because mitral regurgitation is common in cardiac patients, this Doppler-derived T may become a routine diastolic measurement and allow a better understanding of diastolic dysfunction and its management.

References

1. Feigenbaum H. *Echocardiography* (4th ed). Philadelphia: Lea & Febiger, 1986.

2. Hatle L, Angelsen B. *Doppler Ultrasound in Cardiology. Physical Principles and Clinical Applications* (2nd ed). Philadelphia: Lea & Febiger, 1985.

3. Nishimura RA, et al. Doppler echocardiography: theory, instrumentation, technique, and application. *Mayo Clin Proc* 1985;60:321–343.

4. Zoghbi WA, Quinones MA. Determination of cardiac output by Doppler echocardiography: a critical appraisal. *Herz* 1986;11:258.

5. Rokey R, et al. Determination of regurgitant fraction in isolated mitral or aortic regurgitation by pulsed Doppler two-dimensional echocardiography. *J Am Coll Cardiol* 1986;7: 1273–1278.

6. Hatle L, et al. Noninvasive assessment of pressure drop in mitral stenosis by Doppler ultrasound. *Br Heart J* 1978;40:131–140.

7. Callahan MJ, et al. Validation of instantaneous pressure gradients measured by continuous-wave Doppler in experimentally induced aortic stenosis. *Am J Cardiol* 1985;56:989–993.

8. Teirstein PS, Yock PG, Popp RL. The accuracy of Doppler ultrasound measurement of pressure gradients across irregular, dual, and tunnellike obstructions to blood flow. *Circulation* 1985;72:577–584.

9. Currie PJ, et al. Continuous-wave Doppler determination of right ventricular pressure: a simultaneous Doppler-catheterization study in 127 patients. *J Am Coll Cardiol* 1985;6:750–756.

10. Currie PJ, et al. Instantaneous pressure gradient: a simultaneous Doppler and dual catheter correlative study. *J Am Coll Cardiol* 1986;7: 800–806.

11. Burstow DJ, et al. Continuous wave Doppler echocardiographic measurement of prosthetic valve gradients: a simultaneous Doppler-catheter correlative study. *Circulation* 1989;80: 504–514.

12. Fyfe DA, et al. Continuous-wave Doppler determination of the pressure gradient across pulmonary artery bands: hemodynamic correlation in 20 patients. *Mayo Clin Proc* 1984; 59:744–750.

13. Skjaerpe T, Hegrenaes L, Hatle L. Noninvasive estimation of valve area in patients with aortic stenosis by Doppler ultrasound and two-dimensional echocardiography. *Circulation* 1986;73:452–459.

14. Libanoff AJ, Rodbard S. Atrioventricular pressure half-time: measurement of mitral valve area. *Circulation* 1968;38:144.

15. Hatle L, Angelsen B, Tromsdal A. Noninvasive assessment of atrioventricular pressure half-time by Doppler ultrasound. *Circulation* 1979; 60:1096.

16. Thomas JD, Weyman AE. Doppler mitral pressure half-time: a clinical tool in search of theoretical justification. *J Am Coll Cardiol* 1987; 10:923.

17. Samstad S, et al. Half-time of the diastolic aortoventricular pressure difference by continuous-wave Doppler ultrasound: a measure of the severity of aortic regurgitation? *Br Heart J* 1989;61:335–343.

18. Grayburn PA, et al. Quantitative assessment of the hemodynamic consequences of aortic regurgitation by means of continuous wave Doppler recordings. *J Am Coll Cardiol* 1987;10: 135–141.

19. Bargiggia GS, et al. A new method for estimating left ventricular dp/dt by continuous wave Doppler echocardiography: validation studies at catheterization. *Circulation* 1989;80:1287–1292.

20. Chen C, et al. Noninvasive estimation of the instantaneous first derivative of left ventricu-

lar pressure using continuous-wave Doppler echocardiography. *Circulation* 1991;83:2101–2110.

21. Chung N, et al. Measurement of left ventricular dp/dt by simultaneous Doppler echocardiography and cardiac catheterization. *J Am Soc Echocardiogr* 1992;5:147–152.

22. Mulvagh S, et al. Estimation of left ventricular end-diastolic pressure from Doppler transmitral flow velocity in cardiac patients independent of systolic performance. *J Am Coll Cardiol* 1992;20:112–119.

23. Kuecherer HF, et al. Estimation of mean left atrial pressure from transesophageal pulsed Doppler echocardiography of pulmonary venous flow. *Circulation* 1990;82:1127–1139.

24. Nishimura RA, et al. Relationship of pulmonary vein to mitral flow velocities by trans-esophageal Doppler echocardiography: effect of different loading conditions. *Circulation* 1990;81:1488–1497.

25. Rossuoll O, Hatle LK. Pulmonary venous flow velocities recorded by transthoracic Doppler ultrasound: relation to left ventricular diastolic pressures. *J Am Coll Cardiol* 1993;21:1687–1696.

26. Chen C, et al. Nonivasive measurement of the time constant of left ventricular relaxation using the continuous-wave Doppler velocity profile of mitral regurgitation. *Circulation* 1992;86:272–278.

27. Nishimura RA, et al. Noninvasive measurement of rate of left ventricular relaxation by Doppler echocardiography: Validation with simultaneous cardiac catheterization. *Circulation* 1993;88:146–155.

6

Coronary Artery Disease

Coronary artery disease results in more morbidity and mortality than any other disease. Annually, more than 1 million Americans develop acute myocardial infarction, and more than a half-million deaths a year in the United States are related to coronary artery disease. The natural history of coronary artery disease and myocardial infarction is changing, however, with the advent of thrombolytic therapy and coronary angioplasty. Acute reperfusion therapy has become a standard treatment, being administered during the early phase of myocardial infarction. The monitoring of its beneficial effect on myocardial salvage is crucial for subsequent patient management. In this context, echocardiography plays an important role, from the diagnosis of coronary artery disease, early detection of acute myocardial infarction, monitoring of regional wall motion abnormalities following reperfusion therapy, detection of postinfarct complication, and assessment of myocardial viability to prognostic risk stratification.

Regional Wall Motion Analysis

The immediate manifestation of myocardial ischemia is a decrease or cessation of myocardial contractility [1] (systolic thickening) even prior to ST-segment changes or the development of symptoms. Ischemic myocardium may continue to demonstrate forward movement due to a "pulling action" of adjacent nonischemic muscle but the contractility (systolic thickening) of the ischemic myocardial segments is reduced (hypokinesis) or nonexistent (akinesis). Normally, left ventricular (LV) free-wall thickness increases more than 50% during systole. *Hypokinesis* is defined as an increase in systolic wall thickness of less than 40% and *akinesis* is defined as that of less than 10%. *Dyskinesis* is present if the myocardial segment moves outward during systole associated with systolic wall thinning. M-mode echocardiography is useful in recording the temporal changes in wall thickness (Fig. 6-1) and should be obtained by 2D image guidance. With multiple tomographic imaging planes, 2D echocardiography allows the visualization of all the LV wall segments. The LV is conventionally divided into segments for regional wall motion analysis. The American Society of Echocardiography

has recommended a 16-segment model [2] (Fig. 6-2). Each segment is assigned a score based on its contractility: normal = 1; hypokinesis = 2; akinesis = 3; dyskinesis = 4;

Fig. 6-2. A. Schematic drawing of 16 LV wall segments. All 16 segments should be visualized for optimal assessment of regional wall motion, utilizing all the available tomographic planes. Wall segments that can be seen from each tomographic plane are depicted. **B.** All segments can be seen from the parasternal and apical short-axis views: The numbers in the diagram correspond to the wall segments: 1 = basal anteroseptum; 2 = basal anterior wall; 3 = basal anterolateral wall; 4 = basal posterolateral wall; 5 = postero- (or infero-) basal wall; 6 = inferobasal septum; 7 = midanteroseptum; 8 = midanterior wall; 9 = midanterolateral wall; 10 = midposterolateral wall; 11 = midinferior wall; 12 = midinferoseptum; 13 = apical septum; 14 = anteroapex; 15 = lateral apex; 16 = inferoapex.

Fig. 6-1. M-mode echocardiogram of normal **(A)** and abnormal **(B)** ventricular wall thickening. **A.** Normally, wall thickness at end-systole (es) is more than 5 mm greater than that at end-diastole (ed). The arrow indicates the maximal systolic thickening. **B.** The ventricular septum (VS) is thinned and dyskinetic *(arrow)*, moving toward the right ventricle (RV) during end-systole. The thickening of the posterior wall (PW) is normal. This M-mode echocardiogram was obtained from a patient with anterior wall myocardial infarction.

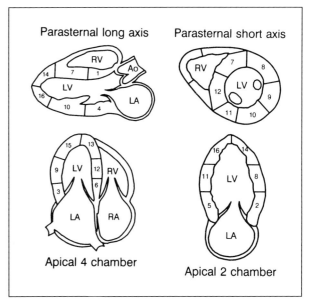

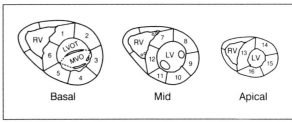

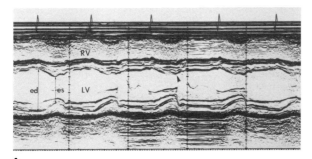

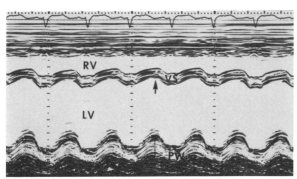

A

B

A

B

and aneurysm = 5. Based on the above wall motion analysis scheme, a *wall motion score index* (WMSI) is calculated to semiquantitate the extent of regional wall motion abnormalities.

$$WMSI = \frac{\text{sum of wall motion scores}}{\text{number of segments visualized}}$$

A normally contracting LV has a WMSI of 1 (each of the 16 segments receives a wall motion score of 1; hence, the total score is 16 and WMSI is 16/16 = 1). The WMSI is higher with larger infarcts as wall motion abnormalities become more extensive.

Technical Caveats

Regional wall motion analysis is among the most challenging tasks in echocardiography. All available windows and tomographic planes should be utilized to visualize the entire LV segment. Apical short- and long-axis views are especially useful to evaluate the apical third of the LV. Continuous scanning from the apical four-chamber to the apical long-axis to the apical two-chamber view allows complete visualization of all LV segments. In patients with chronic obstructive pulmonary disease (COPD) or obesity, a lower-frequency (2.0–2.5-MHz) transducer should be utilized to optimize endocardial definition, and the subcostal window may provide adequate visualization of the LV segments. In patients with a good apical window, use of higher-frequency transducers with adjustment of the focal zone to the near region may enhance the apical endocardial definition, help delineate apical wall motion abnormalities, and differentiate thrombus from apical trabeculation. Occasionally, the supine position may be the best for visualization of apical pathology, using a para-apical window. The apical short-axis view is also useful in the detection of a right ventricular infarct.

Digital Echocardiography

Echocardiographic data (Fig. 6-3) can be digitized for easier and more convenient storage,

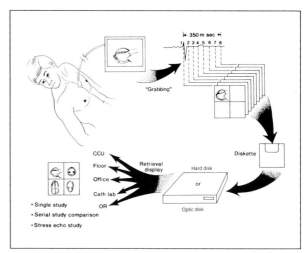

Fig. 6-3. Concept of digital echocardiography. Echo images are digitized and desired segments of a representative cardiac cycle are captured. Eight (in this diagram) separate sequential images (50 msec between two images, seven intervals, giving a total of 350 msec of the cardiac cycle) are "grabbed" onto eight separate cells. Each cell can also be split into two or four compartments to contain multiple views. The onset and the duration of image capture can be manipulated. Once the capturing is completed, the digitized image can be stored on a diskette or in the central hard disk (or optic disk), which can store multiple studies depending on its capacity. The central station is connected to multiple terminals where the digitized study can be retrieved to review or to compare with previous studies. CCU = coronary care unit; OR = operating room.

display, retrieval, and comparison of serial studies [3]. This concept is especially useful in the study of patients with ischemic heart disease. The current technology allows on-line "grabbing" or "capturing" of the entire cardiac cycle or segments of a representative cardiac cycle using a continuous cine loop. Initiation of capturing is triggered by the QRS complex and the programmed length of initial delay. If the initial delay is set at 0 msec, the first image will be grabbed at the onset of the QRS complex when the systolic cycle needs to be stored. Subsequent images are digitized at a preset interval delay, which is usually 50 msec. Eight sequential images (seven intervals) at 50 msec apart provide 350 msec of the cardiac cycle, which is satisfactory to acquire the entire systolic phase at various heart rates. The interval delay may be shortened to 33 msec when the heart rate is extremely fast. The captured image is stored on a floppy or hard disk for archiving and subsequent display. The continuous cine loop can be displayed in a split or a quad-screen for display of multiple views simultaneously or multiple studies for comparison purposes.

Stress Echocardiography

Stress echocardiography is based on the fact that echocardiography in general is a sensitive technique for the detection of wall motion abnormalities at rest as well as those induced by any form of stress. Stress echocardiography is performed either with exercise or after administration of a pharmacologic agent. The exercise protocol includes a standard treadmill exercise test with immediate postexercise echo images obtained within 1.5 minute, or upright or supine bicycle echo images obtained at peak exercise. Since exercise-induced regional wall motion abnormalities usually last for a few minutes after the termination of exercise, immediate postexercise images can be compared to the baseline preexercise images to detect exercise-induced regional wall motion abnormalities [4–12]. Therefore, treadmill exercise with echo images obtained immediately after termination of the exercise is the most frequently utilized form of exercise echocardiogram. Digital echocardiography enhances the capability to acquire satisfactory postexercise images by allowing several successive cardiac cycles to be captured and stored in memory. The most satisfactory postexercise image is selected and compared to the baseline image by side-by-side or quad-screen display (Fig. 6-4). The typical exercise echocardiography protocol at Mayo is shown in Table 6-1. When a patient cannot exercise, stress is induced pharmacologically using dobutamine, dipyridamole, or adenosine [13–16] (Table 6-2). Dobutamine is the agent most commonly used in stress echocardiography.

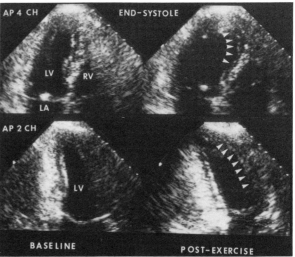

Fig. 6-4. Typical positive exercise echocardiographic images. Baseline end-systolic apical four- and two-chamber views are shown on the left, and postexercise end-systolic frames of the same views are on the right side of the screen. The LV end-systolic cavity is larger after exercise due to exercise-induced ischemia of the anterior wall and the apex *(arrowheads)*. In real time, the ischemic segments are seen as akinetic or dyskinetic segments.

Table 6-1.   Exercise echocardiography protocol

1. Baseline echocardiography. Resting images are digitized and stored.
2. Baseline blood pressure, heart rate, and electrocardiogram.
3. Exercise test according to the patient's and clinician's needs.
4. a. Treadmill exercise, then immediate postexercise echocardiogram, preferably within 1 min.
   b. Bicycle or arm ergometer; images are obtained at low and peak levels of exercise. These images are digitized and stored.
5. Display of baseline, peak exercise (in case of bicycle), and/or postexercise images in a quad-screen using continuous cine loop.
6. Review of exercise-induced heart rate, blood pressure, electrocardiogram, and image changes.

The interpretation of stress echocardiograms is based on the response of LV myocardial wall motion and cavity size (volume). Normally with stress, LV wall motion becomes hyperdynamic and the cavity becomes smaller.

Table 6-2. Pharmacologic stress echocardiography protocol

1. Obtain baseline heart rate, blood pressure, and electrocardiogram.
2. Obtain a baseline echocardiogram. Resting images are digitized and stored.
3. Begin the dobutamine infusion at 5 μg/kg/min.
4. Increase the dobutamine* infusion every 3 min to 10, 20, 30, and 40 μg/kg/min or until patient develops symptoms, side effects, or new regional wall motion abnormalities.
5. In patients on a beta-blocker treatment, the heart rate response to dobutamine may not be satisfactory. If the target rate is not achieved with 40 μg/kg/min of dobutamine, atropine (0.2–1.0 mg IV) is given to increase heart rate.
6. Digitize and store echocardiographic images during the peak infusion and compare baseline and peak infusion images in a quad-screen format.
7. If a patient develops symptoms or persistent tachycardia after the termination of dobutamine, esmolol (2–3 ml, IV) usually terminates the side effects of dobutamine.

*Dipyridamole can be used instead of dobutamine at 0.56 mg/kg × 4 min or 0.84 mg/kg × 10 min, or adenosine beginning at a rate of 50 μg/kg/min and increased every minute to 75, 100, and 140 μg/kg/min × 4 min.

Development of new and the worsening of preexisting regional wall motion abnormalities are the hallmarks of stress-induced myocardial ischemia. The lack of hyperdynamic motion may or may not indicate ischemia. However, if this lack is associated with hyperdynamic motion of other segments after adequate stress, it probably indicates ischemia. The entire LV segments may remain normally contracting (without hyperdynamic motion) when the stress level is inadequate or the patient is taking beta-blockers. When more than 25% of the transmural myocardium is infarcted, it becomes akinetic. Therefore, akinetic myocardium may harbor significant viable myocardium and improve its contractility with exercise or pharmacologic stress. The sensitivity and specificity of stress echocardiography are comparable to those of stress thallium or sestamibi single-photon emission computed tomography. In the largest comparison study of 112 patients, Quinones and his associates reported overall sensitivity and specificity of exercise echocardiography to be 85% and 88%, respectively, compared to 85% and 81% for exercise thallium. The sensitivity of exercise echocardiography and exercise thallium for coronary artery disease in patients with single, double, and triple vessel involvement was also similar (58%, 86%, and 94% versus 61%, 86%, and 94%, respectively) [12].

For interpretations of regional wall motion findings, see Table 6-3.

Table 6-3. Interpretation by regional wall motion (WM) analysis

Rest	Stress	Interpretation
Normal WM and contractility →	Hyperdynamic	Normal
Normal WM →	New WM abnormality, or	Ischemia
	Lack of hyperdynamic WM*	Ischemia
WM abnormality →	Worsening (hypokinesis → akinesis) (akinesis → dyskinesis)	Ischemia
WM abnormality →	Unchanged	Infarct
Akinetic WM →	Improved to hypokinetic, or to normal WM	Viable myocardium

*May not indicate ischemia in the setting of low work load or beta-blockade.

Caveats for Technical and Interpretation Skills

Stress echocardiography is usually performed by a well-trained sonographer, but final interpretation of the study is the echocardiologist's responsibility. The following technical and interpretative caveats ensure the most satisfactory stress echocardiographic examination. For the sonographer:

1. Be thoroughly familiar with the equipment. (There is no time to adjust parameters during the examination, especially after exercise.)
2. Be aware of the most optimal transducer position. Obtain postexercise images from the easier window first. When both parasternal and apical windows are satisfactory, obtain the apical view first.
3. Be as prompt as possible in obtaining postexercise images and record the time interval between the termination of exercise and the completion of imaging. (Try to make the time interval < 1.0 minute).
4. Record all images on videotape as well as digitize them on-line.
5. Do not change field depth during the entire examination.
6. Obtain images on videotape if the patient develops chest pain or significant electrocardiographic changes during the recovery period.

For the cardiologist:

1. Make sure that digitized images are adequate for wall motion analysis (satisfactory endocardial definition).
2. Make sure that the images are grabbed during systole and promptly after exercise.
3. Review the entire videotape, especially in cases where the digitized images are not satisfactory.
4. Be aware of ancillary signs of ischemia such as ventricular volume change and overall contractility. The normal response is decreased end-systolic volume and increased overall contractility.

5. Be aware that normal systolic thickening of the LV wall is different from mere movement (without thickening) of ischemic myocardium, being pulled by adjacent healthy myocardium.

Acute Myocardial Infarction

Echocardiography is widely utilized for the evaluation and management of patients with prolonged chest pain or acute myocardial infarction. It plays an important role in the diagnosis of ischemia or infarction, in the detection of infarct complication, in the evaluation of reperfusion therapy, and for postinfarct risk stratification.

Evaluation of Chest Pain Syndromes

There are many causes of chest pain, most of which can be readily differentiated based on a detailed history and physical examination. However, there are occasions when the pain of myocardial ischemia or infarction cannot be distinguishable from pericarditis, pulmonary embolism, aortic dissection, or pain of noncardiac origin (e.g., cholecystitis, pneumothorax, and esophageal spasm). The initial electrocardiogram is diagnostic of acute myocardial infarction (ST-segment elevation) only in about 50% of patients with infarct. 2D echocardiography for the detection of regional wall motion abnormalities is more sensitive, although not entirely specific for acute myocardial infarction. 2D echocardiography is most useful in differentiating cardiac from noncardiac chest pain. If 2D echocardiography is performed while the patient is experiencing chest pain and it does not reveal any wall motion abnormalities, pain secondary to myocardial ischemia can be virtually excluded [17, 18]. Echocardiography is also extremely useful in detecting or suggesting other cardiovascular abnormalities that mimic acute myocardial infarction, such as aortic dissection, hypertrophic cardiomyopathy, valvular heart disease, pulmonary embolism, and pericardial effusion [19]. Even in patients with an electrocardiogram diagnostic of acute myocardial infarction, 2D echocardiography on admission is useful in documenting not only the precise location of the infarct, but more importantly the extent of regional wall motion abnormalities, which can be compared to subsequent examinations to assess the benefit of reperfusion therapy, infarct expansion, extension, and remodeling [20]. The initial WMSI and Doppler diastolic parameters in patients with acute myocardial infarction on admission can also provide important prognostic information and identify patients at high risk of developing in-hospital complications.

Role of Echocardiography in the Emergency Room

Cardiovascular symptoms (chest pain, dyspnea, syncope, palpitations, and hypotension) are frequent presentations to the emergency room. The triage of patients with chest pain syndrome (prolonged chest pain with nondiagnostic ECG) continues to consume large resources in the emergency room. Since the presence of wall motion abnormalities is a sensitive marker for myocardial ischemia and infarction, 2D echocardiographic examination is useful in categorizing the patients with chest pain syndrome according to their probability (high or low) of having ischemia. If there is no regional wall motion abnormality during or immediately after prolonged chest pain, the chance of myocardial ischemia is very low. The presence of LV hypertrophy occasionally makes the interpretation of subtle wall motion abnormalities (the most frequent clinical setting for a false-negative result) difficult. In patients with no previous myocardial infarction, regional wall motion abnormalities at the time of or soon after prolonged chest pain are specific for myocardial ischemia or infarction. Figure 6-5 demonstrates a proposal for triage of patients with prolonged chest pain using 2D echocardiographic wall motion analysis. The main limitation of widespread use of echocardiography is the lack of adequately trained personnel in the emergency room.

Detection of Complications

Echocardiography is the best means to detect functional and mechanical complications of acute myocardial infarction [21]. The complications of acute myocardial infarction readily recognized by echocardiography are listed in Table 6-4. Doppler and color-flow imaging complement 2D echocardiography in the assessment of the severity of ischemic mitral regurgitation, shunt across infarct ventricular septal defect (VSD), flow in the true or false aneurysm, and the determination of right-side cardiac pressures. Standard transthoracic echocardiography may be difficult to perform in the intensive care unit, especially when the patient is hemodynamically unstable and connected to various life-support devices. Trans-

Fig. 6-5. A proposed scheme for echocardiographic evaluation of patients with prolonged chest pain. When ECG is diagnostic for myocardial infarction (i.e., ST elevation), 2D echocardiogram is not helpful in the diagnosis but may be helpful in determining the extent of infarct, which can be used to estimate myocardial salvage after reperfusion therapy. When ECG is nondiagnostic, absence of regional wall motion abnormalities excludes acute myocardial infarction in nearly all patients and facilitates patient triage to a noncritical care setting or even dismissal with subsequent outpatient evaluation. Unless the patient had a previous infarct, presence of regional wall motion abnormalities indicates myocardial ischemia or infarct. Occasionally, causes other than coronary disease may be found to explain chest pain, such as aortic stenosis, pericarditis, aortic dissection, pulmonary embolism, or cardiomyopathy.

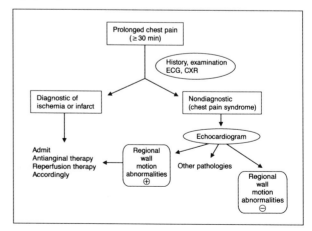

Table 6-4. Complications of myocardial infarction

Acute phase
  Rupture
    Free wall rupture
    Ventricular septal defect
    Papillary muscle rupture
  Mitral regurgitation
    LV dilatation
    Papillary muscle dysfunction
    Papillary muscle rupture
  LV thrombus
  Pericardial effusion/tamponade
  RV infarct

Chronic phase
  Infarct expansion
  Ventricular aneurysm
    True
    Pseudo
  LV thrombus

esophageal echocardiography (TEE) in this situation provides an alternative imaging window. It is well tolerated even by the critically ill patient and offers diagnostic-quality images in nearly all patients [22].

Cardiac Rupture

Cardiac free wall rupture is usually a fatal complication of myocardial infarction and occurs in 1 to 3% of all patients with infarct. In accounts for 8 to 17% of all infarct-related deaths. It typically produces a sudden hemodynamic collapse due to tamponade (see Chap. 12) and electromechanical dissociation. However, patients dying of cardiac rupture have a smaller infarct than those dying of cardiogenic shock. Most ruptures occur within the first week of infarct, the median time being 4 days. It is more common in women and in older patients. Patients with rupture have less severe coronary artery disease and develop infarct expansion. Another clinical situation that potentially enhances cardiac rupture is the use

of thrombolytic therapy (usually more than 10 hours after onset of chest pain), presumably due to hemorrhagic infarct.

Although patients with infarct expansion are at higher risk of cardiac rupture, no specific echocardiographic features have been found to predict this almost always fatal complication. Echocardiographic diagnosis of cardiac rupture is dependent on a high degree of clinical suspicion, a meticulous search for the site of rupture in the region of thinned myocardium, and detection of a small to moderate amount of pericardial effusion leading to tamponade. Rarely, a patient with cardiac rupture survives by pericardial retention of hemopericardium and surgical repair.

Infarct Ventricular Septal Defect

VSD occurs in 1 to 3% of all patients with infarcts and results in progressive hemodynamic deterioration unless surgically corrected. It occurs during the early phase of acute infarct (within the first week). As in free wall rupture, ventricular septal rupture is more common in elderly women without previous myocardial infarction. Nearly half of patients who develop infarct-related VSD have single-vessel coronary artery disease. The most typical clinical presentation is a new systolic murmur with abrupt and progressive hemodynamic deterioration.

The differential diagnosis of a new systolic murmur in patients with acute myocardial infarction includes infarct-related VSD, papillary muscle dysfunction or rupture, pericardial rub, LV outflow tract (LVOT) obstruction, and tricuspid regurgitation. After physical examination, echocardiography should follow as the next logical noninvasive diagnostic procedure in all patients and especially in those with a new murmur who are hemodynamically unstable. Infarct VSD is diagnosed by demonstration of a disrupted ventricular septum with left-to-right shunt (Fig. 6-6). The defect is always located in the region of the thinned myocardium and has dyskinetic motion. The diagnosis can be established 90% of the time by transthoracic 2D echocardiography. TEE may be necessary in a small subgroup of pa-

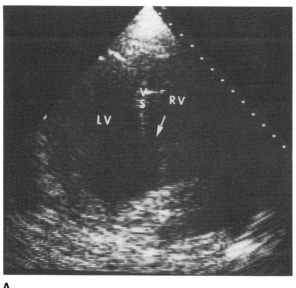

A

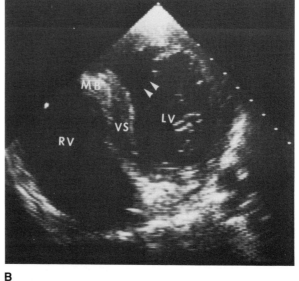

B

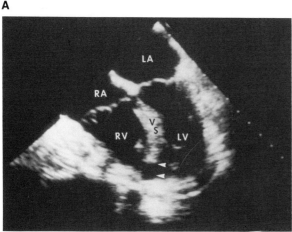

C

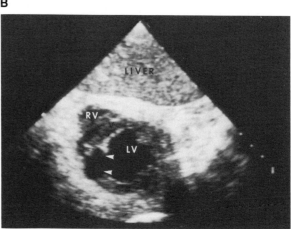

D

Fig. 6-6. Echocardiographic detection of infarct ventricular septal defect (VSD). **A.** Transthoracic modified four-chamber view demonstrating VSD *(arrow)* in a patient with inferior myocardial infarction. The image is not optimal. **B.** Transesophageal transgastric view in the same patient. The cross-sectional view of the LV clearly demonstrates a large inferoseptal defect *(arrowheads)* in the region of moderator band (MB). The right ventricle (RV) is enlarged, which is common in patients with inferoseptal VSD. Due to right ventricular involvement, inferoseptal VSD carries a poorer diagnosis than anteroseptal VSD. **C.** Transesophageal four-chamber view in a patient with anterior wall infarct and new murmur, indicating an apical anteroseptal defect *(arrowheads)*. **D.** Transgastric short-axis view of the LV from the same patient as in **C,** indicating an anteroseptal defect *(arrowheads)*. **E.** Continuous-wave Doppler recording, from the parasternal position, of an infarct VSD. The peak systolic flow velocity is 3 m/sec corresponding to a 36 mm Hg pressure difference between the left and right ventricles. Systolic blood pressure was 90 mm Hg; hence, right ventricular systolic pressure = 90 − 36 = 54 mm Hg. There is continuous shunt through the VSD except during early diastole.

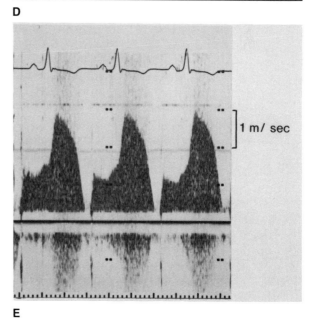

E

75

tients with a suboptimal precordial study [23] (see Fig. 6-6). Peak flow velocity across the VSD measured by continuous-wave Doppler may be used to estimate right ventricular systolic pressure (see Fig. 6-6). When infarct VSD is located at the inferoseptum, the right ventricle is usually involved with myocardial infarction, which renders a poor prognosis. The current therapeutic approach for infarct VSD is urgent surgical intervention. Until the time of surgery, the patient can be stabilized by afterload reduction (nitroprusside) and intraaortic balloon pump counterpulsation.

Papillary Muscle Rupture

Mitral regurgitation is common after acute myocardial infarction. Among 206 patients entering the TIMI (Thrombolysis in Myocardial Infarction) phase I trial, mitral regurgitation was present in 13% [24]. The incidence may be more common (up to 50–60%) if transient mitral regurgitation is included. In that trial, the presence of early mitral regurgitation independently predicted 1-year cardiovascular mortality, but a murmur of mitral regurgitation was heard in less than 10% of the patients.

There are three separate pathophysiologic mechanisms of acute mitral regurgitation after myocardial infarction: (1) LV cavity and mitral annulus dilatation, (2) papillary muscle dysfunction, and (3) papillary muscle rupture. It is therapeutically very important to recognize the exact underlying etiology of ischemic mitral regurgitation since papillary muscle rupture always requires mitral valve replacement or rarely repair, whereas mitral regurgitation due to papillary muscle dysfunction or annulus dilatation may improve with medications, coronary revascularization, or both. It is of interest to note, however, that acute reperfusion with thrombolysis or coronary angioplasty did not reliably reverse severe mitral regurgitation according to a large clinical study [25].

Papillary muscle rupture is the most hemodynamically serious complication involving the mitral valve. The patients usually have a small infarct of right or circumflex coronary distribution. Due to a single coronary supply to the posteromedial papillary muscle (as op-

posed to a dual supply to the anterolateral papillary muscle), rupture of the posteromedial papillary muscle is 6 to 10 times more frequent. Echocardiography is the best way to diagnose papillary muscle dysfunction and rupture (Fig. 6-7). The severity of mitral regurgitation is assessed by Doppler color-flow imaging. Since patients with severe mitral regurgitation usually present with hemodynamic decompensation, TEE may be necessary to clearly establish the diagnosis and assess the severity of mitral regurgitation [23] (Fig. 6-8). Once papillary muscle rupture is diagnosed, urgent mitral valve replacement with or without coronary revascularization is necessary for survival. The long-term survival rate is excellent after successful surgery [26].

Pericardial Effusion and Tamponade

Hemodynamically insignificant pericardial effusion is common after myocardial infarction, especially a large transmural anterior infarct

Fig. 6-7. Apical long-axis view on transthoracic examination demonstrating a partial papillary muscle rupture *(arrow)*. Incidentally, a large amount of pleural effusion (PL) is noted. In real time, the inferolateral wall is akinetic and the anteroseptum is hyperdynamic.

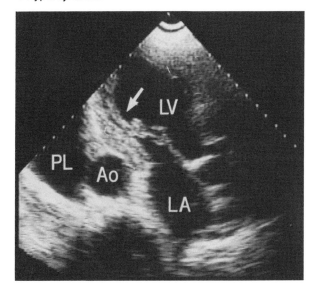

(Fig. 6-9). It is symptomatically treated (e.g., indomethacin [Indocin] therapy for pericarditic chest pain). However, cardiac rupture may present as cardiac tamponade. In this situation, the pericardial sac is seen to be filled with a gelatinous-appearing clot (see Chap. 12). Again, urgent cardiac surgery is needed and emergency pericardiocentesis may be required to stabilize the patient until the time of surgery.

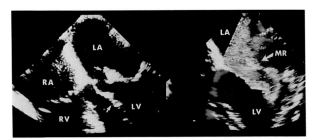

A

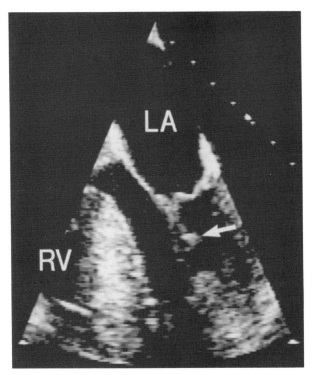

B

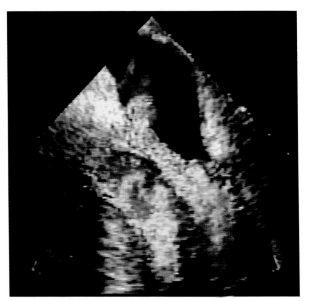

C

Fig. 6-8. TEE demonstrating complete and partial rupture of the papillary muscle. **A.** The left side shows the transesophageal four-chamber view of a completely ruptured papillary muscle prolapsing into the left atrium during systole, and color-flow imaging on the right side shows a broad mitral regurgitation (MR) jet indicating severe mitral regurgitation. (From MP Ashokakumar et al. *Am Heart J* 1989;118: 1330–1334.) **B.** A small portion of papillary muscle head *(arrow)* is partially ruptured, resulting in severe mitral regurgitation in color-flow imaging **(C).**

Right Ventricular Infarct

The right ventricle (RV) is frequently involved in acute myocardial infarction; however, hemodynamically significant RV infarct is infrequent and is almost always associated with inferior wall myocardial infarction. Patients with RV infarct present with an elevated jugular venous pressure, but clear lung fields. They may become hypotensive after nitroglycerin

administration, or develop shock requiring inotropic support and fluid administration. Echocardiographically, the RV is dilated and hypokinetic to akinetic (Fig. 6-10). The right atrium is also large and tricuspid regurgitation may become significant due to tricuspid annulus dilatation. Since RV systolic pressure is not elevated, peak tricuspid regurgitation velocity is not high, actually even lower than 2 m/sec. In patients with a patent foramen ovale (PFO), RV infarct creates an optimal clinical setting for significant right-to-left shunt via PFO due to abnormal RV compliance and markedly increased right atrial pressure. If a patient presents with hypoxemia after inferior wall myocardial infarction, RV infarct and right-to-left shunt via PFO should be strongly considered. This diagnosis can be confirmed by contrast echocardiography (peripheral venous injection of agitated saline). Following opacification of the right atrium, the contrast agent will be seen entering the left atrium via the PFO. This is best assessed by TEE (Fig. 6-11). The PFO and the shunt in this clinical setting can be temporarily closed by inflation of a balloon catheter into the left atrium (using the

Fig. 6-9. Subcostal view showing a moderate amount of pericardial fluid (PF) in a patient with an acute anteroapical infarct. Also noted is a large apical thrombus (T).

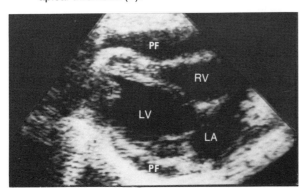

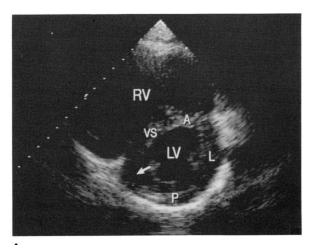

A

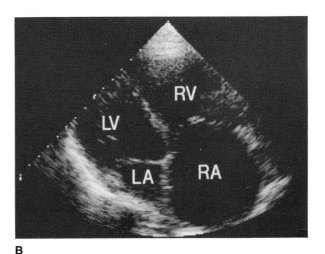

B

Fig. 6-10. Transthoracic parasternal short-axis **(A)** and apical four-chamber **(B)** views showing a dilated right ventricle (RV) and atrium (RA) in a patient with a right ventricular infarct associated with an inferior wall myocardial infarct (MI), indicated by an arrow pointing to thinned akinetic inferior and inferoseptal segments.

Rashkind catheter). The placement of the balloon catheter across the PFO and sufficient inflation of the balloon to obliterate the right-to-left shunt can be guided by TEE (see Chap. 18).

Fig. 6-11. A. Transesophageal four-chamber view demonstrating a right ventricular (RV) infarct. The right chambers are markedly dilated and the atrial septum (AS) is deviated toward the left atrium (LA) due to an increase in right atrial pressure. The patient also has a Swan-Ganz catheter and temporary pacemaker lead, shown in the right atrium (RA) *(arrowheads)*. **B.** Contrast injection via a right-arm vein opacifies the left-side cardiac chambers immediately after opacification of the RA.

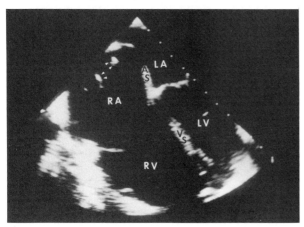

A

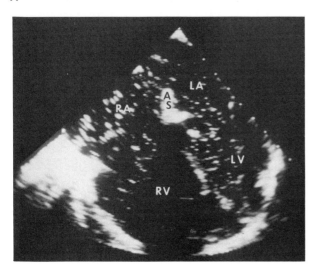

B

Ventricular Aneurysm and Thrombus

Ventricular aneurysm is characterized by myocardial thinning and bulging (outward) motion during diastole and systole. Aneurysm formation is usually related to transmural anterior myocardial infarction and is most commonly found at the apex (85–90%, Fig. 6-12). In a prospective 2D echo study, Visser and coworkers [27] found that LV aneurysm developed in 22% (35/158) of patients with acute myocardial infarction, 32% of those with anterior myocardial infarction, and 9% of those with inferior myocardial infarction. The apical view is the best window to visualize an apical aneurysm and the ventricular aneurysm is a consequence of *infarct expansion* or *"remodeling,"* which indicates a poor prognosis. An infrequent site of ventricular aneurysm is the posterobasal area (10–15%). Ventricular aneurysm frequently harbors thrombus (Figs. 6-13 and 6-14) and can be a focus of malignant ventricular arrhythmias. Because of the concern for a potential embolic event, patients with a large apical infarct or ventricular aneurysm are anticoagulated for at least 3 to 6 months after an

Fig. 6-12. Apex-down, apical four-chamber view showing a large apical aneurysm. The apex is thinned and dilated with dyskinetic motion in real time.

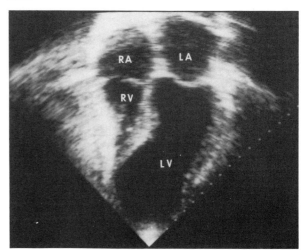

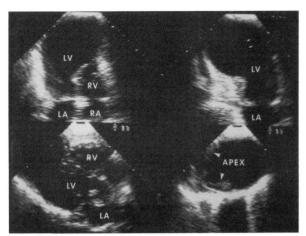

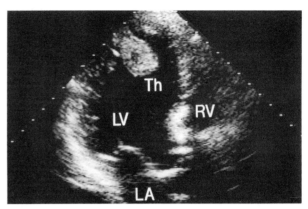

A

Fig. 6-13. A quad-screen display of the LV apical aneurysm. Apical four- and two-chamber views are shown in the upper panel and subcostal long-axis and apical short-axis views are shown in the bottom panel. Due to sluggish blood flow in the apical aneurysm, there was spontaneous echo contrast *(arrows)*. On the apical short-axis view, laminated thrombi are well seen *(arrowheads)*.

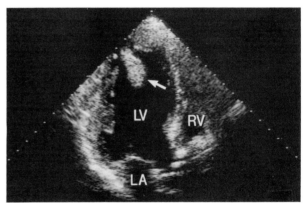

B

Fig. 6-14 A, B.   Example of a pedunculated mobile apical thrombus (Th) in a patient with an anteroapical infarct. The mobile nature of the thrombus can be appreciated by the varying shapes of the thrombus in two separate frames (**A,** Th; **B,** *arrow*). This appearance suggests a high probability of embolization.

infarct when the chance for embolism diminishes. The frequency of apical thrombus has decreased with thrombolytic therapy and therapeutic heparinization during hospitalization. However, unless apical wall motion improves by reperfusion therapy, patients with an apical infarct remain at higher risk of developing thrombus once anticoagulation therapy is stopped. Occasionally, patients survive a cardiac rupture by forming a pseudoaneurysm due to the pericardial retention of the rupture. Pseudoaneurysm is usually characterized by a small "mouth" communication between the LV and aneurysmal cavity (wall formed by the pericardium) but occasionally is difficult to distinguish from true aneurysm. The most frequent location for pseudoaneurysm is the lateral wall due to occlusion of the left circumflex coronary artery. There is to-and-fro blood flow through the rupture site, which can be documented by Doppler and color-flow imaging (Fig. 6-15). Since pseudoaneurysm has a high incidence of rupture as opposed to true aneurysm, surgical repair is always recommended.

Evaluation of Reperfusion Therapy

Timely thrombolytic therapy or balloon angioplasty during acute myocardial infarction minimizes myocardial damage and improves patient survival. However, it is difficult to objectively assess the benefit of reperfusion therapy on myocardial salvage in individual patients. Serial echocardiographic examination can assess the improvement in regional and global LV function after the reestablishment of coronary blood flow. Since the recovery of regional contractility is not immediate, baseline study can be performed within 2 to 5

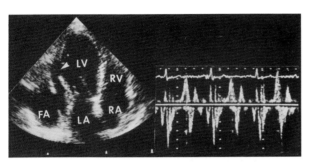

Fig. 6-15. 2D imaging of a free wall rupture *(arrowhead)* resulting in a false aneurysm (FA). The pulsed-wave Doppler shows to-and-fro velocities (right).

hours of intervention. It is safe to assume that reperfusion therapy is successful if serial examinations demonstrate improvement in regional wall motion abnormalities. Serial comparison can be best accomplished by digital echocardiography, utilizing side-by-side review of a continuous cine loop in a quad-screen format. The improvement in regional wall motion abnormalities may occur as early as in the first 24 hours, but complete recovery may take up to 7 to 10 days, occasionally even longer [20, 28].

Not every patient who achieves anatomically successful reperfusion has improved regional myocardial function (i.e., regional wall motion abnormalities). Myocardial salvage has to be substantial enough to decrease the infarcted segment to involve less than 25% of transmural wall thickness ("threshold phenomenon") to regain regional myocardial contractility. If myocardial salvage is less than that (e.g., reduction of 100% transmural involvement to 50%), the myocardium will remain akinetic. However, akinetic segments with viable myocardium are less likely to develop infarct expansion, which is a frequent complication of transmural anterior wall myocardial infarction. Infarct expansion begins soon after acute transmural myocardial infarction develops. The wall becomes thinned and the LV cavity dilates. The process continues for several months and manifests as a gradual increase in LV cavity size and volume along with thinning of the wall on serial 2D echocardiograms. Infarct expansion predisposes the patient to develop an LV aneurysm or ventricular rupture.

Evaluation of Stunned and Hibernating Myocardium

In patients with significant coronary artery disease, LV regional wall motion abnormalities may be reversed after coronary blood flow is restored. There are two pathophysiologic mechanisms for reversible myocardial dysfunction:

1. *Stunned myocardium:* Reversible regional wall motion abnormalities after reperfusion of acute coronary occlusion [29]. Reperfusion can be obtained spontaneously by thrombolytic therapy or coronary angioplasty. Recovery from wall motion abnormalities may take days to weeks.

2. *Hibernating myocardium:* Chronically depressed myocardial function due to chronic myocardial ischemia, which recovers after coronary revascularization [30].

Therefore, both stunned and hibernating myocardium are *viable* with reversible LV dysfunction. Identification of a viable myocardium is clinically important, because coronary revascularization may lead to improved LV function and, hence, survival. Resting 2D echo may help to identify a viable myocardium, by assessing diastolic myocardial wall thickness and evidence of fibrosis. Generally, a myocardial segment of normal or near-normal thickness is considered viable, while a thinned and echo-dense (fibrotic) segment is considered scarred. More frequently than not, however, it is difficult to distinguish a viable from a nonviable myocardium by assessment of LV wall thickness alone.

In animals, it has been shown that beta-adrenergic stimulation improves contractility of a chronically ischemic or postischemic myocardium with regional wall motion abnormalities, whereas it does not improve contractility in an infarcted myocardium. Several studies demonstrated that low-dose dobutamine (5-20 μg/kg/min) induces contractility in viable myocardium whether stunned or hibernating. Dobutamine-responsive wall motion improvement predicts subsequent improvement in regional LV wall thickening after coronary revascularization. This diagnostic test may become clinically useful in deciding whether coronary revascularization will be helpful in patients with LV dysfunction and congestive heart failure as predominant clinical symptoms. Contrast echocardiography may also be helpful in the detection of a viable myocardium, by demonstrating the extent of collateral blood flow within the infarct region. The myocardium may remain viable for a prolonged period in many patients with acute myocardial infarction and an occluded infarct-related coronary artery. The viability of these regions appears to be associated with presence of collateral blood flow, which is best detected by contrast echocardiography [34].

Post–Myocardial Infarction Risk Stratification

The most powerful prognostic indicators after myocardial infarction are the degree of systolic dysfunction, the extent of coronary artery disease, and the presence of heart failure. Therefore, it is logical to predict that patients with a high WMSI have a higher chance of developing subsequent cardiac events. Nishimura and associates [35] demonstrated that patients with post–myocardial infarction complications had a higher WMSI compared to those without complications (2.4 versus 1.7). Furthermore, among the patients with no heart failure (Killip class I) at admission, a subgroup of patients with a WMSI above 2.0 were more likely to develop heart failure during hospitalization. However, in the era of reperfusion therapy, regional myocardial wall motion abnormalities can return to normal contractility after successful reperfusion and in this situation, the high WMSI on the initial echocardiogram may not necessarily predict in-hospital complications.

In addition to the WMSI, diastolic filling parameters derived from mitral inflow velocities correlate well with the incidence of postinfarct heart failure (described in the next section). Stress echocardiography is sensitive in detecting residual ischemia and multivessel disease soon after myocardial infarction occurs. Patients are not, however, able to perform adequate exercise soon after acute myocardial infarction. Preliminary data suggest that stress

echocardiography using dobutamine can be performed safely soon after acute myocardial infarction (3–5 days) and provide predictable stress to the heart.

Diastolic Function

Myocardial ischemia alters diastolic function of the LV. The most prominent initial diastolic abnormality due to ischemia is prolonged and delayed myocardial relaxation. Relaxation becomes slower, resulting in prolongation of IVRT as well as in lower transmitral pressure gradient at the time of mitral valve opening, which decreases early rapid filling (E) of the LV. Deceleration time (DT) of E velocity is prolonged due to continued slow relaxation with an incompletely emptied left atrium. This results in augmented left atrial contraction ($\uparrow$ A velocity).

The typical mitral flow pattern of relaxation abnormality ($\downarrow$E, $\uparrow$DT, $\uparrow$A, $\downarrow$E/A) is seen during transient myocardial ischemia and in patients with coronary artery disease. When a patient sustains myocardial infarction, the mitral flow velocity pattern depends on the interaction of various factors: relaxation abnormalities, ventricular compliance, left atrial pressure, loading conditions, heart rate, medications, and pericardial compliance in the setting of acute cardiac dilatation. No one particular mitral inflow pattern, therefore, is consistently seen in patients with myocardial infarction. Although transmitral Doppler velocities are influenced by multiple factors, increased left atrial pressure is one of the most important determinants and produces a restrictive diastolic filling pattern ($\uparrow$E, $\downarrow$DT, $\downarrow$A, $\uparrow$E/A). Patients with acute myocardial infarction who demonstrate restrictive filling pattern on transmitral Doppler are more likely to experience heart failure (Fig. 6-16) from severe LV systolic dysfunction and/or from severe underlying coronary artery disease [36].

Coronary Artery Visualization

Visualization of coronary arteries has been one of the most challenging tasks for echocardiog-

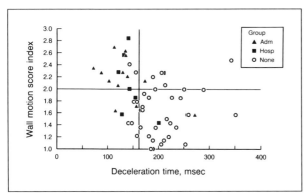

Fig. 6-16. Plot of wall motion score index and deceleration time from mitral inflow velocity in patients with acute myocardial infarction. Patients who had heart failure at admission or during hospitalization are indicated by a darkened triangle or rectangle, respectively. Patients with no heart failure during hospitalization are represented by open circles. It should be noted that many patients with a high WMSI (> 1.8–2.0) are not in heart failure despite the large myocardial infarction. However, most of the patients with a deceleration time of less than 160 msec were in heart failure at the time of admission or developed heart failure during hospitalization. (From JK Oh et al. Restrictive left ventricular diastolic filling identifies patients with heart failure after acute myocardial infarction. *J Am Soc Echocardiogr* 1992;5:497–503.)

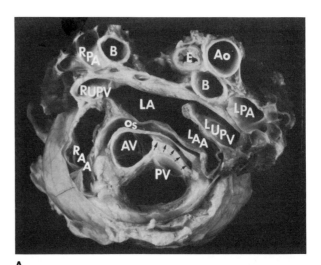

A

B

Fig. 6-17. Anatomic specimen dissected according to the transesophageal view showing the coronary arteries and the corresponding TEE images of the coronary arteries. **A.** Anatomic specimen showing the transesophageal basal short-axis view at the aortic valve level. The left main coronary and a proximal portion of the left anterior descending coronary arteries are shown by black arrows. In this view, the left atrial appendage (LAA) and left upper pulmonary vein (LUPV) are well seen. **B.** Transesophageal basal short-axis view showing the left main ostium *(large arrow)* and the ostium of the right coronary artery *(small arrow)*. Color-flow imaging during diastole shows the left main coronary flow. The coronary flow is indicated by a blue color since the flow is slightly away from the transducer.

raphy. Since Weyman and coauthors [37] first described the feasibility of visualization of the left main coronary artery by transthoracic echocardiography, numerous attempts have been made to improve its sensitivity and specificity. However, it became clear that the transthoracic approach could not adequately, reliably, and consistently visualize the coronary arteries.

The advent of TEE renewed the enthusiasm for echocardiographic visualization of the coronary arteries. As seen in the anatomic specimen sections according to a transesophageal tomographic plane, the left main and proximal portion of the left coronary tree is located within the domain of the basal short-axis view (Fig. 6-17). Preliminary studies reported that the entire left main coronary artery could be visualized in 80 to 90%; the left circumflex in 80%; and the right coronary artery in 15% [38–39]. Further investigations are needed to define the role of TEE in coronary artery visualization. Figure 6-17 shows an example of coronary arteries visualized by TEE. Coronary reserve has been evaluated by interrogating coronary artery flow velocities before and after dipyridamole challenge using pulsed-wave Doppler TEE [40].

Intravascular Ultrasound

Miniaturized high-frequency (20–40-MHz) ultrasound crystals have been incorporated into catheters to image coronary arteries. A small (3.5 French) ultrasound imaging catheter can be manipulated into the coronary arteries. The catheter system allows circumferential tomographic imaging of the artery. Preliminary data suggest that intravascular ultrasound will provide better definition of atherosclerotic plaque thickness and morphology, tissue characterization, and measurement of vascular lumen [41]. This system may be used in conjunction with percutaneous transluminal coronary angioplasty (PTCA), atherectomy, or laser therapy. Another new, exciting development is intracoronary Doppler, which can measure increased flow velocity due to coronary stenosis and can assess coronary flow reserve.

Clinical Impact

Echocardiography has become an essential part of the evaluation of patients presenting with various manifestations of ischemic heart disease. No other imaging technique can provide such a wealth of information readily, noninvasively, and relatively inexpensively at the patient's bedside. Most of adult cardiology practice deals with coronary artery disease: chest pain, stress testing, myocardial infarction, postinfarct complications, risk stratification, and preoperative cardiac evaluation. Echocardiography helps to evaluate every aspect of coronary disease short of visualization of the entire coronary arterial tree and evaluation of the conduction system. Serial regional wall motion analysis utilizing digital echocardiography is an excellent way of evaluating the beneficial effects of thrombolytic therapy on regional myocardial function, and should become a routine part of managing patients with acute myocardial infarction. When patients develop a complication after myocardial infarction, echocardiography should be the first diagnostic procedure of choice so that potentially fatal complications can be diagnosed and intervention started expeditiously to improve the chance of survival. In patients with uncomplicated myocardial infarction, systolic and diastolic function parameters at rest and/or with stress (exercise or pharmacologic stress) determined by 2D Doppler echocardiography provide prognostic information and guide optimal management strategies.

References

1. Tennant R, Wiggers CJ. Effect of coronary occlusion on myocardial contraction. *Am J Physiol* 1935;112:351–361.
2. American Society of Echocardiography Committee on Standards. Recommendations for quantification of the left ventricle by two-dimensional echocardiography. *J Am Soc Echocardiogr* 1989;2:358–367.
3. Feigenbaum H. Digital recording, display, and storage of echocardiograms. *J Am Soc Echocardiogr* 1988;5:378–383.
4. Wann LS, et al. Exercise cross-sectional echocardiography in ischemic heart disease. *Circulation* 1979;60:1300–1308.
5. Robertson WS, et al. Exercise echocardiography: A clinically practical addition in the evaluation of coronary artery disease. *J Am Coll Cardiol* 1983;2:1085–1091.
6. Maurer G, Nanda NC. Two-dimensional echocardiographic evaluation of exercise-induced left and right ventricular asynergy: correlation with thallium scanning. *Am J Cardiol* 1981;48:720–727.
7. Limacher MC, et al. Detection of coronary artery disease with exercise two-dimensional echocardiography: description of a clinically applicable method and comparison with radionuclide ventriculography. *Circulation* 1983;67:1211–1218.
8. Armstrong WF, et al. Complementary value of two-dimensional exercise echocardiography to routine treadmill exercise testing. *Ann Intern Med* 1986;105:829–835.
9. Sawada SG, et al. Exercise echocardiography detection of coronary artery disease in women. *J Am Coll Cardiol* 1989;14:140–147.
10. Sawada SG, et al. Prognostic value of a normal exercise echocardiogram. *Am Heart J* 1990;120:49–55.

11. Crouse LJ, Harbrecht JJ, Vacek JL. Exercise echocardiography as a screening test for coronary artery disease and correlation with coronary angiography. *Am J Cardiol* 1991; 67:1213–1218.

12. Quinones MA, et al. Exercise echocardiography versus 201-Tl single-photon emission computed tomography in evaluation of coronary artery disease: analysis of 292 patients. *Circulation* 1992;85:1026–1031.

13. Picano E, Lattanzi F, L'Abbate A. Present application, practical aspects, and future issues on dipyridamole echocardiography. *Circulation* 1991;83(suppl III):111–115.

14. Berthe C, Pierard LA, Hiernaux M. Predicting the extent and location of coronary artery disease in acute myocardial infarction by echocardiography during dobutamine infusion. *Am J Cardiol* 1986;58:1167–1172.

15. Pierard LA, Berthe C, Albert A. Haemodynamic alterations during ischaemia induced by dobutamine stress testing. *Eur Heart J* 1989;10:783–790.

16. Sawada SG, Segar DS, Ryan T. Echocardiographic detection of coronary artery disease during dobutamine infusion. *Circulation* 1991;83:1605–1614.

17. Oh JK, et al. Role of two-dimensional echocardiography in the emergency room. *Echocardiography* 1985;3:217–226.

18. Sabia P, et al. Value of regional wall motion abnormality in the emergency room diagnosis of acute myocardial infarction: a prospective study using two-dimensional echocardiography. *Circulation* 1991;84 (Suppl I):85–92.

19. Oh JK, et al. Evaluation of acute chest pain syndrome by two-dimensional echocardiography: its potential application in the selection of patients for acute reperfusion therapy. *Mayo Clin Proc* 1987;62:59–66.

20. Oh JK, et al. Effects of acute reperfusion on regional myocardial function: serial two-dimensional echocardiography assessment. *Int J Cardiol* 1989;22:161–168.

21. Nishimura RA. *The Role of Echocardiography in Acute Myocardial Infarction.* New York: Elsevier Science, 1990.

22. Oh JK, et al. Transesophageal echocardiography in critically ill patients. *Am J Cardiol* 1990;66:1492–1495.

23. Kishon Y, et al. Evolution of echocardiographic modalities in detection of postmyocardial infarction ventricular septal defect and papillary muscle rupture: study of 62 patients. *Am Heart J* [in press].

24. Lehmann KG, et al. Mitral regurgitation in early myocardial infarction: incidence, clinical detection, and prognostic implications. *Ann Intern Med* 1992:117:10–17.

25. Tcheng JE, et al. Outcome of patients sustaining acute ischemic mitral regurgitation during myocardial infarction. *Ann Intern Med* 1992;117:18–24.

26. Kishon Y, et al. Mitral valve operation in postinfarction rupture of a papillary muscle: immediate results and long-term follow-up of 22 patients. *Mayo Clin Proc* 1992;67:1023–1030.

27. Visser CA, et al. Incidence, timing, and prognostic value of left ventricular aneurysm formation after myocardial infarction: a prospective, serial echocardiographic study of 158 patients. *Am J Cardiol* 1986;57:729–732.

28. Broderick TM, et al. Comparison of regional and global left ventricular function by serial echocardiograms after reperfusion in acute myocardial infarction. *J Am Soc Echocardiogr* 1989;2:315–323.

29. Braunwald E, Kloner RA. The stunned myocardium: prolonged, post-ischemic ventricular dysfunction. *Circulation* 1982;66:1146–1149.

30. Rahimtoola SH. The hibernating myocardium. *Am Heart J* 1989;117:211–221.

31. Pierard LA, et al. Identification of viable myocardium by echocardiography during dobutamine infusion in patients with myocardial infarction after thrombolytic therapy: comparison with positron emission tomography. *J Am Coll Cardiol* 1990;15:1021–1031.

32. Smart SC, et al. Low-dose dobutamine echocardiography detects reversible dysfunction after thrombolytic therapy of acute myocardial infarction. *Circulation* 1993;88:405–415.

33. Cigarroa CG, et al. Dobutamine stress echocardiography identifies hibernating myocardium and predicts recovery of left ventricular function after coronary revascularization. *Circulation* 1993;88:430–436.

34. Sabia PJ, et al. An association between collateral blood flow and myocardial viability in patients with recent myocardial infarction. *N Engl J Med* 1992;327:1825–31.

35. Nishimura RA, et al. Role of two-dimensional

echocardiography in the prediction of in-hospital complications after acute myocardial infarction. *J Am Coll Cardiol* 1984;4:1080–1087.

36. Oh JK, et al. Restrictive left ventricular diastolic filling identifies patients with heart failure after acute myocardial infarction. *J Am Soc Echocardiogr* 1992;5:497–503.

37. Weyman AE, et al. Noninvasive visualization of the left main coronary artery by cross-sectional echocardiography. *Circulation* 1976; 54:169–174.

38. Taams MA, et al. Detection of left coronary artery stenosis by transesophageal echocardiography. *Eur Heart J* 1988;9:1162–1166.

39. Yoshida K, Yoshikawa J, Hozumi T. Detection of left main coronary artery stenosis by transesophageal color Doppler and two-dimensional echocardiography. *Circulation* 1990; 81:1271–1276.

40. Iliceto S, et al. Transesophageal Doppler echocardiography evaluation of coronary blood flow velocity in baseline conditions and during dipyridamole-induced coronary vasodilation. *Circulation* 1991;83:61–69.

41. Nishimura RA, et al. Intravascular ultrasound imaging: in vitro validation and pathologic correlation. *J Am Coll Cardiol* 1990; 16:145–154.

7

Valvular Heart Disease

Prior to the clinical application of Doppler, echocardiography was limited to a qualitative description of valvular abnormalities. Most of the patients with severe valvular heart disease underwent cardiac catheterization before surgical intervention. Doppler, however, has changed the role of echocardiography in the evaluation of valvular disease. Pressure gradients, cardiac output, stenotic valve area, regurgitant fraction, and severity of valvular regurgitation are now determined reliably by Doppler echocardiography and color-flow imaging. In the majority of patients with valvular heart disease, echocardiographic evaluation should provide comprehensive data regarding left ventricular (LV) dimension and global systolic function, valvular morphology, valvular hemodynamics, and pulmonary pressures. Based on this information in conjunction with the patient's history and physical examination, clinicians can determine the most optimal treatment strategy including surgical intervention. In this chapter, comprehensive echocardiographic evaluation of valvular heart diseases is discussed in a step-by-step manner.

Evaluation of Valvular Stenosis

A stenotic valve is generally thickened and calcified, and its opening is restricted. All of these features can be visualized by 2D echocardiography. 2D echocardiographic examination is helpful in identifying the underlying etiologies of valvular stenosis such as bicuspid aortic valve, rheumatic mitral valve, and carcinoid heart disease. 2D echocardiographic assessment, however, is at best semiquantitative. To obtain hemodynamic data, all patients with valvular stenosis should have a comprehensive Doppler examination.

Blood flow velocity across a stenotic valve increases as the orifice area becomes smaller. From Doppler velocity (V), transvalvular pressure gradients can be derived based on the modified Bernoulli equation (see Chap. 5):

$$\text{Pressure gradient} = 4 \times V^2$$

All available transducer windows should be utilized to be certain that the Doppler ultrasound beam is parallel with the direction of the stenotic jet. A nonimaging continuous-wave Doppler transducer is smaller and therefore easier to manipulate between the ribs and suprasternal notch, compared to a duplex transducer. Occasionally, color-flow imaging is useful in aligning the continuous-wave Doppler beam parallel with the direction of the blood flow jet.

The accuracy of the Doppler-derived pressure gradient has been validated by cardiac catheterization data obtained in simultaneous correlation studies [1–3]. It should be emphasized that for a given valve area, the flow velocity, hence, the pressure gradient, will vary with changes in cardiac output. Therefore, the cardiac output should be taken into consideration in determining the severity of valvular stenosis. The *continuity equation,* derived from the same basic hydraulic formula on which the Gorlin formula is based [4], can reliably estimate valve area by calculating stroke volume from another cardiac orifice. Excellent correlations between 2D/Doppler values and catheter-derived aortic valve areas have been reported [5–9]. *Pressure half-time* (PHT), which is the time interval required for the peak pressure gradient to reach one-half of its initial value, is another useful Doppler parameter to assess the severity of mitral stenosis [10]. The rate of pressure fall is slower as the mitral orifice becomes smaller; hence, the PHT is prolonged. However, PHT can falsely underesti-

mate the severity of mitral stenosis since it can be shortened by concomitant aortic regurgitation (AR), by decreased ventricular compliance, or immediately after mitral balloon valvuloplasty [11–14]. Evaluation of pulmonary and tricuspid stenosis utilizes methods similar to those described above for aortic and mitral stenosis, respectively. A comprehensive echocardiographic evaluation of individual valvular stenosis is illustrated in the following section.

Aortic Stenosis

2D and M-mode Echocardiography

A normal aortic valve has thin cusps and an unrestrictive systolic opening, as seen in Figure 7-1. The normal aortic valve area is 3–4 cm^2 and normal opening excursion generally produces 2.0 cm of leaflet separation (Fig. 7-1A). The same degree of separation is maintained during most of systole unless the patient has a low cardiac output (Fig. 7-1B) or left ventricular outflow tract (LVOT) obstruction. The most common form of aortic valvular stenosis is due to degenerative calcification. Therefore, the leaflets are thickened and the cusp opening is reduced (Fig. 7-2A). Multiple echoes in the aortic root are also a common finding (Fig. 7-2B). However, the M-mode echocardiogram may appear normal in patients with a noncalcific stenotic valve with systolic doming, as in congenital aortic stenosis, since the restriction of valve opening occurs at the distal portion with doming. 2D echocardiography visualizes the entire aortic valve structure and is helpful to identify noncalcific as well as calcific aortic stenosis (Fig. 7-3). Although occasionally difficult, the number of aortic cusps can be determined by 2D echocardiography, especially from the parasternal short-axis view at the aortic valvular level (Fig. 7-4). In addition, the degree of valvular calcification, size of aortic annulus and supravalvular ascending aorta, and the presence of secondary subvalvular obstruction are easily evaluated. 2D echocardiography is also useful to determine the degree of LV hypertrophy (wall thickness and

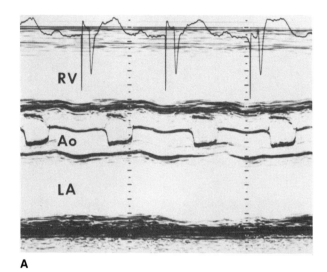

A

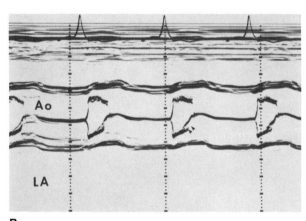

B

Fig. 7-1. M-mode echocardiograms of a normal aortic valve. The aortic cusps are thin and their opening is not limited, having a maximal separation of 2 cm. Normally, the maximal opening is maintained throughout systole **(A)**, but tapers off during midsystole *(double arrowheads)* when cardiac output is severely reduced **(B)**. In patients with dynamic LVOT obstruction, the aortic valve opening is interrupted during midsystole but resumes again at late systole (see Fig. 5-2).

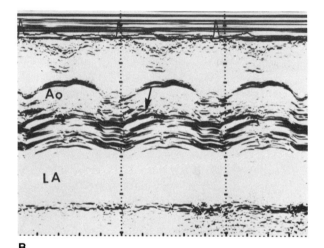

Fig. 7-2. M-mode echocardiogram of a calcific aortic valve. The aortic cusps are thickened *(arrowhead* in **A**; *arrow* in **B**) and the opening is reduced (8–10 mm in **A**; 4 mm in **B**). Also, multiple dense echoes are noted in the aortic root during systole and diastole. These findings suggest significant aortic stenosis but a Doppler study is required to determine how significant the stenosis is.

mass), left atrial enlargement, ventricular function, and the integrity of other valves.

Doppler Echocardiography

The hemodynamic severity of aortic stenosis determined by Doppler is based on *peak aortic velocity, mean pressure gradient, aortic valve area,* and *LVOT–aortic valve (AV) time velocity integral (TVI) ratio* [5–9, 15]. A meticulous search for the maximum aortic velocity is essential since all the above parameters are derived from the peak aortic velocity. The methods and interpretations of Doppler examinations are discussed in a stepwise manner.

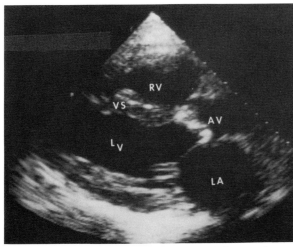

Fig. 7-3. 2D echocardiography still-frame of calcific aortic stenosis. The aortic valve (AV) is calcified and LV wall thickness is increased due to LV hypertrophy. The left atrium (LA) is enlarged.

Method

Step 1. Obtain the maximum aortic jet velocity by systematic search utilizing multiple windows (Figs. 7-5 and 7-6).

Step 2. Calculate the mean aortic gradient and TVI by tracing the maximum velocity jet.

Step 3. Determine stroke volume and cardiac output from LVOT diameter and velocity (Fig. 7-7).

Step 4. Calculate aortic valve area using the continuity equation (Fig. 7-8 and 7-9).

See also Chapter 5 for a detailed discussion of Doppler hemodynamics.

Definition of Severe Aortic Stenosis

When LV systolic function and cardiac output are normal, severe aortic stenosis is defined by

1. A peak aortic valve velocity of 4.5 m/sec or greater (Fig. 7-10)
2. A mean pressure gradient of 50 mm Hg or higher (Fig. 7-10)
3. An aortic valve area of 0.75 cm² or smaller

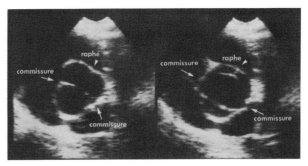

A

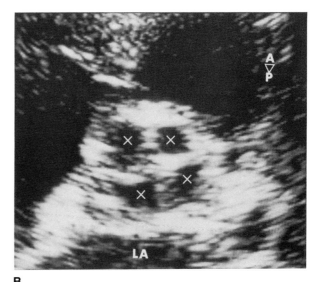

B

Fig. 7-4. Still-frame 2D echocardiogram of a bicuspid **(A)** and quadricuspid **(B)** aortic valve. **A.** On the left is a diastolic frame showing commissures at 4 and 10 o'clock positions. On the right is a "fish mouth" opening during systole. The raphe is at the 1 o'clock position. (From R Brandenburg, et al. *Am J Cardiol* 1983;51:1469–1473.) **B.** Diastolic frame showing four aortic cusps (x). (From B Feldman, et al. *Am J Cardiol* 1990;65:937–938.)

4. An LVOT/AV TVI or velocity ratio of 0.2 or lower (Fig. 7-11)

When LV systolic function and cardiac output are altered, the following should be considered. Peak velocity and mean aortic gradient vary with changes in stroke volume. If LV function or stroke volume is decreased, the peak aortic velocity and mean gradient may be lower than 4.5 m/sec and 50 mm Hg, respec-

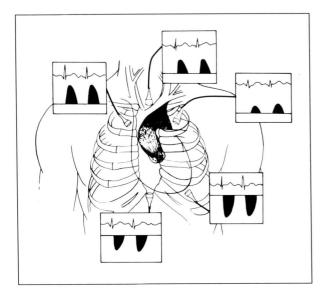

Fig. 7-5. Schematic drawing of multiple transducer positions used to obtain aortic stenosis jet velocity. The maximum velocity is usually obtained from the apex (85% of the time), but all the transducer positions should be utilized to ensure securing the maximum velocity. (Modified from RA Nishimura, et al. *Mayo Clin Proc* 1985;60:321–343.)

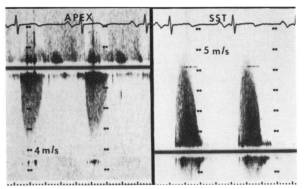

Fig. 7-6. Continuous-wave Doppler spectra from a patient with aortic stenosis. The velocity from the suprasternal notch (SST) is higher (4.5 m/sec) than that from the apical window (3.5 m/sec), making a difference of 32 mm Hg (81 − 49 mm Hg) in maximum instantaneous gradient. Aortic regurgitation jet was better documented from the apex in this patient.

tively, in patients with severe aortic stenosis. However, the velocity or TVI ratio should be independent of any change in stroke volume since the LVOT and aortic valve velocities change proportionally (see Fig. 7-11). In the setting of low cardiac output (hence, low gradient), the calculated aortic valve area may indicate a decreased effective orifice area and overestimate the true severity of aortic stenosis. A gradual low-dose infusion of dobutamine (up to 20 μg/kg/min) to increase cardiac output may be helpful in differentiating morphologically severe aortic stenosis from decreased effective orifice area due to low cardiac output (pseudo-severe aortic stenosis). In patients with true severe aortic stenosis, dobutamine infusion will increase the peak velocity and TVI of both the LVOT and the aortic valve proportionally (hence, the LVOT/AV TVI ratio remains the same), whereas an increase in velocity and TVI of the LVOT is far greater than that of the aortic valve (whose area becomes

larger with higher output; hence, the LVOT/AV TVI ratio increases) in patients with pseudo-severe aortic stenosis. Dobutamine can be infused gradually from 5 μg/kg/min in 5-μg increments every 3 minutes until the LVOT velocity or TVI reaches a normal value—0.8 to 1.0 m/sec or 20 to 25 cm, respectively. Maximum stroke volume is usually obtained with 15–20 μg/kg/min. In patients with increased cardiac output (as in AR or anemia) across the aortic valve, aortic stenosis may not be severe even when the peak velocity is 4.5 m/sec or greater and the mean gradient is 50 mm Hg or higher. Again, LVOT/AV velocity (or TVI) ratio and aortic valve area should be helpful in determining the severity of aortic stenosis.

To calculate aortic valve area in the presence of significant AR, the following should be considered. Flow across the aortic valve increases with AR as does aortic gradient. However, the increase is reflected in the LVOT and aortic valve velocities proportionally and their TVI ratio remains the same for a given aortic valve area. Cardiac catheterization is unreliable in this situation and tends to result in a lower calculated aortic valve area, mainly due to an underestimation of cardiac output.

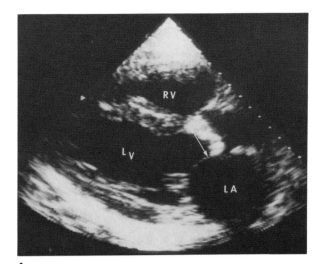

A

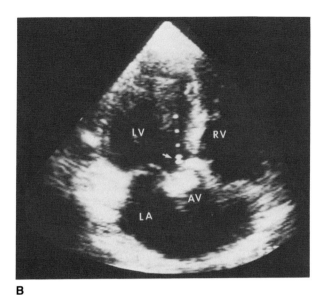

B

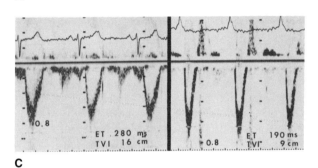

C

Fig. 7-7. Stroke volume across the aortic valve needs to be calculated to determine aortic valve area. This is done by measuring the LVOT diameter and flow velocity. **A.** Measurement of LVOT diameter: from the systolic freeze-frame of the parasternal long-axis view, the distance from where the anterior aortic cusp meets the ventricular septum to the point where the posterior cusp meets the anterior mitral leaflet. The line between the two cusps is almost perpendicular to the anterior wall of the aortic root. **B.** Measurement of LVOT velocity from the apical long-axis view; the pulsed-wave sample volume *(arrow)* is located 3 to 5 mm proximal to the aortic valve (AV). If it is too close to the aortic valve, prestenotic acceleration jet velocity may be recorded. **C.** Determination of LVOT TVI. Two examples of LVOT velocity spectra are shown. TVI is determined by tracing the velocity envelope, and

is equal to the sum of individual velocities of the Doppler spectrum. Although both spectra show a similar peak velocity (0.8 m/sec), the TVI is markedly different due to the difference in ejection time (ET). Once the LVOT diameter (D) and TVI are determined, flow across the LVOT is calculated as follows:

$$
\begin{aligned}
LVOT &= LVOT\ area \times LVOT\ TVI \\
&= (D/2)^2 \times \pi \times LVOT\ TVI \\
&= D^2 \times 0.785 \times LVOT\ TVI
\end{aligned}
$$

The following table shows LVOT areas calculated from various LVOT diameters.

LVOT diameter (D) (cm)	Area ($D^2 \times 0.785$) (cm^2)
1.5	1.77
1.6	2.01
1.7	2.27
1.8	2.54
1.9	2.84
2.0	3.14
2.1	3.46
2.2	3.80
2.3	4.15
2.4	4.52
2.5	4.90

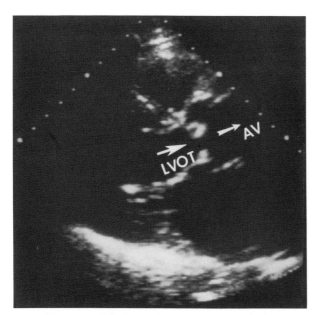

Fig. 7-8. Still-frame from a 2D echocardiogram showing the LVOT and the stenotic aortic valve (AV). The continuity equation states that the flow across the LVOT is the same as the flow across the aortic valve ("what goes in must come out"). Therefore,

LVOT flow = AV flow

LVOT D^2 × 0.785 × LVOT TVI = AVA × AV TVI

$$AVA = LVOT\ D^2 \times 0.785 \times \frac{LVOT\ TVI}{AV\ TVI}$$

where D = diameter, and AVA = aortic valve area.

Since flow duration across the LVOT and the aortic valve is the same, the TVI ratio is similar to their peak velocity (V) ratio. Therefore, the continuity equation can be simplified to

$$AVA = D^2 \times 0.785 \times \frac{LVOT\ V}{AV\ V}$$

It should be noted that TVI or peak velocity ratio is inversely proportional to the area ratio of the LVOT and the aortic valve. For example, a TVI ratio of 0.3 indicates that the aortic valve area is about 30% of the LVOT area. This ratio is also useful in the determination of aortic stenosis severity (see Fig. 7-11).

Limitations and Pitfalls

The limitations and pitfalls of Doppler echocardiography in assessing aortic stenosis are as follows.

1. The aortic stenosis jet must be differentiated from other systolic Doppler findings

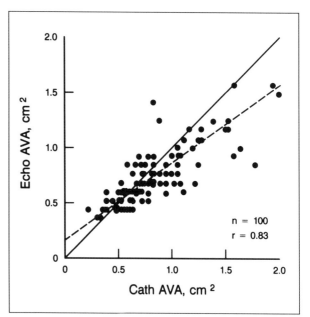

Fig. 7-9. Correlation between Doppler-derived (by the continuity equation) and catheter-derived (by the Gorlin formula) aortic valve areas (AVA) in 100 patients. It should be noted that the difference between the two methods is greater when the aortic valve area is more than 1.0 cm². (From JK Oh et al. Prediction of the severity of aortic stenosis by Doppler aortic valve area determination: prospective Doppler-catheterization correlation in 100 patients. *J Am Coll Cardiol* 1988;11:1227–1234.)

(Fig. 7-12) including mitral regurgitation, LVOT obstruction, tricuspid regurgitation, and pulmonary stenosis.

2. It may be difficult to measure LVOT diameter due to heavy calcification of the aortic valve and annulus. In this situation, one should use the other nonregurgitant orifice (right ventricular outflow tract or mitral valve) to calculate stroke volume. In this case, the TVI ratio, not the peak velocity ratio, must be used since flow ejection periods are different.

3. It may be difficult to obtain satisfactory LVOT velocity due to coexisting LVOT obstruction due to basal septal hypertrophy.

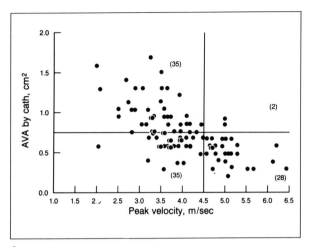
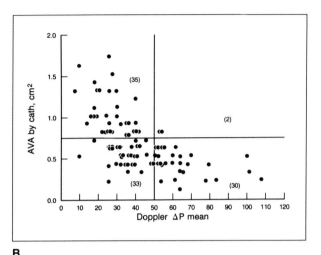

A   **B**

Fig. 7-10. Plot of catheter-derived aortic valve area (AVA) versus Doppler peak velocity **(A)**, and versus Doppler-derived mean pressure gradients **(B)**. The aortic valve area is 0.75 cm^2 or smaller when the peak velocity and mean pressure gradient are at least 4.5 m/sec and 50 mm Hg, respectively, in essentially all patients. However, half of the patients with lower Doppler peak velocities and mean gradients also had an aortic valve area of 0.75 cm^2 or smaller, especially in the setting of low cardiac output. (From JK Oh et al. Prediction of the severity of aortic stenosis by Doppler aortic valve area determination: prospective Doppler-catheterization correlation in 100 patients. *J Am Coll Cardiol* 1988;11:1227–1234.)

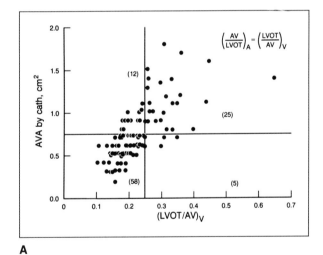
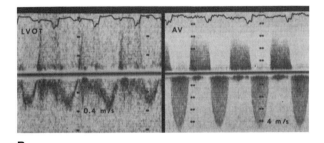

A   **B**

Fig. 7-11. **A.** Correlation of the LVOT/AV velocity ratio with catheter-derived aortic valve area (AVA). The LVOT/AV velocity or TVI ratio is inversely proportional to their area ratio. When the ratio is greater than 0.25 (i.e., aortic valve area > 25% of LVOT area), the aortic valve area is greater than 0.75 cm^2. Most of the patients with a ratio less than 0.2 (i.e., aortic valve area < 20% of LVOT area) have severe aortic stenosis (i.e., aortic valve area ≤ 0.75 cm^2). The ratio is independent of cardiac output status. (From JK Oh et al. Prediction of the severity of aortic stenosis by Doppler aortic valve area determination: prospective Doppler-catheterization correlation in 100 patients. *J Am Coll Cardiol* 1988;11:1227–1234.) **B.** An example of critical aortic stenosis in the setting of low cardiac output. The aortic valve velocity is 4.2 m/sec and the LVOT flow velocity is 0.4 m/sec, indicating a marked decrease in cardiac output. The LVOT/AV velocity ratio is less than 0.1.

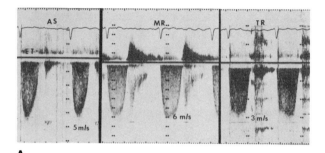

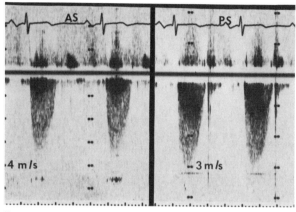

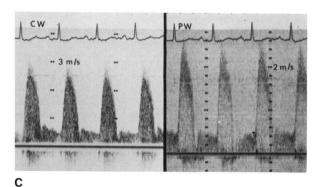

Fig. 7-12. Differentiation of aortic stenosis Doppler spectrum from other systolic Doppler spectra. Systolic flow velocities by continuous-wave Doppler echocardiography need to be analyzed on the following bases: (1) peak velocity, (2) flow duration or ejection time (ET), (3) location of Doppler window, (4) accompanying diastolic flow signals, and (5) Doppler flow configuration. **A.** The duration of mitral (MR) and tricuspid (TR) regurgitations is longer than that of aortic stenosis (AS) since there is no ejection through the aortic valve during isovolumic relaxation and contraction, whereas regurgitation flow occurs during those periods. The mitral regurgitation jet velocity is usually more than 4 m/sec unless the left atrial pressure is markedly elevated. The peak velocity of mitral regurgitation flow is always higher than that of aortic stenosis when present together in the same patient. Tricuspid valve inflow velocity is lower than mitral inflow velocity unless there is severe tricuspid regurgitation. The AR jet also is frequently documented together with the aortic stenosis velocity pattern. **B.** The Doppler spectrum of pulmonary stenosis (PS) is almost identical to that of aortic stenosis (AS). The pulmonary stenosis signal is best obtained from the subcostal or left upper parasternal window, whereas an aortic stenosis jet is most easily evaluated from the apex or right parasternal window. The flow velocity from the LVOT obstruction produces a late-peaking, dagger-shaped velocity spectrum, which can be easily recognized and differentiated from other Doppler spectra. **C.** Occasionally, stenosis of the innominate or subclavian artery produces a systolic flow velocity resembling that of aortic stenosis from the suprasternal notch. However, velocity from a stenotic cerebrovascular vessel has a diastolic component. The origin of the 3 m/sec jet by continuous-wave Doppler can be located by pulsed-wave Doppler echocardiography by placing the sample volume in the left common carotid artery.

4. If the patient's rhythm is other than sinus, the aortic and LVOT velocities will vary with each cardiac cycle depending on the preceding R-R interval. In this case, one should use the average velocities from 8 to 10 cardiac cycles, and/or match the R-R intervals for LVOT and aortic valve velocity to obtain the TVI or velocity ratio (Fig. 7-13).

Clinical Implications

Echocardiography provides a comprehensive evaluation of patients with aortic stenosis and based on this information, precise management decisions can be made. In patients with severe aortic stenosis (mean gradient > 50 mm Hg and/or aortic valve area ≤ 0.75 cm²), we now perform and recommend aortic valve replacement with preoperative coronary angi-

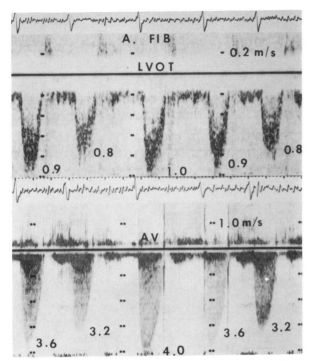

Fig. 7-13. Determination of aortic valve area in atrial fibrillation. Even in atrial fibrillation, one can match up similar R-R intervals between LVOT velocities and the aortic valve flow velocities, as seen here. With similar cardiac cycle length, the LVOT/AV velocity ratio remains quite constant. In this example, the LVOT velocities are 0.9, 0.8, 1.0, 0.9, and 0.8 m/sec. The aortic valve velocities with similar cardiac cycle length are 3.6, 3.2, 4.0, 3.6, and 3.2 m/sec, respectively. Therefore, their velocity ratio remains 1 : 4, and it can be used to calculate aortic valve area from the continuity equation.

ography, but without LV angiography or invasive hemodynamic determination.

Mitral Stenosis

2D and M-mode Echocardiography
In almost all patients, mitral stenosis is caused by rheumatic involvement of the mitral valve. Typical 2D/M-mode echocardiographic features (Fig. 7-14) include

1. Thickened mitral leaflets and subvalvular apparatus

2. "Hockey stick" appearance of the anterior mitral leaflet in diastole (long-axis view)
3. "Fish mouth" orifice in short-axis view
4. Decreased E-F slope (M-mode)
5. Anterior motion of the posterior mitral leaflet (M-mode)
6. Increased left atrial size with the potential of thrombus formation

The mitral valve area can be measured by planimetry from the parasternal short-axis view (Fig. 7-14B). It may be difficult in patients with a previous commissurotomy or heavy calcification. In patients undergoing mitral balloon valvuloplasty, the *echocardiography score* based on valve thickness, calcification, mobility, and subvalvular thickening (Table 7-1) predicts the outcome of the procedure [16]. Patients with an echo score of 8 or lower have a more favorable result from mitral balloon valvuloplasty than do patients with a higher score, but an echo score higher than 8 does not preclude the option of valvuloplasty.

Doppler and Color-Flow Imaging
Doppler echocardiography evaluates several important hemodynamic parameters for estimating the severity of mitral stenosis [10, 17, 18]. These include *mitral pressure gradients, PHT, mitral valve area, pulmonary artery pressure,* and *associated regurgitation.* As the obstruction increases, not only does the pressure gradient increase but also the rate of pressure decay is prolonged.

Estimation of Mitral Stenosis Severity
The method used to estimate the severity of mitral stenosis is as follows.

Step 1. Determine the pressure gradient by obtaining maximum velocity using continuous-wave Doppler from the apical and paraapical positions (Fig. 7-15).

Step 2. Obtain the mean gradient and TVI (Figs. 7-16 and 7-17).

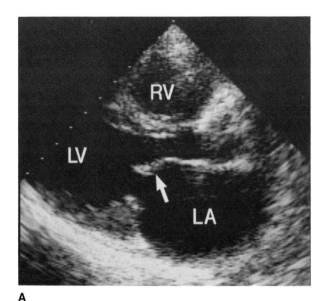

A

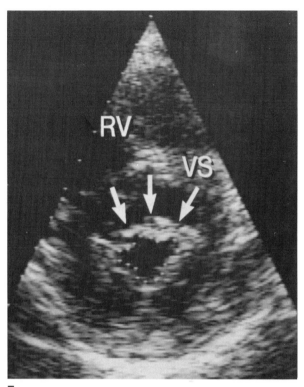

B

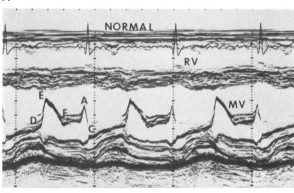

C

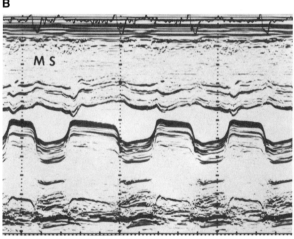

D

Fig. 7-14.   A. 2D echocardiogram of the parasternal long-axis view during diastole in a patient with mitral stenosis. The mitral leaflets are thickened with the typical "hockey stick" appearance *(arrow).* The left atrium (LA) is enlarged. **B.** 2D echocardiogram of the parasternal short-axis view showing the "fish mouth" orifice *(arrows)* of the stenotic mitral valve. The orifice area is measured by manual tracing. **C.** M-mode echocardiogram of a normal mitral valve. **D.** M-mode echocardiogram of typical mitral stenosis. The mitral leaflet is thickened and the E-F slope is decreased.

Step 3. Calculate mitral valve area (MVA). By the PHT method:

$$MVA = 220/PHT$$

By the continuity equation:

$$MVA = LVOT\ D^2 \times 0.785 \times \frac{LVOT\ TVI}{MV\ TVI}$$

Step 4. Determine the pulmonary artery pressure by utilizing the tricuspid regurgitation velocity (see Chap. 13).

Table 7-1. Echocardiographic score used to predict outcome of mitral balloon valvuloplasty*

Grade	Mobility	Subvalvular thickening	Thickening	Calcification
1	Highly mobile valve with only leaflet tips restricted	Minimal thickening just below the mitral leaflets	Leaflets near normal in thickness (4–5 mm)	A single area of increased echo brightness
2	Leaflet mid and base portions have normal mobility	Thickening of chordal structures extending up to one-third of the chordal length	Midleaflets normal, considerable thickening of margins (5–8 mm)	Scattered areas of brightness confined to leaflet margins
3	Valve continues to move forward in diastole, mainly from the base	Thickening extending to the distal third of the chords	Thickening extending through the entire leaflet (5–8 mm)	Brightness extending into the midportion of the leaflets
4	No or minimal forward movement of the leaflets in diastole	Extensive thickening and shortening of all chordal structures extending down to the papillary muscles	Considerable thickening of all leaflet tissue (>8–10 mm)	Extensive brightness throughout much of the leaflet tissue

*The total echocardiographic score was derived from an analysis of mitral leaflet mobility, valvular and subvalvular thickening, and calcification, which were graded from 0 to 4 according to the above criteria. This gave a total score of 0 to 16.

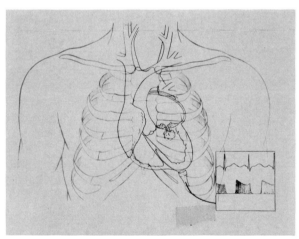

Fig. 7-15. Schematic diagram of stenotic mitral valve and Doppler velocity measurement from the apex. The mitral velocity is obtained from the apex 100% of the time. The mitral flow can be eccentric and color-flow imaging can occasionally guide the continuous-wave Doppler beam to minimize the angle of θ. (From RA Nishimura, et al. *Mayo Clin Proc* 1985;60:325.)

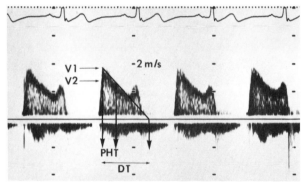

Fig. 7-16. PHT calculation from continuous-wave Doppler spectrum of mitral stenosis. V2 is where the pressure gradient is one-half of the peak pressure gradient at V1 and is calculated as V1/1.4. PHT is the time interval from V1 to V2. PHT is always 29% of the deceleration time (DT), which is the time interval for peak velocity (V1) to reach the baseline. In this case example, DT is 600 msec, PHT is 174 msec, mitral valve area is 220/174, which equals 1.26 cm² (≈ 1.3 cm²).

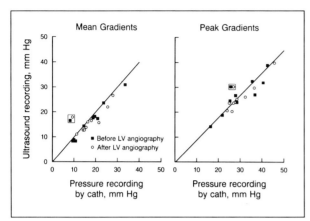

Fig. 7-17. Doppler-derived peak (maximum) and mean gradients correlated very well with respective pressure gradients measured by cardiac catheterization. (From L Hatle, et al. Noninvasive assessment of pressure drop in mitral stenosis by Doppler ultrasound. *Br Heart J* 1978;40:138.)

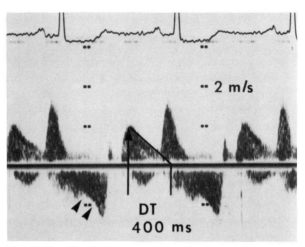

Fig. 7-18. Continuous-wave Doppler from the apex. Mitral DT and PHT (= 0.29 × DT) are prolonged. The mitral valve was normal in this patient, and the main cardiac pathology was LV hypertrophy. The prolonged DT (or PHT) is related to abnormal relaxation of the myocardium. The E velocity is not increased. The patient also had a mild degree of LVOT obstruction *(double arrowheads)*, which is not unusual in patients with LV hypertrophy.

Definition of Mitral Stenosis Severity

The following categorizes the severity of mitral stenosis according to the mitral valve area.

Normal: 4 to 6 cm²

Mild: 1.6 to 2.0 cm²

Moderate: 1.1 to 1.5 cm²

Severe: 1.0 cm² or smaller

Mitral stenosis is considered severe when: (1) mean pressure gradient is 12 mm Hg or higher, (2) mitral valve area is 1.0 cm² or smaller, and (3) PHT is 220 msec or longer.

In summary, mitral valve area can be determined directly by planimetry on 2D echocardiograms and the continuity equation, or indirectly by the PHT method. All three methods should be utilized in every patient, but the direct methods are more reliable than the PHT method.

Limitations and Pitfalls

The limitations and pitfalls in assessing mitral stenosis are as follows.

1. Not all prolonged PHTs indicate mitral stenosis. Patients with abnormal myocardial relaxation have a prolonged PHT, but the peak E velocity is not increased (Fig. 7-18).

2. The PHT is affected by concomitant AR or a decreased compliance state. A rapid elevation in LV diastolic pressure in these conditions may shorten the PHT and underestimate the severity of mitral stenosis. Mitral valve area should be estimated by 2D planimetry, the continuity equation, and the PHT method. Any significant difference among various determinations should be explained.

3. Concomitant mitral regurgitation may overestimate the severity of mitral stenosis when the continuity equation is used to calculate mitral valve area.

4. Patients with low cardiac output or bradycardia may have a low mean gradient even in the presence of severe mitral stenosis.

5. The mitral stenosis jet may be quite eccentric. It may be helpful to guide the continuous-wave Doppler beam using color-flow imaging.

Exercise Hemodynamics

For patients who have mainly exertional symptoms and in whom resting hemodynamics do not clearly indicate severe mitral stenosis, it is useful to perform the Doppler study during or immediately after exercise (i.e., on a bicycle or treadmill). Although the mitral valve area may change mildly with exercise, the increased cardiac output and heart rate will result in a significant increase in gradient, left atrial pressure, and pulmonary artery pressure (Fig. 7-19). Therefore, a significant worsening of hemodynamics with exercise can be helpful in explaining the patient's symptoms in the face of a mild to moderate resting hemodynamic abnormality. The PHT has been shown to decrease with exercise, suggesting that PHT is influenced by other factors in addition to mitral valve area. Therefore, in most patients with mitral stenosis, exercise Doppler hemodynamics is helpful in explaining symptomatology when the resting study shows a less than severe degree of mitral stenosis.

Clinical Implications

Echocardiography is now the gold standard for evaluation of mitral stenosis, obviating the need for cardiac catheterization. This noninvasive technique is well suited for serial examination to assess progression. When percutaneous mitral balloon valvuloplasty is considered transesophageal echocardiography is needed to exclude left atrial thrombus.

Evaluation of Valvular Regurgitation

2D/M-mode echocardiography is useful in the assessment of valvular regurgitation by dem-

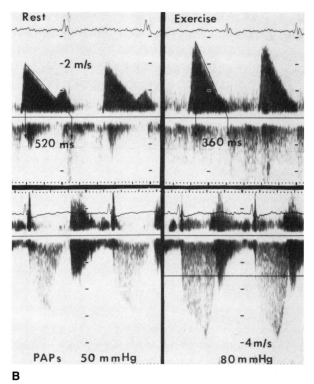

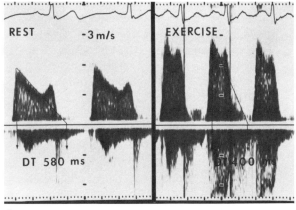

A   **B**

Fig. 7-19.   A. Continuous-wave Doppler of patient at rest and after exercise. The heart rate increased from 65 to 110 beats/min. The peak and mean gradients increased, but the PHT is shorter (from 220 to 180 msec) with exercise. **B.** Continuous-wave Doppler recordings of the mitral and tricuspid valves in a patient with mitral stenosis and exertional dyspnea, at rest and with exercise (10 sit-ups). By the PHT method, the mitral stenosis is moderate in severity: PHT = 520 × 0.29 = 150 m/sec; mitral valve area = 220/150 = 1.47 cm². Systolic pulmonary artery pressure (PAP) at rest is 50 mm Hg, since the tricuspid regurgitation peak velocity is 3 m/sec. With mild exercise, the mitral peak velocity increases to 3 m/sec (= 36 mm Hg) and the tricuspid regurgitant velocity to 4 m/sec, providing a systolic pulmonary artery pressure of about 80 mm Hg.

onstrating the structural substrate for regurgitation (i.e., mitral valve prolapse, endocarditis, bicuspid aortic valve, annulus dilatation, carcinoid, etc.), measuring LV size and global systolic function, and occasionally revealing the hemodynamic impact of regurgitation (Fig. 7-20). However, the severity of valvular regurgitation cannot be assessed reliably by 2D echocardiography alone.

The primary semiquantitative echocardiographic modality to assess valvular regurgitation is color-flow imaging, which displays the intracavitary blood flow similar to qualitative angiography. The criteria for determining regurgitation severity on color-flow imaging are based on the width and area of the regurgitant jet. However, the assessment of severity of valvular regurgitation should be based not only on color-flow imaging but also on hemodynamic data collected by continuous- and pulsed-wave Doppler echocardiography. This *integrated approach* for the assessment of valvular regurgitation is discussed in detail in the following section. Newer and more quantitative methods of determining regurgitant volume, regurgitant fraction, and regurgitant orifice using *proximal isovelocity surface area* (PISA) and the basic hydraulic orifice formula (i.e., flow = area × velocity) are also described in this chapter.

Aortic Regurgitation

2D/M-mode Echocardiography

The etiology of AR varies widely and includes congenitally abnormal valve, dilated aortic root, Marfan's syndrome, endocarditis, aortic dissection, prosthetic valve dysfunction, and most commonly, degenerative calcific aortic valve. These structural abnormalities are easily detected by 2D transthoracic and transesophageal (TEE) echocardiography. M-mode is occasionally helpful in demonstrating premature mitral valve closure or diastolic opening of the aortic valve as a sign of severe, usually acute, AR, and marked elevation of LV diastolic pressure. However, Doppler color M-mode has virtually replaced standard M-mode studies as a method of assessing the severity of AR.

Doppler/Color-Flow Imaging

Echocardiographic evaluation of the severity of AR requires meticulous *color-flow imaging, continuous-wave Doppler of the AR jet,* and *pulsed-wave Doppler of the descending thoracic aorta* and *mitral inflow.* Color-flow imaging of AR is best performed from the parasternal long- and short-axis views (by transthoracic echo window) or from the LVOT view (by TEE window).

When color-flow imaging was compared with aortic angiography, the maximal extent or length of the AR jet was poorly correlated with the angiographic severity of AR. The regurgitant jet area obtained from the parasternal short-axis view relative to the short-axis area of the LVOT at the level of the aortic annulus correlated best with angiographic severity of AR [19]. The width of the AR jet at its origin relative to the size of the LVOT was found to be also a good predictor of the angiographic AR severity (Fig. 7-21). There are other Doppler features that should be used in the determination of regurgitation severity. In AR, PHT of the AR signals [20, 21] (Fig. 7-22),

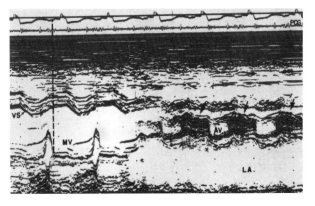

Fig. 7-20. M-mode echocardiogram of the mitral valve (MV) and the aortic valve (AV) in a patient with severe acute AR due to aortic endocarditis. Mitral valve closure is premature (prior to the QRS complex) and echo-dense mass is recorded at the aortic valve *(arrows)* during diastole due to a large vegetation. (From Roy, et al. *Circulation* 1976;53:474–482.)

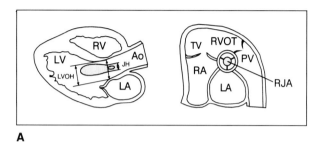

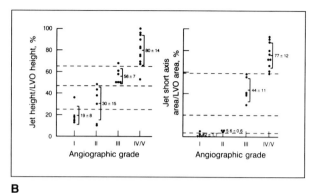

A   **B**

Fig. 7-21. A. Schematics of color-flow imaging to estimate the severity of AR, from the parasternal long- (left) and short- (right) axis views. LV outflow height (LVOH) and jet height (JH) are determined from the parasternal long-axis view. Regurgitant jet area (RJA) is measured from the parasternal short-axis view at the aortic valve level. **B.** Jet height/LVO height ratio (left) and RJA/LVO area ratio (right) are plotted against angiographic grade of AR. When the ratios are greater than 60 to 65%, the AR is severe; when less than 30%, it is mild. (**A, B:** From GJ Perry et al. Evaluation of aortic insufficiency by Doppler color flow mapping. *J Am Coll Cardiol* 1987;9:952–959.)

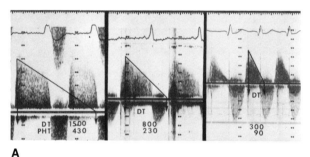

A

Fig. 7-22. A. Continuous-wave Doppler spectra of AR from three patients are shown to illustrate the decreased PHT with more severe AR. The left panel indicates mild AR with a PHT of 430 msec; the right panel indicates severe AR with a PHT of 90 msec, and the middle one indicates moderately severe AR. **B.** The reason for shorter DT (or PHT) with severe AR is shown in the schematic of LV and aortic (AO) pressure curves. With more significant AR, the aortic pressure drop is more rapid as is the LV diastolic pressure rise with more regurgitant volume back into the LV. **C.** Continuous-wave spectrum of the aortic valve demonstrating two separate slopes of the AR velocity curve. DT should not be measured from the initial steeper slope. Therefore, DT is the interval from a to c, not from a to b.

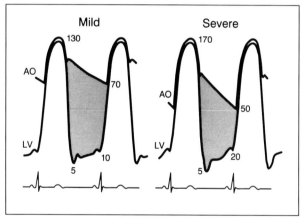

B

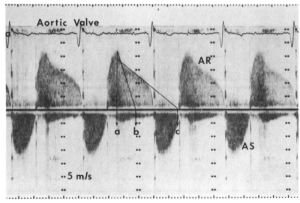

C

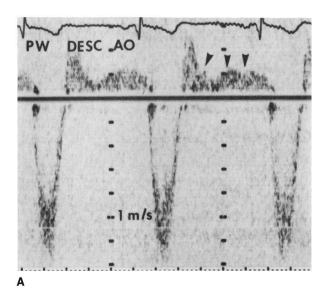

A

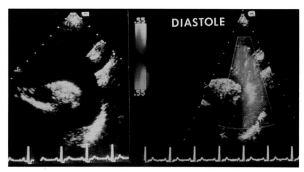

B

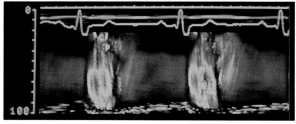

C

Fig. 7-23. **A.** Holodiastolic reversal flow *(arrowheads)* in the descending aorta indicates severe AR. Similar diastolic reversal can be seen in descending thoracic aneurysm or shunt into the aorta during diastole (as in the Blalock procedure). The sample volume is usually located near the takeoff of the left subclavian artery. **B.** 2D color-flow imaging of the descending thoracic aorta during diastole. The orange-red flow in the descending aorta indicates flow toward the transducer, that is, reversal flow due to severe AR. **C.** Color M-mode from the descending thoracic aorta shows holodiastolic reversal flow. Systolic flow has orange islands inside the blue forward flow, indicating aliasing; that is, the velocity of the center flow is greater than the Nyquist limit of 0.55 m/sec (shown in **B**).

diastolic reversal flow in the descending aorta (Fig. 7-23), and deceleration time (DT) of early mitral flow velocity (Fig. 7-24) should be measured [22]. With an increasing amount of AR, LV diastolic pressure becomes elevated, resulting in shortened PHT of the AR Doppler signal and mitral DT. Regurgitant volume and fraction can be quantitated as described in Chapter 5. If there is no significant mitral regurgitation, mitral valve (MV) inflow can be used to represent systemic flow volume:

$$\text{MV flow} = \text{MV annulus area} \times \text{MV TVI}$$

where MV annulus area is determined by annulus diameter^2 × 0.785, and MV TVI by placing a sample volume at the MV annulus.

Regurgitant volume is the difference between stroke volume across the LVOT and mitral valve inflow, and regurgitant fraction (RF) is obtained by the following equation:

$$\text{RF} = \frac{\text{Regurgitant volume}}{\text{LVOT stroke volume}} \times 100$$

Based on the collective data from 2D Doppler and color-flow imaging, the severity of AR is determined as follows.

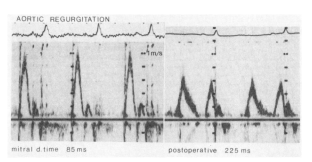

Fig. 7-24. Mitral inflow pulsed-wave Doppler in severe acute AR before (left) and after (right) aortic valve replacement. In acute severe AR, LV diastolic pressure rises quickly and produces restrictive mitral inflow pattern, with high E velocity, low A velocity, increased E/A ratio, and occasionally diastolic mitral regurgitation.

103

Severe AR is defined by

1. AR jet width/LVOT diameter ratio of 60% or more
2. AR jet area/LVOT area ratio of 60% or more
3. AR PHT less than 250 msec
4. Restrictive mitral flow pattern (in acute setting)
5. Holodiastolic flow reversal in the descending aorta
6. Dense continuous-wave Doppler signal
7. Regurgitant fraction of 55% or more
8. Regurgitant volume of 60 ml or more
9. LV diastolic dimension of 7.5 cm or more (chronic AR)

Mild AR is defined by

1. AR jet width/LVOT diameter ratio less than 30%
2. AR jet area/LVOT diameter less than 30%
3. AR PHT more than 400 msec
4. Mild early diastolic flow reversal in the descending aorta
5. Faint continuous-wave Doppler signal
6. Regurgitant fraction less than 30%
7. LV diastolic dimension (chronic) of 6.0 cm or less

Mitral Regurgitation

2D/M-mode Echocardiography

As in AR, 2D/M-mode is useful in detecting the underlying etiology for mitral regurgitation such as mitral valve prolapse (Fig. 7-25), flail mitral leaflet with or without ruptured chordae, mitral annulus calcification, papillary muscle dysfunction or rupture, rheumatic valve, cleft mitral valve, endocarditis, and perforation. It is also useful in following LV cavity size and function, major determinants for the timing of surgical intervention for mitral regurgitation.

Doppler/Color-Flow Imaging

In color-flow imaging of mitral regurgitation, the area of regurgitant jet relative to the left atrial size is most predictive of regurgitant severity determined by angiography [23, 24] (Fig. 7-26). However, color-flow imaging of valvular regurgitation is dependent on gain setting, pulsed repetition frequency, field depth, direction of jet, and loading conditions. Adjacent cardiac walls influence the size of the regurgitant color flow if the regurgitant jet is eccentric. A flow jet directed against the atrial wall appears smaller than a free jet of the same

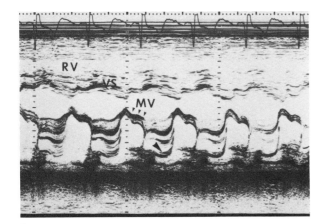

A

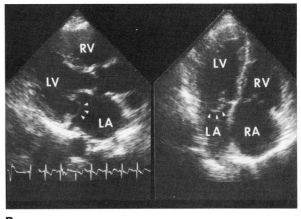

B

Fig. 7-25. M-mode and 2D echocardiograms of mitral valve prolapse (MVP). **A.** The M-mode study shows a thickened mitral valve *(arrowheads)* and systolic prolapse of the posterior mitral leaflet *(large arrowhead)*. **B.** The parasternal long-axis view (left) shows myxomatous mitral leaflets and prolapse of the posterior leaflet *(arrowheads)*. The apical four-chamber view (right) shows similar findings. Due to a saddle shape of the mitral annulus, bowing of mitral leaflets is frequently observed in the apical views. To make a definite diagnosis of mitral valve prolapse, prolapse should be recognized from the parasternal long-axis view.

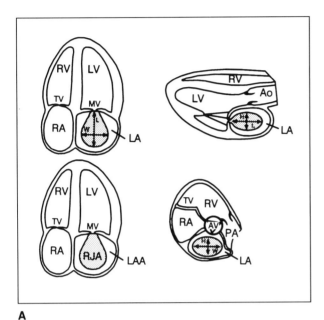

A

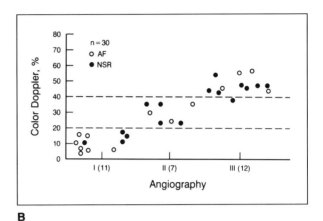

B

Fig. 7-26. **A.** Schematic drawings of color-flow imaging of mitral regurgitation from the apical four-chamber and parasternal long- and short-axis views. Left atrial area (LAA) and regurgitant jet area (RJA) are measured by planimetry. **B.** RJA/LAA ratios from the three planes are plotted against the angiographic severity of mitral regurgitation. When the ratio is more than 40%, mitral regurgitation is severe. (From F Helmcke et al. Color Doppler assessment of mitral regurgitation with orthogonal planes. *Circulation* 1987;75:175–183.) **C.** Systolic frame of apical four-chamber view showing color-flow imaging of severe mitral regurgitation *(arrows).* The regurgitant area appears to occupy more than 50% of left atrial area.

C

regurgitant volume (Coanda effect). Therefore, jet size on color-flow imaging should be interpreted in the context of jet geometry and surrounding solid boundaries [25] (Fig. 7-27).

In mitral regurgitation, antegrade flow (mitral inflow) velocity may increase with severe regurgitation (especially with a prosthesis with a fixed orifice area), and the continuous-wave Doppler spectrum may have a characteristic configuration (due to the "V" wave) with in-creased intensity. Mitral regurgitation Doppler velocity tends to be lower (4–5 m/sec) with increasing severity because of higher left atrial pressure reducing the transmitral systolic gradient (Fig. 7-28), unless LV pressure is markedly elevated (as in aortic stenosis or hypertrophic obstructive cardiomyopathy). In severe mitral regurgitation, there may be a systolic flow reversal in the pulmonary vein [26, 27] (Fig. 7-29).

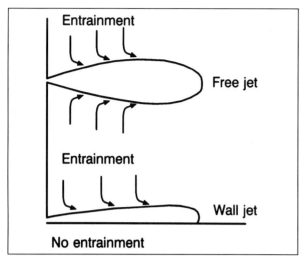

Fig. 7-27. Varying relations between the orifice and the chamber wall to create different jet geometries. Flow traveling along the wall produces a thin-layer, small-sized jet. This kind of jet was 34 ± 5% smaller in area than corresponding free jets without the Coanda effect. (From EG Cape et al. Adjacent solid boundaries alter the size of regurgitant jets on Doppler color flow maps. *J Am Coll Cardiol* 1991;17:1094–1102.)

Regurgitant volume and fraction can be calculated to assess the severity of mitral regurgitation using 2D/Doppler studies [28] (Fig. 7-30). In the absence of significant AR, the difference between flow across the mitral valve and flow across the LVOT is mitral regurgitant volume. Flow across the mitral valve is calculated by the product of the mitral annulus area and the TVI of flow obtained by placing the sample volume at the mitral annulus. Flow across the LVOT is calculated by the product of the aortic annulus area and the TVI of flow obtained by placing the sample volume at the aortic annulus. Regurgitant fraction is calculated by dividing regurgitant volume by flow across the mitral valve (MV) and multiplying by 100.

$$MV\ RV = MV\ flow - LVOT\ flow$$

$$MV\ regurgitant\ fraction = \frac{MV\ RV}{MV\ flow} \times 100(\%)$$

where MV RV = MV regurgitant volume.

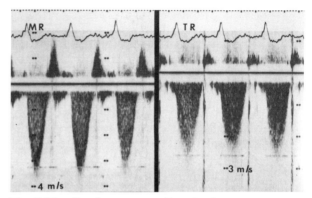

Fig. 7-28. Continuous-wave Doppler from the apex toward the mitral valve. The mitral regurgitation (MR) peak velocity is 3.5 m/sec (= transmitral gradient of 50 mm Hg). This was obtained in a patient with cardiogenic shock from severe mitral regurgitation and LV dysfunction. His pulmonary capillary wedge pressure was 54 mm Hg and systolic blood pressure was 100 mm Hg on inotropic support. The mitral regurgitant jet configuration is different from the tricuspid regurgitant jet from the same patient. Mitral inflow velocity is increased to 1.8 m/sec and tricuspid inflow velocity is about 0.6 m/sec.

Newer Quantitative Approaches

Several investigators have tried to quantitate regurgitant volume flow rate using the PISA by color-flow mapping and the principle of flow continuity [29, 30]. When (regurgitant) flow goes through a fixed orifice, flow converges as lines of increasing velocity proximal to the orifice. A series of isovelocity lines can be drawn tangential to the radial streamlines. Doppler color-flow imaging can identify a series of PISAs as red-blue aliasing interfaces corresponding to the isovelocities. Volume flow rate (ml/sec) can be calculated as

$$2\pi r^2\ (cm^2) \times Vr\ (cm/sec) = 6.28r^2 \times Vr$$

where $2\pi r^2$ = the proximal isovelocity hemispheric surface area at a radial distance r from the orifice, and

  Vr = the aliasing velocity at the radial distance r.

Using various Vr values, the best correlation between measured flow rates and PISA was found when the lowest Vr and the correspond-

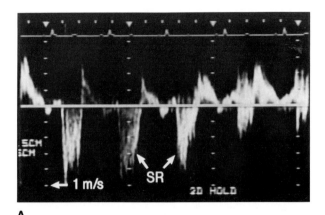

A

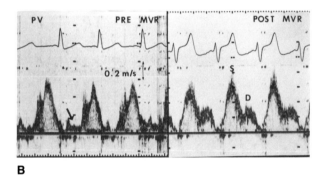

B

Fig. 7-29. A. Pulsed-wave Doppler velocity in the pulmonary vein in a patient with severe mitral regurgitation. There is significant systolic flow reversal (SR) in the pulmonary vein due to severe mitral regurgitation. **B.** Pulmonary vein (PV) pulsed-wave Doppler using TEE in the operating room. The baseline study (left) shows severe mitral regurgitation with decreased and reversed systolic pulmonary vein flow *(arrow)*, which was restored (right) after mitral valve repair (MVR). Postoperatively, systolic (S) forward flow in the pulmonary vein is greater than diastolic (D) flow.

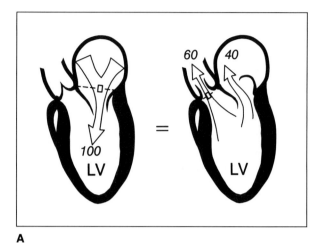

A

B

Fig. 7-30. Schematic drawing of how to calculate mitral regurgitant (MR) volume and regurgitant fraction (RF). **A.** The calculation is based on the conservation of flow ("what goes in must come out"). Inflow through the mitral valve during diastole (100 ml, for example) should be equal to the sum of outflow through the LVOT (60 ml) and mitral regurgitant volume (40 ml). **B.** Therefore, mitral regurgitant volume is calculated by subtracting the volume of flow across the LVOT from mitral inflow volume during diastole. Regurgitant fraction (RF) is mitral regurgitant volume divided by mitral inflow and multiplied by 100.

$$\text{Mitral RF} = \frac{MR}{(MV\ D^2 \times 0.785 \times MV\ TVI)} \times 100(\%)$$

where MR = mitral regurgitant volume, and
MV = mitral valve.

ingly largest radial distance (r) were used. The calculated volume flow rate is not affected by the shape of the orifice and machine factors such as gain, filter, frame rate, and packet size. PISA can be obtained by a hemispheric or hemielliptic model. Although the hemielliptic model appears to correlate better with actual flow rate and the hemispheric model underestimates the rate, the latter method is simpler to calculate. This method may become a routine part of the estimation of regurgitant vol-

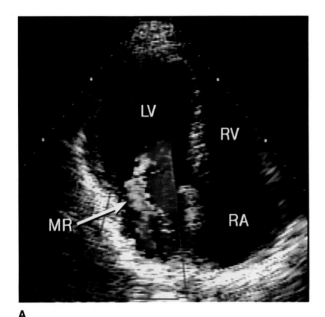

A

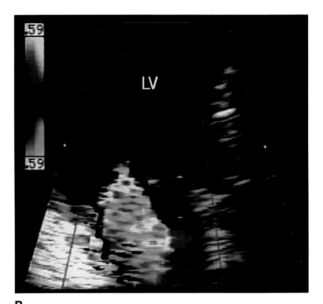

B

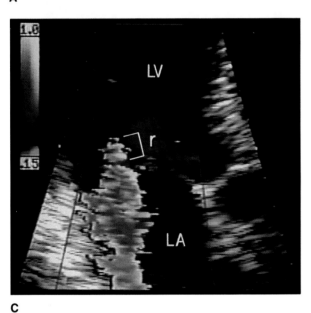

C

Fig. 7-31.   Calculation of mitral regurgitation peak flow rate, effective regurgitant orifice (ERO) area, and regurgitant volume (RV) using PISA method. **A.** Apical four-chamber view with optimal color flow imaging of mitral regurgitation (MR). **B.** Expanded image of the mitral valve and MR jet. Color bar (left upper corner) indicates the aliasing velocity of 0.59 m/sec or 59 cm/sec. **C.** Color flow baseline is shifted downward so that the negative aliasing velocity (Vr) is 15 cm/sec. The proximal isovelocity line is well defined with the radius (r) of 0.85 cm. If peak MR velocity (V) and TVI are 6 m/sec (600 cm/sec) and 130 cm, respectively,

$$
\begin{aligned}
\text{Flow rate} &= 6.28 \times (0.85)^2 \times 15 \\
&= 68 \text{ ml/sec} \\
\text{ERO} &= 68/600 \\
&= 0.11 \text{ cm}^2 \\
\text{RV} &= 0.11 \times 130 \\
&= 15 \text{ ml}
\end{aligned}
$$

These values indicate a mild degree of mitral regurgitation.

ume flow rate, regurgitant volume, and effective regurgitant orifice (ERO), but more clinical correlations are required.

The stepwise method of obtaining regurgitant flow rate, ERO size, and regurgitant volume is as follows (Fig. 7-31).

1. Optimize color-flow imaging of mitral regurgitation from an apical window (Fig. 7-31A).

2. Expand the image of the regurgitant mitral valve (Fig. 7-31B); use zoom or regional expansion selection (RES) mode.

3. Shift color-flow baseline downward to 15 to 30 cm/sec as the negative aliasing velocity (Vr) (Fig. 7-31C). The knob to control Doppler baseline shift also controls color-flow baseline.

4. Measure the radius (r) of the proximal isovelocity hemisphere (Fig. 7-31C).

5. Obtain peak velocity (V) and TVI of mitral regurgitation jet (in cm/sec and cm, respectively) by continuous-wave Doppler.

6. Calculate mitral regurgitation flow rate, volume, and orifice size.

$$\text{Flow rate (ml/sec)} = 2\pi r^2 \times Vr$$
$$= 6.28 \times r^2 \times Vr$$

$$\text{ERO (cm}^2) = \text{flow rate}/V \text{ (cm/sec)}$$

$$\text{Regurgitant volume (ml)} = \text{ERO} \times \text{TVI} \text{ (ml)}$$

Another newer quantitative method to measure mitral regurgitation fraction using the amplitude-weighted mean velocity from continuous-wave Doppler spectra has promise. Although this new technique has a potential limitation in the patient with an enlarged valvular annulus (compared to the width of the continuous-wave beam), it is independent of the need to measure the area of the LV inflow and outflow tracts [31].

After the above data are obtained, the following criteria suggest severe mitral regurgitation:

1. Color-flow area larger than 8.0 cm² or more than one-third of left atrial area
2. Regurgitant volume of 60 ml or more
3. Regurgitant fraction of 55% or more
4. ERO larger than 0.35 cm²
5. Pulmonary vein systolic flow reversals
6. Dense continuous-wave Doppler signal
7. Tapering of continuous-wave Doppler configuration
8. Increased E velocity ($\geq$ 1.5 m/sec)
9. LV diastolic dimension of 7.0 cm or larger (chronic)
10. Left atrial size of 5.5 cm or larger

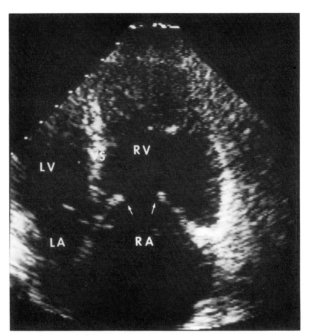

Fig. 7-32. Right ventricular inflow view showing a systolic frame of the tricuspid valve *(arrows)*. It is held open due to carcinoid involvement of the valve.

Tricuspid Regurgitation

2D/M-mode Echocardiography

2D/M-mode echocardiography detects the underlying etiology of tricuspid regurgitation such as rheumatic valve, prolapse, carcinoid (Fig. 7-32), Ebstein's anomaly, annular dilatation, right ventricular infarct, and tricuspid valve rupture.

Doppler/Color-Flow Imaging

Aforementioned Doppler features of mitral regurgitation should be systematically looked for and applied to tricuspid regurgitation. However, instead of pulmonary vein flow reversal, severe tricuspid regurgitation results in systolic flow reversal in the hepatic vein (Fig. 7-33). The tricuspid continuous-wave Doppler signal is characteristic when the regurgitation is severe: increased forward flow velocity, relatively decreased tricuspid regurgitation velocity, and concave late systolic configuration of tricuspid regurgitation due to a large right atrial "V" wave (see Fig. 7-33).

Severe tricuspid regurgitation is diagnosed when the following criteria are present:

1. Color-flow regurgitant jet area 30% or more of right atrial area
2. Dense continuous-wave Doppler signal
3. Annulus dilatation (≥ 4 cm) or inadequate cusp coaptation
4. Late systolic concave configuration of continuous-wave signal
5. Increased tricuspid inflow velocity (≥ 1.0 m/sec)
6. Systolic flow reversals in the hepatic vein

Valvular Regurgitation in Normal Subjects

It should be pointed out that trivial to mild degrees of valvular regurgitation are common in the normal population and its prevalence increases with age [32, 33] (Table 7-2). The Doppler color-flow imaging technique is so sensitive that it detects trivial to mild degrees of valvular regurgitation, frequently not appreciated even by careful auscultation. Klein and colleagues [33] assessed age-related prevalence of valvular regurgitation in 118 normal volunteers by comprehensive color-flow imaging. Regurgitation of mitral, aortic, tricuspid, and pulmonary valves was detected in 48%, 11%, 65%, and 31% of subjects, respectively (see Table 7-2). Aortic regurgitation was absent in the volunteers who were younger than 50 years old. There was no influence of gender on the frequency of valvular regurgitation. Although hemodynamically not important, Doppler detection of valvular regurgitation is useful in estimating right-sided intracardiac pressures. Doppler-detectable trivial regurgitation does not warrant prophylaxis for subacute bacterial endocarditis.

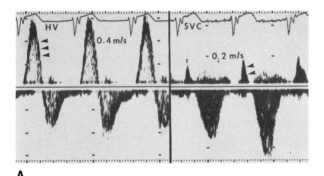

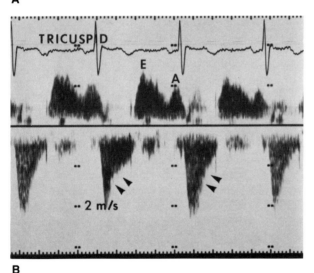

Fig. 7-33. **A.** Hepatic vein (HV) pulsed-wave Doppler shows marked systolic reversal *(arrowheads)* due to severe tricuspid regurgitation. The systolic reversal *(arrowheads)* is less prominent in the superior vena cava (SVC) of the same patient. **B.** Cardiovascular Doppler spectrum of the tricuspid valve in a patient with severe tricuspid regurgitation. Forward inflow velocity is increased (E; 1.4 m/sec) and tricuspid regurgitant peak velocity is relatively decreased due to a smaller pressure gradient. A large "V" wave makes the Doppler spectrum dented during mid to late systole *(arrowheads)*.

Transesophageal Echocardiography

The diagnosis of valvular stenosis does not usually require help from the transesophageal approach since continuous-wave Doppler is the primary mode of assessing the severity of stenotic lesions. Even when 2D imaging of the

Table 7-2. Prevalence (%) of valvular regurgitation by decade of life

Age (yr) (n)	Mitral	Aortic	Tricuspid	Pulmonary
20–29 (23)	35	0	43	23
30–39 (20)	40	0	70	20
40–49 (18)	44	0	61	23
50–59 (21)	48	14	52	42
60–69 (21)	67	24	81	31
≥ 70 (15)	60	33	93	50
Overall (118)	48	11	65	31

Source: Modified from AL Klein et al. Age-related prevalence of valvular regurgitation in normal subjects: a comprehensive color flow examination of 118 volunteers. *J Am Soc Echocardiogr* 1990;2:57.

valve structure is suboptimal, the continuous-wave Doppler examination can be quite satisfactory to assess the hemodynamic severity of the stenotic valve. Recently, continuous-wave Doppler has been incorporated into the transesophageal echocardiography (TEE) probe and it will aid the hemodynamic assessment of stenotic valves, especially the mitral and pulmonic valves since their flow jet is usually parallel with the direction of the transesophageal ultrasound beam (Fig. 7-34). This modality is especially helpful during an intraoperative procedure (i.e., determination of mitral valve gradient after mitral valve repair and annuloplasty) or an interventional procedure (i.e., mitral balloon valvuloplasty for mitral stenosis). Planimetry to determine stenotic aortic valve area may be feasible from transesophageal 2D imaging. The biplane or multiplane tomographic approach will make the short-axis view of the aortic valve more easily available for this purpose. TEE is essential in the evaluation of valvular regurgitation in certain patients. In some patients, dense annular calcification frequently prevents optimal visualization of the color-flow jet in the atrial cavity from precordial windows. However, regurgitant jet characteristics depend on jet velocities and instrumental factors. Color-flow imaging of regurgitant jet by TEE produces jet characteristics different from those obtained by transthoracic echocardiography. When the same patients with mitral regurgitation were studied by both transthoracic and transesophageal echocardiography, the transthoracic approach usually revealed regurgitation jets with a smaller mosaic pattern (47% of the total regurgitation area), whereas the mosaic area detected by TEE constituted 70% of the regurgitation jet [34]. The best correlation with angiographic severity of mitral regurgitation was obtained by transthoracic total regurgitation area and transesophageal mosaic area. With monoplane TEE, a mosaic regurgitation area less than 3 cm² predicted mild mitral regurgitation (96% sensitivity and 100% specificity) and a mosaic regurgitation area greater than 6 cm² predicted severe mitral regurgitation [35] (91% sensitivity and 100% specificity). The transesophageal approach is better than the transthoracic approach in the evaluation of pulmonary vein systolic flow reversals, which suggest severe mitral regurgitation (see Fig. 7-29). The transesophageal approach is also ideal in the evaluation of mitral and tricuspid valve morphology [36]. Therefore, when the etiology or degree of valvular regurgitation is in doubt, TEE should be the natural next step (Figs. 7-35 and 7-36). In all patients who are considered for mitral balloon valvuloplasty, TEE should be performed to exclude thrombus in the left atrium or in the left atrial appendage [36, 37]. Figure 7-37 shows a large left atrium and left atrial appendage thrombi visualized by TEE, but not by transthoracic examination.

TEE plays an important role intraoperatively in valvular repair [38–41]. This is discussed in more detail in Chapter 17.

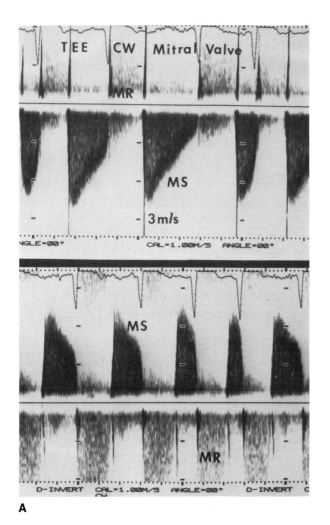

A

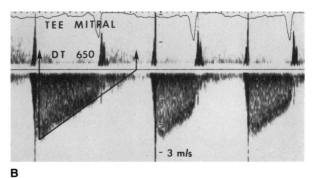

B

Fig. 7-34. **A.** Continuous-wave Doppler of the stenotic mitral valve obtained from transesophageal examination. The top tracing shows a mitral stenosis (MS) jet recorded below the baseline since mitral inflow is going away from the TEE probe. The Doppler spectrum can be electronically inverted to the opposite direction, identical to ones from transthoracic continuous-wave examination (bottom). **B.** The DT is 650 msec; hence, the PHT is 190 msec and mitral valve area is 1.15 cm².

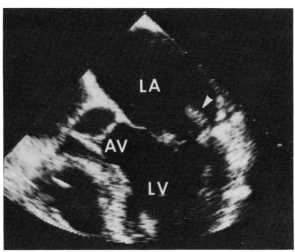

A

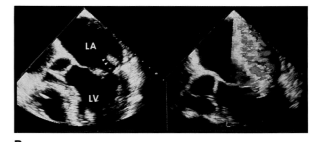

B

Fig. 7-35. **A.** TEE view of flail posterior mitral valve *(arrowhead)*. TEE is better than any other imaging technique in characterizing morphology of the mitral valve. **B.** Color-flow imaging shows severe mitral regurgitation.

Clinical Impact

When a patient undergoes an echocardiographic evaluation for valvular heart disease, the parameters listed below should be assessed using the *integrated approach* of 2D, continuous- and pulsed-wave Doppler, and color-flow imaging. In some patients, TEE may be necessary.

1. LV dimension and systolic function
2. LV wall thickness and mass
3. Valvular morphology
4. Valvular hemodynamics
   a. Stroke volume and cardiac output
   b. Pressure gradients
   c. Valve area
5. Valvular regurgitation
   a. Semiquantitative approach (color-flow): mild = grade I; moderate = grade II; moderately severe = grade III; severe = grade IV
   b. Quantitative approach: regurgitant volume; regurgitant fraction; effective orifice area
6. Pulmonary artery pressure

It should be emphasized that the determination of severity of valvular lesions is based on all the available echocardiographic data (integrated approach). Any discrepancies between different parameters of severity should be explained. For example: A patient has a mean aortic pressure gradient of 55 mm Hg but the aortic valve does not appear to be severely stenotic on 2D imaging. Further evaluation shows that cardiac output is increased due to significant anemia, reflected as an increase in LVOT velocity and TVI. Using the integrated echocardiographic approach, assessment of valvular heart disease should be complete in the majority of patients. When surgical intervention is needed, patients with suspected coronary artery disease or at high risk will need coronary angiography. Hemodynamic evaluation by cardiac catheterization is necessary only in those patients in whom adequate and reliable 2D/Doppler and color-flow imaging cannot be performed (approximately 5%), or in those patients in whom there is marked discrepancy between clinical 2D/Doppler findings (clinically severe versus Doppler-mild), which are unresolved by repeat studies by a more experienced member of the team.

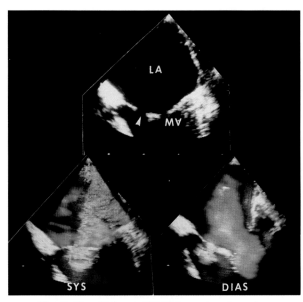

Fig. 7-36. Enlarged TEE four-chamber view demonstrating a perforation of the anterior mitral leaflet *(arrowhead, top)*. Color-flow imaging demonstrates mitral regurgitation through the perforation during systole and forward flow during diastole (smaller blue jet).

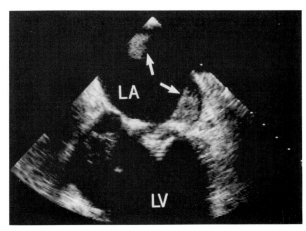

Fig. 7-37. TEE basal short-axis view showing thrombi in the left atrium (LA) and left atrial appendage *(arrows)*.

References

1. Callahan MJ, et al. Validation of instantaneous pressure gradients measured by continuous-wave Doppler in experimentally induced aortic stenosis. *Am J Cardiol* 1985:56:989–993.

2. Smith MD, et al. Correlation of continuous wave Doppler velocities with cardiac catheterization gradients: an experimental model of aortic stenosis. *J Am Coll Cardiol* 1985; 6:1306–1314.

3. Currie PJ, et al. Continuous-wave Doppler echocardiographic assessment of severity of calcific aortic stenosis: simultaneous Doppler-catheter correlative study in 100 adult patients. *Circulation* 1985;71:1162–1169.

4. Gorlin, R, Gorlin SG. Hydraulic formula for calculation of the area of the stenotic mitral valve, other cardiac valves, and central circulatory shunts. *Am Heart J* 1951;41:1–45.

5. Skjaerpe T, Hegrenaes L, Hatle L. Noninvasive estimation of valve area in patients with aortic stenosis by Doppler ultrasound and two-dimensional echocardiography. *Circulation* 1985;72:810–818.

6. Zoghbi WA, et al. Accurate noninvasive quantification of stenotic aortic valve area by Doppler echocardiography. *Circulation* 1986; 73:452–459.

7. Otto CM, et al. Determination of the stenotic aortic valve area in adults using Doppler echocardiography. *J Am Coll Cardiol* 1986; 7:509–517.

8. Teirstein P, et al. Doppler echocardiographic measurement of aortic valve area in aortic stenosis: a noninvasive application of the Gorlin formula. *J Am Coll Cardiol* 1986;8:1059–1065.

9. Oh JK, et al. Prediction of the severity of aortic stenosis by Doppler aortic valve area determination: prospective Doppler-catheterization correlation in 100 patients. *J Am Coll Cardiol* 1988;11:1227–1234.

10. Hatle L, et al. Noninvasive assessment of pressure drop in mitral stenosis by Doppler ultrasound. *Br Heart J* 1978;40:131–140.

11. Nakatani S, et al. Value and limitations of Doppler echocardiography in the quantification of stenotic mitral valve area: comparison of the pressure half-time and the continuity equation methods. *Circulation* 1988;77:78–85.

12. Nakatani S, et al. Time related changes in mi-

tral valve area after balloon mitral valvuloplasty assessed by Doppler continuity equation method. *Circulation* 1988(Suppl II);78:487–495.

13. Thomas JD, et al. Inaccuracy of mitral pressure half-time immediately after percutaneous mitral valvulotomy. *Circulation* 1988;78:980–993.

14. Chen C, et al. Reliability of the Doppler pressure half-time method for assessing effects of percutaneous mitral balloon valvuloplasty. *J Am Coll Cardiol* 1989;13:1309–1313.

15. Hegrenaes L, Hatle L. Aortic stenosis in adults: noninvasive estimation of pressure differences by continuous wave Doppler echocardiography. *Br Heart J* 1985;54:396–404.

16. Abascal V, et al. Echocardiographic evaluation of mitral valve structure and function in patients followed for at least 6 months after percutaneous balloon mitral valvuloplasty. *J Am Coll Cardiol* 1988;12:606–615.

17. Holen J, et al. Determination of pressure gradient in mitral stenosis with a noninvasive ultrasound Doppler technique. *Acta Med Scand* 1976;199:455–460.

18. Come P, et al. Noninvasive assessment of mitral stenosis before and after percutaneous balloon mitral valvuloplasty. *Am J Cardiol* 1988;61:817–825.

19. Perry GJ, et al. Evaluation of aortic insufficiency by Doppler color flow mapping. *J Am Coll Cardiol* 1987;9:952–959.

20. Teague SM, et al. Quantification of aortic regurgitation utilizing continuous wave Doppler ultrasound. *J Am Coll Cardiol* 1986;8:592–599.

21. Samstad SO, et al. Half time of the diastolic aortoventricular pressure difference by continuous wave Doppler ultrasound: a measure of the severity of aortic regurgitation? *Br Heart J* 1989;61:336–343.

22. Oh JK, et al. Characteristic Doppler echocardiographic pattern of mitral inflow velocity in severe aortic regurgitation. *J Am Coll Cardiol* 1989;14:1712–1717.

23. Helmcke F, et al. Color Doppler assessment of mitral regurgitation with orthogonal planes. *Circulation* 1987;75:175–183.

24. Spain MG, et al. Quantitative assessment of mitral regurgitation by Doppler color flow imaging: angiographic and hemodynamic correlations. *J Am Coll Cardiol* 1989;13:585–590.

25. Cape EG, et al. Adjacent solid boundaries alter

the size of regurgitant jets on Doppler color flow maps. *J Am Coll Cardiol* 1991; 17:1094–1102.

26. Klein AL, Tajik AJ. Doppler assessment of pulmonary venous flow in healthy subjects and in patients with heart disease. *J Am Soc Echocardiogr* 1991;4:379–392.

27. Castello R, et al. Effect of mitral regurgitation on pulmonary venous velocities derived from transesophageal echocardiography color-guided pulsed Doppler imaging. *J Am Coll Cardiol* 1991;17:1499–1506.

28. Kaneshige AM, Enriquez-Sarano ME. Mitral regurgitation: Echocardiographic assessment of its severity and the optimal timing of operation *Cardio* 1993;41–48.

29. Utsunomiya T, et al. Doppler color flow "proximal isovelocity surface area" method for estimating volume flow rate: effects of orifice shape and machine factors. *J Am Coll Cardiol* 1991;17:1103–1111.

30. Recusani F, et al. A new method for quantification of regurgitant flow rate using color Doppler flow imaging of the flow convergence region proximal to a discrete orifice. *Circulation* 1991;83:594–604.

31. Jenni R, et al. Quantification of mitral regurgitation with amplitude-weighted mean velocity from continuous wave Doppler spectra. *Circulation* 1989;79:1294–1299.

32. Yoshida K, et al. Color Doppler evaluation of valvular regurgitation in normal subjects. *Circulation* 1988;78:840–847.

33. Klein AL, et al. Age-related prevalence of valvular regurgitation in normal subjects: a comprehensive color flow examination of 118 volunteers. *J Am Soc Echocardiogr* 1990; 2:54–63.

34. Castello R, et al. Variability in the quantitation of mitral regurgitation by Doppler color flow mapping: comparison of transthoracic and transesophageal studies. *J Am Coll Cardiol* 1992;20:433–438.

35. Castello R, et al. Quantitation of mitral regurgitation by transesophageal echocardiography with Doppler color flow mapping: correlation with cardiac catheterization. *J Am Coll Cardiol* 1992;19:1516–1521.

36. Sochowski RA, et al. Comparison of accuracy of transesophageal versus transthoracic echocardiography for the detection of mitral valve prolapse with ruptured chordae tendineae (flail mitral leaflet). *Am J Cardiol* 1991; 67:1251–1255.

37. Jaarsma W, et al. Transesophageal echocardiography during percutaneous balloon mitral valvuloplasty. *J Am Soc Echocardiogr* 1990; 3:384–391.

38. Kleinman JP, et al. A quantitative comparison of transesophageal and epicardial color Doppler echocardiography in the intraoperative assessment of mitral regurgitation. *Am J Cardiol* 1989;64:1168–1172.

39. Sheikh KH, et al. The utility of transesophageal echocardiography and Doppler color flow imaging in patients undergoing cardiac valve surgery. *J Am Coll Cardiol* 1990;15:363–372.

40. Stewart WJ, Salcedo EE, Cosgrove DM. The value of echocardiography in mitral valve repair. *Cleve Clin J Med* 1991;58:177–183.

41. Freeman WK, et al. Intraoperative evaluation of mitral valve regurgitation and repair by transesophageal echocardiography: incidence and significance of systolic anterior motion. *J Am Coll Cardiol* 1992;20:599–609.

8

Prosthetic Valve Evaluation

Valve replacement is usually required for symptomatic severe valvular heart disease, although valve repair is increasingly utilized for a regurgitant lesion. No prosthetic valve is perfect and a significant portion of the cardiology practice is dedicated to following patients with a prosthetic valve and evaluating prosthetic valvular dysfunction when they present with cardiovascular symptoms. Prosthetic valves can be classified either as tissue or nontissue (or mechanical). A tissue valve is an actual valve or one made of biologic tissue from an animal or human. A mechanical valve is made up of nonbiologic material (e.g., pyrolitic carbon, Silastic, or titanium) as in a ball-cage (Starr-Edwards) or tilting disk (St. Jude Medical). Blood flow characteristics, hemodynamics, durability, and thromboembolic tendency vary depending on the type and size of each prosthesis and more importantly on patient characteristics. The physical examination of patients with prosthetic valves is different from that of patients with native valves since prosthetic valves are inherently stenotic and may produce additional prosthetic sounds (due to the ball movement or disk closure). Therefore, it can be a clinical challenge to distinguish abnormal from normal prosthetic valve sounds.

Prosthetic valve dysfunction includes obstruction, regurgitation, thromboembolism, and endocarditis or ring abscess. These pathologies of the prosthesis are readily detected by comprehensive (transthoracic [TTE] and transesophageal [TEE]) echocardiographic examination. 2D echocardiography can identify gross structural abnormalities of a prosthesis (Fig. 8-1) but its sensitivity for cardiac prosthetic dysfunction is hampered by difficulty visualizing structures around and behind the cardiac

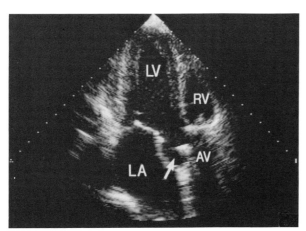

Fig. 8-1. Apical long-axis view demonstrating dehisced aortic prosthesis (AV). There is a large echo-free space *(arrow)* between the posterior aortic wall and the aortic prosthesis.

prosthesis due to the high degree of echo reflectance of the prosthetic material that results in attenuation of the ultrasound beam. Multiple ultrasound reverberations from the prosthesis also result in difficulties in interpretation. On the other hand, Doppler echocardiography reliably detects flow velocity across a prosthetic valve, which permits determination of pressure gradients using the modified Bernoulli equation (pressure gradient = 4 × velocity²). Simultaneous Doppler and invasive dual-catheter pressure measurements across various prosthetic valves have shown an excellent correlation with each other [1] (Fig. 8-2). However, several in vitro models of a normal disk prosthesis demonstrated an "overestimation" of aortic prosthetic gradients determined by Doppler velocities compared to catheter-derived gradients [2, 3]. The highest catheter-derived gradient was found within the central orifice of the valve of the St. Jude prosthesis and it decreased rapidly when the catheter was moved downstream ("pressure recovery" phenomenon). The discrepancy is smaller in a prosthesis with a larger ring and in a tissue prosthesis. The potential source of difference between Doppler-derived and catheter-derived prosthetic pressure gradients should be kept in mind, but it has not been a major problem in the clinical setting of a dysfunctional

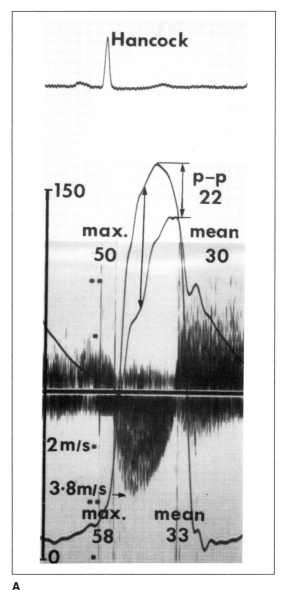

A

Fig. 8-2.   A. Simultaneous Doppler and catheterization study in a patient with a Hancock aortic prosthesis. Good correlation exists between the Doppler-derived and the catheter-derived maximum (58 versus 50 mm Hg) and mean (33 versus 30 mm Hg) pressure gradients. Similar good correlation was also noted for the mechanical aortic prosthesis. Note that the peak-to-peak (p-p) gradient, which is a nonphysiologic assessment, underestimates the severity of obstruction (p-p gradient, 22 mm Hg; catheter-derived mean gradient, 30 mm Hg).

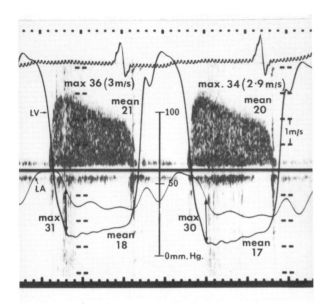

B

Fig. 8-2. (cont.).
B. Simultaneous continuous-wave Doppler and catheter pressure measurements (left ventricle and atrium) in a patient with an obstructed Hancock mitral prosthesis. The maximum (36 versus 31 mm Hg) and mean (21 versus 18 mm Hg by Doppler and catheter, respectively) gradients derived from these two techniques correlate well. **C, D.** Overall correlation between Doppler- and catheter-derived pressure gradients in various prosthetic valves. Both maximum instantaneous **(C)** and mean **(D)** gradients derived from the two methods correlate excellently. (**A–D:** From DJ Burstow et al. Continuous wave Doppler echocardiographic measurement of prosthetic valve gradients: a simultaneous Doppler-catheter correlative study. *Circulation* 1989;80:504–514.)

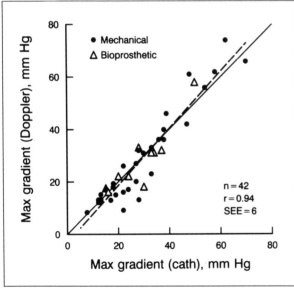

C

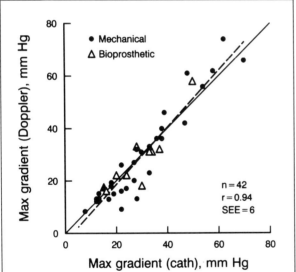

D

prosthesis. The continuity equation can be utilized to estimate the functional orifice area of prosthetic aortic and mitral valves [4–6]. The prosthetic valve is inherently stenotic in varying degrees compared to the respective native valve; therefore, flow velocity across a normal prosthetic valve is higher than that expected for a native valve. Normal prosthetic flow velocity (hence, maximum and mean pressure gradients) varies based on its type, size, and location and the cardiac output. Hence, it is important to know the normal ranges of flow velocities across a particular prosthesis for comparison with measured values. The Mayo echocardiography laboratory determined prospectively a range of normal Doppler values for each type of aortic, mitral, and tricuspid prosthesis based on large numbers of patients: 609, 456, and 86, respectively [7–9] (Tables 8-1 through 8-3).

Table 8-1. Doppler hemodynamic profiles of 609 normal aortic valve prostheses

	No.	Peak velocity (m/sec)	Mean gradient (mm Hg)	LVOT TVI/AV TVI
Heterograft	214	2.4 ± 0.5	13.3 ± 6.1	0.44 ± 0.21
Ball-cage	160	3.2 ± 0.6	23.0 ± 8.8	0.32 ± 0.09
Bjork-Shiley	141	2.5 ± 0.6	13.9 ± 7.0	0.40 ± 0.10
St. Jude	44	2.5 ± 0.6	14.4 ± 7.7	0.41 ± 0.12
Homograft	30	1.9 ± 0.4	7.7 ± 2.7	0.56 ± 0.10
Medtronic Hall	20	2.4 ± 0.2	13.6 ± 3.3	0.39 ± 0.09
Total	609	2.6 ± 0.7	15.8 ± 8.3	0.40 ± 0.16

LVOT = left ventricular outflow tract; AV = aortic valve; TVI = time velocity integral.
Source: Modified from FA Miller et al. Normal aortic valve prosthesis hemodynamics: 609 prospective Doppler examinations (Abstract). *Circulation* 1989;80(suppl II):169.

Table 8-2. Doppler hemodynamic profiles of 456 normal mitral valve prostheses

	No.	Peak velocity (m/sec)	Mean gradient (mm Hg)	Effective area (cm²)
Heterograft	150	1.6 ± 0.3	4.1 ± 1.5	2.3 ± 0.7
Ball-cage	161	1.8 ± 0.3	4.9 ± 1.8	2.4 ± 0.7
Bjork-Shiley	79	1.7 ± 0.3	4.1 ± 1.6	2.6 ± 0.6
St. Jude	66	1.6 ± 0.4	4.0 ± 1.8	3.0 ± 0.8

Source: Modified from M Lengyel et al. Doppler hemodynamic profiles of 456 clinically and echo-normal mitral valve prostheses (Abstract). *Circulation* 1990;82(suppl III):43.

Table 8-3. Doppler hemodynamic profiles of 86 normal tricuspid valve prostheses

	No.	Peak velocity (m/sec)	Mean gradient (mm Hg)	Pressure half-time (m/sec)
Ball-cage	35	1.3 ± 0.2	3.2 ± 0.8	140 ± 48
Heterograft	43	1.3 ± 0.2	3.2 ± 1.1	145 ± 37
St. Jude	7	1.2 ± 0.3	2.7 ± 1.1	108 ± 32
Bjork-Shiley	1	1.3	2.2	144
Total	86	1.3 ± 0.2	3.1 ± 1.0	140 ± 42

Source: Modified from HM Connolly et al. Doppler hemodynamic profiles of eighty-six normal tricuspid valve prostheses (Abstract). *J Am Coll Cardiol* 1991;17:69A.

Since the hemodynamics of a prosthesis depend on various factors, it is recommended that a baseline Doppler study be done in the early postoperative period so that it can be used as a reference for later comparisons. In one study, a repeat Doppler examination 3 to 5 months later found clinically insignificant changes in pressure gradients across an aortic prosthesis [10].

Obstruction

When a prosthetic valve becomes obstructed, the motion of the disk, ball, or leaflets de-

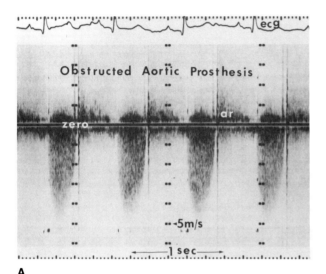

A

B

Fig. 8-3. Obstructed Bjork-Shiley aortic prosthesis. **A.** The continuous-wave Doppler examination revealed a high velocity of 5 m/sec, corresponding to a maximum instantaneous gradient of 100 mm Hg ($= 4 \times 5^2$). **B.** At operation, a fibrin clot along the sewing ring was found to be the cause of the obstruction.

creases. However, it is difficult to visualize and yet more difficult to quantitate the restriction of excursion by surface 2D echo examination. The most accurate method to detect and quantitate the degree of prosthetic obstruction is Doppler echocardiography (Fig. 8-3 and 8-4). The Doppler study must be performed using various transducer positions in order to ascertain that maximum jet velocity across the stenotic prosthesis has been recorded. From the

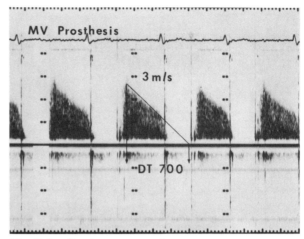

Fig. 8-4. Continuous-wave Doppler spectrum of an obstructed mitral disk prosthesis. Both peak velocity (2.8 m/sec) and pressure half-time (PHT) (DT $\times$ 0.29 = 203 msec) are increased. The peak velocity corresponds to a maximum instantaneous gradient of 31 mm Hg. The transesophageal image of obstructed disk motion is shown in Figure 8-7.

Doppler velocity tracing, maximum and mean pressure gradients and the effective valve area can be calculated using the same formulae and equations described for the native valve (see Chap. 7). It is, however, important to remember that the increased flow velocity per se does not always indicate prosthetic obstruction. The velocity can be increased without stenosis, in a high-output state, and in the presence of severe prosthetic regurgitation. In order to derive accurate maximum and mean gradients in such situations, it is imperative that upstream velocity (V_1) also be obtained using pulsed-wave Doppler and entered into the Bernoulli equation. For example, if maximum velocity of flow through the left ventricular (LV) outflow tract (LVOT) is 1.8 m/sec and flow velocity through the aortic prosthesis is 4 m/sec, the maximum gradient is 51 mm Hg ($= 4 \times 4^2 - 4 \times 1.8^2$). In patients with a mitral prosthesis, the pressure half-time (PHT) is useful to determine whether increased velocity (i.e., gradient) is secondary to increased flow or to obstruction, although the effective orifice area is most reliably determined by the continuity

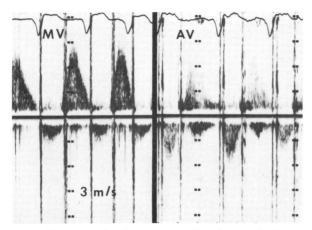

Fig. 8-5. Continuous-wave Doppler spectra in a patient with severe mitral prosthetic regurgitation who has mitral and aortic prostheses (both of the Bjork-Shiley type). **A.** The mitral velocity is increased to 3 m/sec, but its PHT is normal (60 msec), indicating increased flow across the mitral prosthesis without obstruction. **B.** The velocity through the aortic prosthesis is relatively low (1.6 m/sec), indicating that the increased mitral flow velocity is due to mitral regurgitation rather than a high systemic cardiac output. In the latter case, peak velocity through the aortic prosthesis is expected to increase. (see Table 8-1 for expected normal velocity). TEE imaging of the mitral prosthesis in this patient is shown in Figure 8-6.

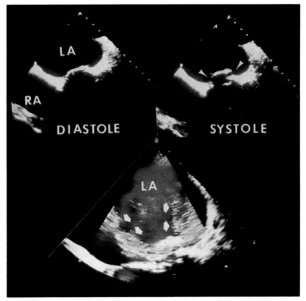

Fig. 8-6. TEE horizontal plane image of the same patient as in Figure 8-5. (Top) Diastolic and systolic frame of TEE of a mitral disk prosthesis. During systole, the sewing ring *(arrowheads)* becomes detached from the annulus. (Bottom) Color-flow imaging shows severe mitral regurgitation (MR) *(arrows)* due to the dehisced mitral prosthesis, with two discrete large jets directed medially and laterally into a dilated left atrium. At surgery, near complete dehiscence of the Bjork-Shiley mitral prosthesis was found.

equation. Figure 8-5 demonstrates a continuous-wave Doppler tracing of mechanical mitral and aortic prostheses in a patient with symptoms of dyspnea on exertion. The peak mitral prosthetic flow velocity was markedly increased along with an increase in maximum and mean pressure gradients. However, the PHT was not prolonged, indicating no obstruction of the prosthesis, and increased transmitral velocity was solely due to increased flow across the mitral orifice (either overall increase in cardiac output or severe prosthetic regurgitation). The LVOT velocity can be utilized to distinguish a generalized increase in cardiac output (as in anemia) from severe mitral regurgitation. It increases in the former and decreases with the latter (it was reduced in this patient). TEE demonstrated a dehisced mitral prosthesis with severe (grade 4/4) regurgita-

tion (Fig. 8-6). The PHT as well as peak flow velocity are expected to increase when a mitral or tricuspid prosthesis is obstructed (see Fig. 8-4).

If an aortic prosthesis is obstructed, flow velocity (hence, pressure gradient) increases unless cardiac output decreases (see Fig. 8-3). Increased aortic prosthetic flow velocity is also expected with severe prosthetic regurgitation (hence, increased flow through the aortic prosthesis). However, LV flow velocity is normal to slightly decreased with aortic obstruction (as in aortic stenosis), and it increases with aortic regurgitation. The LVOT and aortic prosthesis velocity or time velocity integral (TVI) ratio is helpful to differentiate increased aortic prosthesis flow velocity due to a prosthetic obstruction (the ratio decreases, ≤ 0.2) from increased velocity due to regurgitation (ratio remains normal, ≥ 0.3); see Table 8-1.

Calculation of Effective Prosthetic Orifice Area

PHT may grossly overestimate the area of the mitral prosthesis. The constant 220 was derived for stenotic lesions of the native mitral valve, not for calculating effective orifice area of a mitral prosthesis. When there is no significant aortic or mitral regurgitation, the continuity equation is a valid and better method for determining the area of mitral as well as aortic prostheses [4]:

$$MP\ area = LVOT\ area \times (LVOT\ TVI/MP\ TVI)$$
$$= LVOT\ diameter^2 \times 0.785 \times (LVOT\ TVI/MP\ TVI)$$

where MP = mitral prosthesis,
 LVOT TVI = left ventricular outflow tract time velocity integral, and
 MP TVI = time velocity integral of mitral prosthesis velocity obtained by continuous-wave Doppler.

The area of the aortic prosthesis can be estimated by the product of the TVI ratio (between LVOT and aortic prosthesis) and the area of LVOT, using the continuity equation.

$$AP\ area = LVOT\ area \times (LVOT\ TVI/AP\ TVI)$$
$$= SRID^2 \times 0.785 \times (LVOT\ TVI/AP\ TVI)$$

where AP = aortic prosthesis, and
 SRID = sewing-ring inner diameter.

LVOT area is calculated from the inner diameter of the sewing ring. Aortic prosthesis TVI is obtained from continuous-wave Doppler velocity of the aortic prosthesis.

Regurgitation

Color-flow imaging is the principal technique utilized to detect prosthetic valvular regurgitation. The same criteria used for native valvular regurgitation are utilized for the semiquantitation of prosthetic valvular regurgitation. However, color-flow imaging of a mitral prosthesis by the transthoracic approach is frequently unsatisfactory (especially for a mechanical prosthesis) because of the marked attenuation of the ultrasound beam by the prosthesis and reverberations in the left atrium. TEE circumvents the above limitations.

It should be noted that a small amount of "built-in" regurgitation is normal for all types of prostheses. By transthoracic color-flow imaging, regurgitant flow is detected in about 30% of normally functioning prostheses. The detection rate increases to 44% and 95% for aortic and mitral prostheses, respectively, when transesophageal color-flow imaging is used. The "normal" prosthetic regurgitant flow has the following characteristics [9]:

1. Regurgitant jet area of less than 2 cm^2 and a jet length of less than 2.5 cm in the mitral position
2. A jet area of less than 1 cm^2 and a length of less than 1.5 cm in the aortic position

Pathologic regurgitation should be distinguished from the "normal" regurgitation of a prosthetic valve using the above criteria, morphology of the valve, and the location of regurgitant jet.

As in the assessment of regurgitation of native valves, an "integrated approach" is required for the evaluation of prosthetic valvular regurgitation, color-flow imaging being one of several determinants. Since transthoracic color-flow imaging has more limitations with prosthetic valves, it is essential to obtain complete hemodynamic data using pulsed-wave and continuous-wave Doppler before considering TEE. For aortic prosthetic regurgitation, the following should be determined: PHT of the jet, mitral inflow pattern, diastolic reversal flow in the descending thoracic aorta, and regurgitant fraction. For mitral prosthetic regurgitation, the following should be determined: mitral inflow peak velocity and PHT, intensity of the mitral regurgitant continuous-wave signal, and regurgitant fraction. These parameters can be assessed and interpreted as in the native valves (see Chap. 7). The following indicate severe aortic prosthetic regurgitation:

1. PHT of regurgitant jet is 250 m/sec or lower

2. Restrictive mitral inflow pattern (in acute aortic regurgitation)
3. Holodiastolic reversals in the descending thoracic aorta
4. Regurgitant fraction of 55% or higher

The following indicate severe mitral prosthetic regurgitation:

1. Increased mitral inflow peak velocity ($\geq$ 2.5 m/sec) *and* normal mitral inflow PHT ($\leq$ 150 m/sec)
2. Dense mitral regurgitant continuous-wave Doppler signal
3. Regurgitant fraction of 55% or higher

Transesophageal Echocardiography

Prosthetic valve stenosis (or obstruction) is usually diagnosed by detecting increased flow velocity by precordial continuous-wave Doppler; it is difficult to actually visualize the decreased motion of the prosthetic valve by precordial 2D echocardiography. The motion of the prosthetic valve, especially mitral and tricuspid prosthetic valves, is more clearly seen by TEE. Figure 8-7 demonstrates a TEE view of decreased disk opening motion in a patient with obstruction of a mitral disk prosthesis.

Fig. 8-7. TEE (horizontal basal view) of an obstructed mitral disk prosthesis. The systolic (left) and diastolic (right) frames demonstrate a marked decrease in the opening angle of mitral disk (approximately 30 degrees). Normally an angle of 60 degrees is expected. The continuous-wave Doppler velocity across this mitral prosthesis is shown in Figure 8-4 with increased peak velocity and PHT.

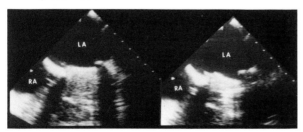

Disk motion may become intermittently abnormal and prolonged TEE observation may be necessary if such intermittent abnormality is clinically suspected (Fig. 8-8). Most current TEE probes are equipped with continuous-wave Doppler and are able to measure transmitral flow velocities and pressure gradients reliably.

TEE is essential in the evaluation of mitral and tricuspid prosthetic regurgitation and sometimes aortic prosthetic regurgitation [11–14] (Figs. 8-8 through 8-10). The transesophageal view of the atria is not hindered by the prosthesis, and the origin and extent of mitral or tricuspid prosthetic regurgitation are clearly demonstrated by TEE. When aortic prosthetic regurgitation originates from the posterior aspect of the prosthesis, TEE is also quite helpful, but anteriorly located aortic prosthetic regurgitation may not be seen from the transesophageal window, especially in the presence of a mitral prosthesis.

TEE is also useful in the evaluation of endocarditis, ring abscess, thromboembolic event, and intracardiac (especially atrial) mass or thrombi in the presence of a prosthetic valve. These applications are discussed separately in subsequent chapters (see Chaps. 9 and 14).

Clinical Impact

Hemodynamic cardiac catheterization is now rarely necessary to evaluate prosthetic valvular dysfunction. With 2D, Doppler, color-flow, and transesophageal imaging if necessary, a comprehensive evaluation of prosthetic valves is feasible. However, it should be emphasized that the "integrated approach" is the key for the most comprehensive evaluation (by transthoracic and transesophageal examination) to provide the following information:

1. Ventricular size and function
2. Structural integrity of the prosthesis
3. Hemodynamic data
   a. Peak flow velocity
   b. Maximum and mean gradients
   c. PHT (or deceleration time)
   d. Effective valve area

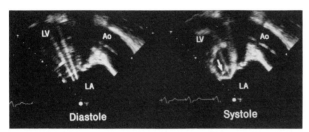

A

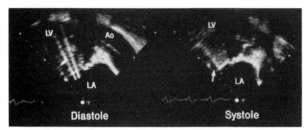

B

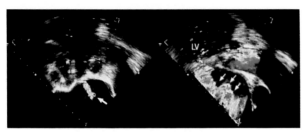

C

Fig. 8-8. Intermittent failure to close one of the mitral prosthesis disks resulting in intermittent severe mitral regurgitation, detected by TEE.
A. Normal motion of a St. Jude mitral prosthesis seen from the TEE longitudinal plane. During diastole, the two disks are almost parallel. Each disk moves about 85 degrees toward the left atrium (LA) during systole. A small echo-dense structure *(arrow)* was seen.
B. Intermittently, one of the disks failed to close during systole *(arrow)*. **C.** Color-flow imaging during normal closure showed a mild degree of periprosthetic regurgitation *(arrow, left)*, but during a failed closure (right), there was severe prosthetic mitral regurgitation *(arrows)*. At surgery, a small fibrin-thrombus material was found to be caught between the two disks. The prosthesis was replaced with a Starr-Edwards prosthesis.

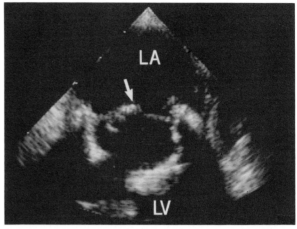

A

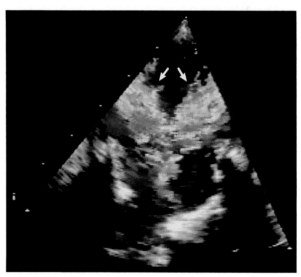

B

Fig. 8-9. **A.** Horizontal TEE basal view on 2D and color-flow imaging of a degenerative mitral bioprosthesis. The cusps are thickened and prolapsed *(arrow)*, allowing severe mitral prosthetic regurgitation. **B.** Color-flow imaging shows two wide separate mitral regurgitation jets *(arrows)*.

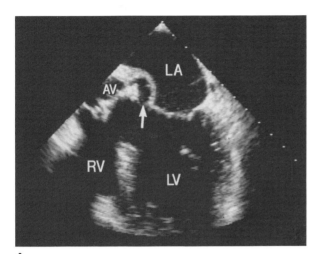

A

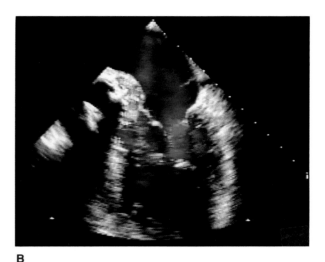

B

Fig. 8-10.   A. Horizontal TEE view demonstrating a dehisced aortic prosthesis. The echo-free space *(arrow)* during systole suggests an old abscess cavity. **B.** During diastole, color-flow imaging shows regurgitant flow in the echo-free space.

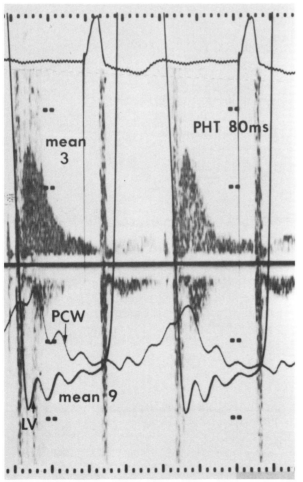

A

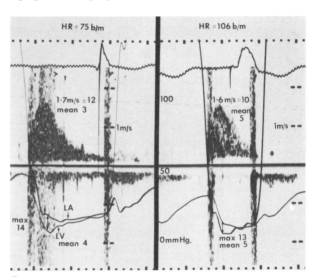

B

Fig. 8-11.   A. Simultaneous continuous-wave Doppler of flow through a mitral prosthesis and pressure recordings from the LV and the pulmonary capillary wedge (PCW). The catheter-derived mean gradient was much higher than the Doppler-derived mean gradient (9 versus 3 mm Hg). **B.** When direct left atrial (LA) pressure was measured by the transseptal approach, the mean gradient across the mitral prosthesis was essentially identical to the Doppler-derived mean pressure gradient (top left).

e. Pulmonary artery pressure
f. Diastolic filling profile
g. Color-flow jet area
h. Pulmonary vein (for mitral regurgitation) or descending aorta (for aortic regurgitation) flow reversals
i. Regurgitant fraction

With these collective data obtained by comprehensive echocardiographic examination, the most appropriate management plan can be formulated in most patients with a dysfunctional prosthetic valve.

Caveat

Occasionally, there is a significant discrepancy between Doppler-derived and catheter-derived pressure gradients across a prosthetic valve. For a mitral prosthesis, the catheter-derived gradient can be an overestimate of the actual transmitral gradient, as illustrated in Figure 8-11. When pulmonary capillary wedge pressure is utilized as a surrogate of left atrial pressure instead of transseptal catheterization for direct measurement of left atrial pressure, the transmitral pressure gradient may be overestimated due to phase shift and damped contour. For an aortic disk prosthesis, the Doppler-derived maximum instantaneous gradient may be higher than the catheter-derived maximum gradient since the pressure within the prosthetic orifice is higher than that in the ascending aorta (pressure recovery). However, the duration of peak Doppler velocity is quite short and the mean pressure gradients determined by the two methods should be similar.

References

1. Burstow DJ, et al. Continuous wave Doppler echocardiographic measurement of prosthetic valve gradients: a simultaneous Doppler-catheter correlative study. *Circulation* 1989; 80:504–514.

2. Baumgartner H, et al. Discrepancies between Doppler and catheter gradients in aortic prosthetic valves in vitro: a manifestation of localized gradients and pressure recovery. *Circulation* 1990;82:1467–1475.

3. Stewart SFC, et al. Errors in pressure gradient measurement by continuous wave Doppler ultrasound: type, size and age effects of bioprosthetic aortic valves. *J Am Coll Cardiol* 1991;18:769–779.

4. Dumesnil JG, et al. Validation and applications of mitral prosthetic valvular areas calculated by Doppler echocardiography. *Am J Cardiol* 1990;65:1443–1448.

5. Dumesnil JG, et al. Validation and applications of indexed aortic prosthetic valve areas calculated by Doppler echocardiography. *J Am Coll Cardiol* 1990;16:637–643.

6. Chafizadeh ER, Zoghbi WA. Doppler echocardiographic assessment of the St. Jude medical prosthetic valve in the aortic position using the continuity equation. *Circulation* 1991; 83:213–223.

7. Miller FA, et al. Normal aortic valve prosthesis hemodynamics: 609 prospective Doppler examinations (Abstract). *Circulation* 1989; 80(suppl II):169.

8. Lengyel M, et al. Doppler hemodynamic profiles of 456 clinically and echo-normal mitral valve prostheses (Abstract). *Circulation* 1990;82(suppl III):43.

9. Connolly HM, et al. Doppler hemodynamic profiles of eighty-six normal tricuspid valve prostheses (Abstract). *J Am Coll Cardiol* 1991; 17:69A.

10. Wiseth R, et al. Validity of an early postoperative baseline Doppler recording after aortic valve replacement. *Am J Cardiol* 1991; 67:869–872.

11. Mohr-Kahaly S, et al. Regurgitant flow in apparently normal valve prostheses: improved detection and semiquantitative analysis by transesophageal two-dimensional color-coded Doppler echocardiography. *J Am Soc Echocardiogr* 1990;3:187–195.

12. Nellessen U, et al. Transesophageal two-dimensional echocardiography and color Doppler flow velocity mapping in the evaluation of cardiac valve prostheses. *Circulation* 1988;78:848–855.

13. Taams MA, et al. Transesophageal Doppler color flow imaging in the detection of native and Bjork-Shiley mitral valve regurgitation. *J Am Coll Cardiol* 1989;13:95–99.

14. Khandheria BK, et al. Value and limitations of transesophageal echocardiography in assessment of mitral valve prostheses. *Circulation* 1991;83:1956–1968.

9

Infective Endocarditis

Infective endocarditis represents protean clinical manifestations of infection of endocardial structures, most commonly involving the native or prosthetic cardiac valve. As the population lives longer and is increasingly subject to surgical, pharmacologic, and habitual manipulations, it is exposed to various microorganisms that can cause infective endocarditis. The incidence of endocarditis varies depending on the type of population; in a population-based study in Olmsted County, Minnesota, the incidence was 4.9 per 100,000 person-years [1]. The incidence is higher in patients who have a preexisting valvular heart disease (rheumatic valve, bicuspid aortic valve, myxomatous mitral valve), a cardiac prosthesis, or congenital heart disease, or who are intravenous (IV) drug users. The mitral and aortic valves are most commonly involved with endocarditis but right-side cardiac valve involvement is not uncommon in IV drug users. Infective endocarditis is rarely cured without optimal antibiotic treatment. Since the consequence of untreated endocarditis is devastating and often fatal, it is of utmost importance to promptly recognize and appropriately treat the underlying infection and its complications. In this clinical context, echocardiography has become an essential part of evaluating patients with infective endocarditis. It plays a vital role in the diagnosis, assessment of structural and hemodynamic complications, and monitoring of treatment of endocarditis.

Diagnosis

Since the first M-mode echocardiographic observation of valvular vegetation in 1973 [2], the role of echocardiography in infective endocarditis has changed, along with the improvements in resolution and technologic advances including Doppler, color-flow imaging, and transesophageal echocardiography (TEE). Currently, echocardiography is the diagnostic procedure of choice in detecting valvular vegetation. With the changing social environments and behaviors, it is not uncommon to have culture-negative endocarditis. Therefore, the diagnosis of infective endocarditis may be suggested on the basis of echocardiography even in the absence of or certainly prior to positive findings on blood culture.

A vegetation appears as an echogenic mobile mass (or masses) attached to the valvular cusp or leaflet (Figs. 9-1 and 9-2) or the prosthetic valve (Fig. 9-3). The usual initial attachment site to the mitral and tricuspid valves is on the atrial side, but aortic vegetations can involve either the aortic or ventricular valve surface. Vegetation can be linear, round, or irregular (shaggy) and frequently may show high-frequency flutter or oscillation [3].

The sensitivity of 2D echocardiography for detection of vegetation depends on its size, location, and the echocardiographic window used. The smallest vegetation detectable by transthoracic examination is 3 to 5 mm in diameter. The sensitivity of detecting vegetation is 65 to 80% with transthoracic 2D echocardiography, and has improved to 90 to 95% with TEE [4–7] (Figs. 9-3 through 9-6). The diagnostic yield of transthoracic echocardiography is especially poor in prosthetic valve endocarditis (sensitivity of about 25%); however, TEE has improved the sensitivity of detecting vegetation from 85 to 90% in this clinical setting.

The noninvasive detection of valvular vegetation, the hallmark of endocarditis, is one of the major diagnostic contributions of echocardiography. Furthermore, echo examination is essential for the assessment of structural and hemodynamic complications of endocarditis (Table 9-1). Any patient with or suspected to have endocarditis should undergo a baseline comprehensive echocardiographic examination (including TEE if necessary) and serial ex-

Fig. 9-1. Mitral valve vegetation in an elderly patient with streptococcal viridans endocarditis. The transthoracic parasternal long-axis view demonstrates a large shaggy vegetation *(arrowheads)* attached to the atrial surface of the mitral valve. In real time, the mass moved back and forth across the mitral annulus.

Fig. 9-2. The subcostal long-axis view shows a vegetation attached to the tricuspid valve on the atrial side *(arrow)*. This was obtained from an 81-year-old man with enterococcal endocarditis. The vegetation remained unchanged after treatment with penicillin and gentamicin.

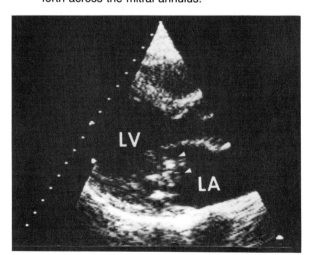

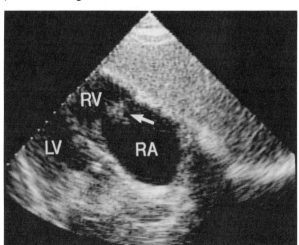

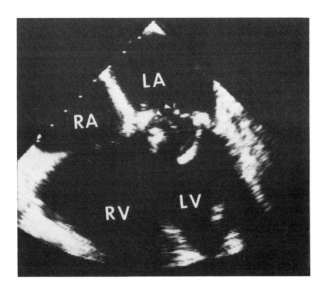

Fig. 9-3. TEE four-chamber view. Small linear mobile masses *(arrowheads)* (in real time) are attached to the mitral bioprosthesis. These lesions were not seen by transthoracic study. Blood culture did not identify an organism since the patient was partially treated with multiple antibiotics.

Fig. 9-4. (Top) On the left, TEE demonstrates aortic valve (AV) vegetation *(arrowhead)* involving the left or noncoronary cusp. On the right, the systolic frame on color-flow examination shows normal flow across the left ventricular outflow tract (LVOT) and mild mitral regurgitation. (Bottom) On the left, the diastolic frame shows prolapse of the aortic valve *(arrowhead)* into the LVOT. On the right, color-flow imaging shows severe aortic regurgitation, the blue mosaic color jet filling the entire LVOT area.

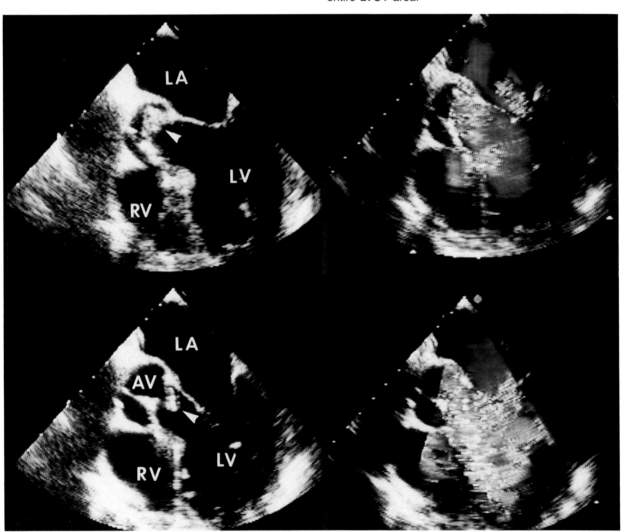

131

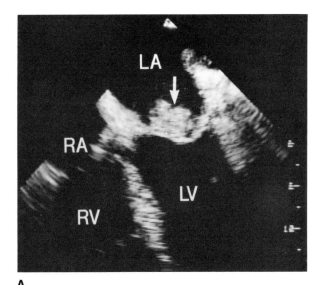

A

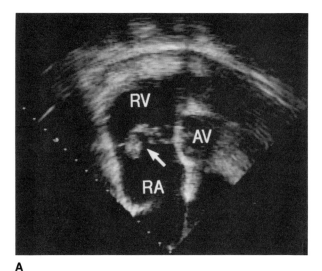

A

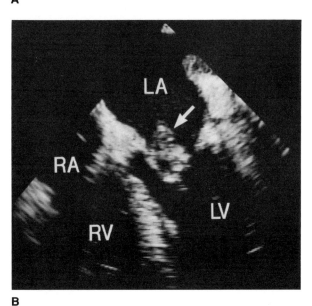

B

Fig. 9-5. TEE demonstrates a large mitral valve vegetation *(arrow)* in the systolic **(A)** and diastolic **(B)** phase. The vegetation is attached to the atrial side of the mitral valve. It was not clearly visualized on the transthoracic echocardiogram.

B

Fig. 9-6. **A.** Longitudinal TEE view of the tricuspid valve vegetation *(arrow)* from the same patient as in Figure 9-2. The anterior leaflet prolapses and valve coaptation is not satisfactory. **B.** Color-flow imaging demonstrates significant tricuspid regurgitation.

aminations as dictated by the clinical and hemodynamic status of the patient.

Complications

Complications of endocarditis arise primarily from vegetation, destruction of valvular or in-

tracardiac structures, and subsequent hemodynamic deteriorations. Therefore, the presence and the characteristics of the vegetation affect the prognosis and clinical course of patients with infective endocarditis. In a comprehensive prospective study of 204 patients with documented infective endocarditis [8], clinical complications were correlated with

Table 9-1. Complications of endocarditis

Structural
  Cusp or leaflet rupture/flail
  Perforation
  Abscess
  Aneurysm
  Fistula
  Dehiscence of prosthetic valve
  Pericardial effusion (more frequent with abscess)
Hemodynamic
  Valvular regurgitation
    Acute mitral regurgitation
    Acute aortic regurgitation
      Premature mitral valve closure
      Restrictive mitral inflow pattern
  Valvular stenosis
  Shunt
  Congestive heart failure
Embolization

transthoracic echocardiographic findings and characteristics of vegetations. When no significant valvular abnormalities were detected by echocardiography, no one developed congestive heart failure, required valve replacement, or failed to improve with antibiotic treatment. Peripheral and cerebral emboli occurred in 15% of patients with no detectable vegetations. In left-side valve endocarditis, the frequency of clinical complications increased with greater mobility, extent, consistency (less calcific), and size of vegetation. When the vegetation was larger than 11 mm, 50% of patients or more developed at least one complication of infective endocarditis. In patients with tricuspid valve endocarditis, pulmonary embolism was the most common complication (69%).

Mugge and colleagues [5], utilizing TEE, also noted that the patients with a large (> 10 mm) vegetation involving or attached to the mitral valve were at increased risk for embolic events, but vegetation size was not correlated with the degree of heart failure and patient survival. Echocardiography is useful not only in diagnosing endocarditis, but also in predicting potential complications by characterizing valvular vegetation. Valve replacement is required in one-third of patients with left-side endocarditis and in less than 10% of patients

with right-side involvement. Therefore, detection of valvular vegetation does not necessarily indicate valvular replacement. Surgery is indicated when the patient's hemodynamic condition deteriorates, high-degree conduction abnormalities develop, mobile vegetation persists after an embolic event, or when vegetation becomes larger while being treated with antibiotics.

Transesophageal Echocardiography

Due to improved resolution, the sensitivity of TEE for detecting vegetation or complications of endocarditis is much higher than that of the transthoracic approach. It has been suggested that TEE should be performed in all patients with suspected or diagnosed endocarditis, but the clinical impact of such an approach certainly requires further evaluation. One clinical caveat is that endocarditis prophylaxis should not be given prior to TEE examination when endocarditis is suspected since it will interfere with future blood culture results. The sensitivity of transthoracic echocardiography in detecting the complications of endocarditis (see Table 9-1) is quite low [9] (Fig. 9-7). Since TEE improves the diagnostic sensitivity of detecting these complications [10, 11] (Fig. 9-8), it should be performed in all patients suspected to have such abnormalities (these patients usually have persistent fever, heart failure without a demonstrable etiology, persistent positive findings on blood cultures) or in patients in whom transthoracic echocardiography was nondiagnostic.

Anatomic complications of endocarditis were found to be much more common than previously appreciated when consecutive patients with aortic valve endocarditis were examined by TEE [12]. Forty-four percent of patients with aortic valve endocarditis had involvement of subaortic structures: mitral-aortic intervalvular fibrosa aneurysm and/or perforation with communication into the left atrium, aortic annular abscess, and perforation of the mitral leaflet. This is an important obser-

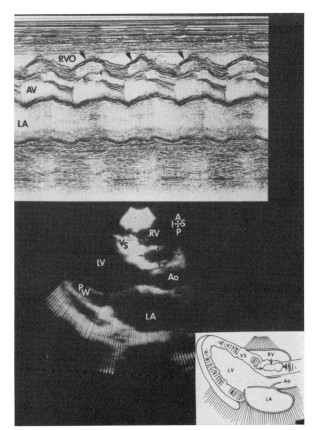

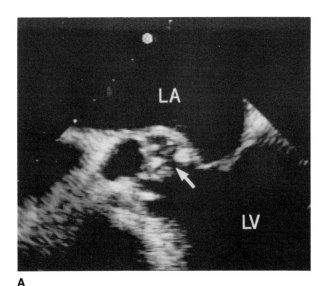

A

Fig. 9-7. M-mode echocardiogram (top) and 2D parasternal long-axis view (bottom) showing an aortic root abscess. (Top) An echo-free space *(arrows)* anterior to the aortic valve (AV) is recorded. (Bottom) 2D echo image shows a cavity in the anterior aortic root extending into the upper ventricular septum (VS). A small pericardial effusion is present behind the posterior wall (PW); this occurs frequently with cardiac abscess.

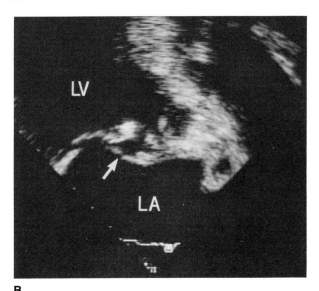

B

Fig. 9-8.   Horizontal **(A)** and longitudinal **(B)** TEE views of aortic valve endocarditis forming an abscess posteriorly (*arrow* in **A**). The abscess involves the mitral-aortic intervalvular fibrosa, which had a rupture (*arrow* in **B**) best seen from the longitudinal view, resulting in LVOT to left atrial shunt.

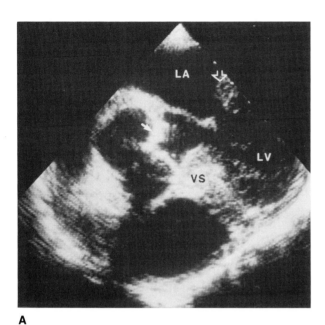

A

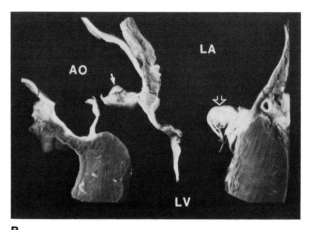

B

Fig. 9-9.   A. Still-frame of horizontal TEE showing nodular echo density on the posterior mitral leaflet *(open arrow)* and another density on the aortic valve *(arrow)*. **B.** Anatomic specimen from the same patient, dissected through the same tomographic plane as seen in **A.** Vegetation is seen on the mitral valve *(open arrow)* and the aortic valve *(arrow)*. (From E Klodas, WD Edwards, BK Khandheria. Use of transesophageal echocardiography for improving detection of valvular vegetations in subacute bacterial endocarditis. *J Am Soc Echocardiogr* 1989;2:386–389.)

vation since these complications may be responsible for unexplained hemodynamic compromise. Only in half of these patients were the subaortic complications suggested by transthoracic examination.

Echocardiographic-Pathologic Correlation

A published case report from the Mayo Clinic provided an opportunity to correlate TEE findings of aortic and mitral valve vegetations with anatomic findings on autopsy of an 81-year-old man [13] (Fig. 9-9). The vegetations could not be detected by transthoracic echocardiography.

Limitations and Pitfalls

There are several limitations and pitfalls to the echocardiographic detection of valvular vegetation. Other valvular lesions such as marked myxomatous degeneration of the mitral valve (Fig. 9-10), noninfective vegetations (Libman-Sacks or marantic endocarditis), and tumor or thrombus attached to a valve (e.g., papilloma) may simulate or mask vegetations. When a valve is sclerotic, calcified, or prosthetic, visualization of a vegetation is more difficult. TEE may be useful under these circumstances. Since vegetation is usually mobile and may not be seen in certain imaging planes, multiple tomographic planes should be utilized. Clinical presentations and other laboratory data (blood culture results, sedimentation rate, and other systemic symptoms) need to be incorporated in the interpretation of echocardiographic findings. Healed (old) vegetation is more fibrotic and refractile than new fresh vegetation. The differentiation may be possible by echocardiographic tissue characterization [14].

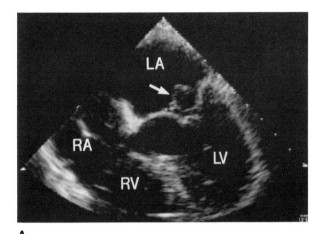

A

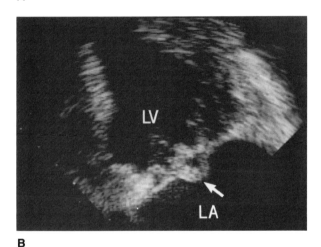

B

Fig. 9-10. Horizontal **(A)** and longitudinal **(B)** TEE images of myxomatous flail posterior mitral leaflet *(arrow)* mimicking mitral valve vegetation. Careful examination of the structure in real-time study can usually differentiate this from vegetation. Flail mitral leaflet is frequently accompanied by ruptured chordae tendineae.

References

1. Steckelberg JM, et al. Influence of referral bias on the apparent clinical spectrum of infective endocarditis. *Am J Med* 1990;88:582–588.

2. Dillon JC, et al. Echocardiographic manifestations of valvular vegetations. *Am Heart J* 1973;86:698–704.

3. Roy P, et al. Spectrum of echocardiographic findings in bacterial endocarditis. *Circulation* 1976;53:474–482.

4. Rohmann RE, et al. Improved diagnostic value of echocardiography in patients with infective endocarditis by transesophageal approach. A prospective study. *Eur Heart J* 1988;9:43–53.

5. Mugge A, et al. Echocardiography in infective endocarditis: reassessment of prognostic implications of vegetation size determined by the transthoracic and the transesophageal approach. *J Am Coll Cardiol* 1989;14:631–638.

6. Shively BK, et al. Diagnostic value of transesophageal compared with transthoracic echocardiography in infective endocarditis. *J Am Coll Cardiol* 1991;18:391–397.

7. Taams MA, et al. Enhanced morphological diagnosis in infective endocarditis by transesophageal echocardiography. *Br Heart J* 1990;63:109–113.

8. Sanfilippo AJ, et al. Echocardiographic assessment of patients with infectious endocarditis: prediction of risk for complications. *J Am Coll Cardiol* 1991;18:1191–1199.

9. Scanlon JG, Seward JB, Tajik AJ. Valve ring abscess in infective endocarditis: visualization with wide angle two-dimensional echocardiography. *Am J Cardiol* 1982;49:1794–1800.

10. Daniel WG, et al. Improvements in the diagnosis of abscesses associated with endocarditis by transesophageal echocardiography. *N Engl J Med* 1991;324:795–800.

11. Bansal RC, Graham BM, Jutzy KR. Left ventricular outflow tract to left atrial communication secondary to rupture of mitral-aortic intervalvular fibrosa in infective endocarditis: diagnosis by transesophageal echocardiography and color flow imaging. *J Am Coll Cardiol* 1990;15:499–504.

12. Karalis DG, et al. Transesophageal echocardiographic recognition of subaortic complications in aortic valve endocarditis. Clinical and surgical implications. *Circulation* 1992;86:353–362.

13. Klodas E, Edwards WD, Khandheria BK. Use of transesophageal echocardiography for improving detection of valvular vegetations in subacute bacterial endocarditis. *J Am Soc Echocardiogr* 1989;2:386–389.

14. Tak T, et al. Value of digital image processing of two-dimensional echocardiograms in differentiating active from chronic vegetations of infective endocarditis. *Circulation* 1988;78:116–123.

10

Cardiomyopathies

Broadly, the cardiomyopathies (CMs) are classified into three types: (1) dilated, (2) hypertrophic, and (3) restrictive. They usually have distinct morphologic and functional characteristics. In dilated CM, the left ventricle (LV) is enlarged and systolic function is decreased. Hypertrophic CM is characterized by varying degrees of ventricular hypertrophy, most notably of the ventricular septum. Ventricular systolic function is usually hyperdynamic in hypertrophic and normal in restrictive CM. The atria are markedly dilated in restrictive CM due to stiff ventricles causing restrictive diastolic filling. The CMs can also be subgrouped as primary or secondary, depending on whether the CM is related to a systemic disease (secondary) or involves the heart primarily with an undetermined cause (primary). The definition and classification of the CMs as reported by the World Health Organization (WHO) task force is shown in Table 10-1. In this chapter, only primary CMs are discussed; other cardiac diseases due to a systemic illness are dealt with in the next chapter.

Dilated Cardiomyopathy

2D Echocardiography

Dilated CM is characterized by a dilated LV cavity and decreased global systolic function (Fig. 10-1). Both end-diastolic and end-systolic dimensions and volumes are moderately to markedly increased, and systolic functional parameters (ejection fraction, fractional shortening, stroke volume, and cardiac output) are uniformly reduced [1]. The wall thickness is variable but typically is within normal limits.

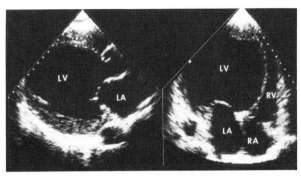

A

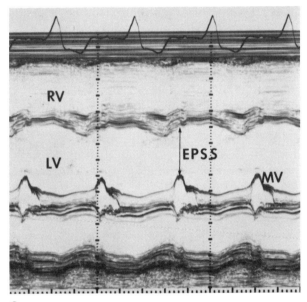

C

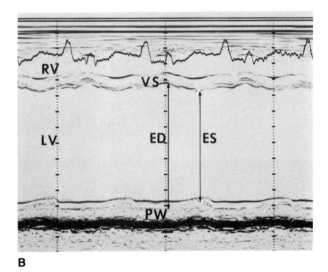

B

Fig. 10-1.   A. Typical 2D echocardiogram of dilated CM: systolic frame from parasternal long-axis (left) and apical four-chamber views (right). The LV cavity is markedly dilated, wall thickness is normal, and function is severely reduced. The right ventricle (RV) and right atrium (RA) are normal in size. **B.** Typical M-mode echocardiogram of dilated CM at the midventricular (or papillary muscle) level. Both end-diastolic (ED) and end-systolic (ES) dimensions are increased (78 mm and 68 mm, respectively). Ejection fraction is calculated from these dimensions: $(ED^2 - ES^2)/ED^2 \times 100\% = 24\%$. Wall thickening is globally reduced. **C.** At the mitral valve (MV) level, valve opening is reduced due to low cardiac output, and increased E-point septal separation (EPSS) of 30 mm indicates decreased systolic function.

Table 10-1.   Report of the WHO/ISFC task force on the definition and classification of cardiomyopathies

Primary Cardiomyopathies
  Definition
    Heart muscle diseases of unknown cause
  Classification
    Dilated cardiomyopathy
    Hypertrophic cardiomyopathy
    Restrictive cardiomyopathy
Specific heart muscle disease
  Definition
    Heart muscle disease of known cause or associated
      with disorders of other systems
    Disorders of the myocardium due to systemic or
      pulmonary hypertension, coronary artery disease,
      valvular heart disease, or congenital cardiac
      anomalies have been excluded
  Classification
    Infective
    Metabolic
      Endocrine
      Familial storage and infiltration
      Deficiency
      Amyloid
    Systemic diseases
      Systemic lupus erythematosus, sarcoidosis,
        muscular dystrophies
      Friedreich's ataxia
    Toxic
      Ethanol, radiation, doxorubicin

Source: From Report of the WHO/ISFC task force on the definition and classification of cardiomyopathies. *Br Heart J* 1980; 44:672–673.

The LV mass, however, is uniformly increased. Usually, contractility is reduced in global fashion, but superimposed regional wall motion abnormalities can also be present. Similar findings are seen in patients with extensive myocardial ischemia, myocarditis, alcoholic CM, hemochromatosis, sarcoidosis, or doxorubicin (Adriamycin) toxicity.

Secondary features in dilated CM include dilated mitral annulus and incomplete coaptation of mitral leaflets responsible for the associated mitral regurgitation, evidence of low cardiac output (decreased excursion of mitral leaflet), enlarged atrial cavities, right ventricle enlargement, and apical mural thrombus.

Doppler (Pulsed-Wave, Continuous-Wave) and Color-Flow Imaging

Doppler is useful for determining cardiac output, pulmonary artery pressure, and mitral inflow filling pattern (i.e., diastolic function). Cardiac output is routinely measured using the LV outflow tract (LVOT) time velocity integral (TVI) and diameter (see Chap. 5). Mitral inflow filling patterns provide useful insight into LV filling pressures as well as diastolic function. In general, the pattern of abnormal relaxation (decreased E velocity, increased A velocity, decreased E/A ratio, prolonged deceleration time [DT], and increased isovolumic relaxation time [IVRT]) is associated with normal to mildly elevated filling pressures and minimal symptoms (class I–II), while the restrictive pattern (increased E, decreased A, increased E/A, shortened DT, decreased IVRT) is associated with moderately to markedly increased LV end-diastolic and left atrial pressures and symptoms of congestive heart failure (class III–IV) [2,3] (Fig. 10-2). The status of pulmonary artery pressure estimated from tricuspid regurgitation velocity was found to be prognostic in dilated CM [4]. The patients with a tricuspid regurgitation velocity of 3.0 m/sec or higher had much higher mortality, higher incidence of heart failure, and more frequent hospitalization than did the patients with lower velocities. Therefore, restrictive diastolic filling pattern and high tricuspid regurgitation

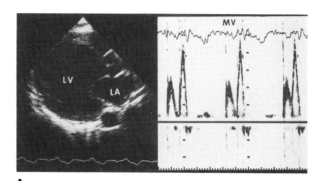

A

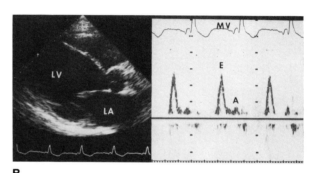

B

Fig. 10-2. **A.** 2D parasternal long-axis view of typical dilated CM (left) and pulsed-wave Doppler velocity recording (right) of mitral valve (MV) inflow showing a relaxation abnormality pattern with increased A velocity. Patients with this type of diastolic filling pattern usually have minimal to mild symptoms, despite severe LV systolic dysfunction. **B.** 2D parasternal long-axis view of another typical dilated CM (left) and mitral valve inflow velocity pattern (right) of restrictive physiology with a markedly decreased A velocity and an increased E/A ratio. Patients with this type of diastolic filling have increased filling pressure and symptomatic congestive heart failure.

velocity identify the patients with increased risk, in addition to the global systolic functional parameter [5].

Familial Dilated Cardiomyopathy and Arrhythmogenic Right Ventricular Dysplasia

It is recommended that echocardiographic screening of immediate family members of a patient with dilated CM be performed because

of the high incidence (20.3%) of familial dilated CM [6]. Familial association was also
noted in patients with arrhythmogenic right
ventricular dysplasia (ARVD) or Uhl's anomaly. It is primarily a right ventricular CM due
to fatty displacement of the right ventricular
free wall. Echocardiographically, the right ventricle is dilated with poor contractility out of
proportion to the degree of LV dilatation and
dysfunction, which is not uncommon in
ARVD. Due to right ventricular failure, right
ventricular systolic pressure is usually in the
low-normal range; hence, tricuspid regurgitation velocity is usually less than 2 m/sec. The
main clinical concern in patients with ARVD
is malignant ventricular arrhythmias.

Hypertrophic Cardiomyopathy

2D/M-mode Echocardiography

Although *asymmetric septal hypertrophy* is the
most common type of morphology, hypertrophic CM (Fig. 10-3) can present with concentric, apical, or free wall LV hypertrophy [7–10].
When the basal septum is hypertrophied and
bulging, the LVOT becomes narrowed, which
provides a substrate for dynamic obstruction.
The blood flow velocity across the narrowed
LVOT is increased and produces the "venturi"
effect. Consequently, the mitral leaflets and
support apparatus are drawn toward the septum (i.e., *systolic anterior motion*) producing obstruction to the LVOT (Fig. 10-4). The LVOT
obstruction is dynamic and depends on the
loading conditions and contractility of the LV.
When the aortic flow is interrupted because
of the development of LVOT obstruction, the
aortic valve develops premature midsystolic
closure. Systolic anterior motion of the mitral
valve distorts the configuration of the mitral
valve, resulting in mitral regurgitation. Therefore, varying degrees of mitral regurgitation
almost invariably accompany the obstructive
form of hypertrophic CM.

M-mode echocardiography is useful to doc-

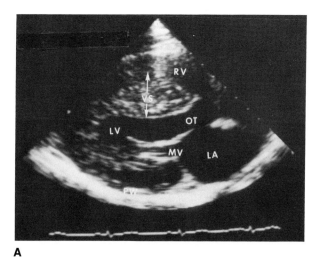

A

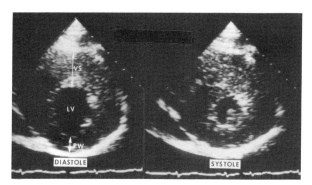

B

Fig. 10-3.   A. Parasternal long-axis view of
hypertrophic CM (nonobstructive variant). The
ventricular septum (VS) is asymmetrically
hypertrophied compared to the posterior wall (PW).
The left atrium (LA) is mildly enlarged. **B.** Diastolic
and systolic frames of the parasternal short-axis
view. Note that the entire ventricular septum is
uniformly and markedly hypertrophied. Furthermore,
the anterolateral LV free wall is also markedly
hypertrophied while the posteroinferior wall is of
normal thickness. Note also the abnormal texture of
the involved myocardium.

ument asymmetric septal hypertrophy, systolic
anterior motion of the mitral valve, and midsystolic aortic valve closure [11–13] (Fig.
10-5). However, the M-mode findings are not
specific for hypertrophic CM. Asymmetric septal hypertrophy is also seen in right ventricular
hypertrophy, hypertension, and inferior wall
myocardial infarction with preceding LV hy-

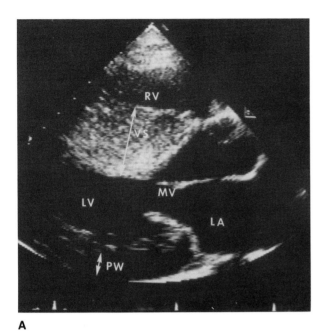

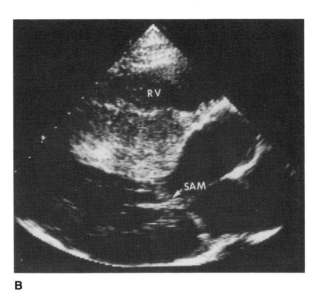

Fig. 10-4. 2D echocardiogram showing hypertrophic obstructive CM. **A.** Diastolic frame. The ventricular septum (VS) is markedly hypertrophic (34 mm) and has abnormal myocardial texture. **B.** Systolic frame. Systolic anterior motion (SAM) of the anterior mitral leaflet is shown, obstructing the LVOT.

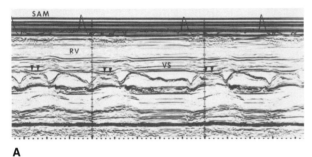

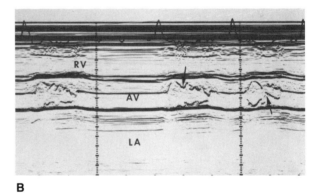

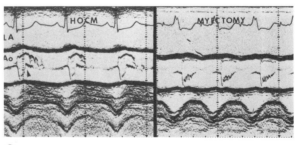

Fig. 10-5. **A.** M-mode echocardiogram showing systolic anterior motion (SAM, *double arrowheads*) of the anterior mitral leaflet. **B.** M-mode echocardiogram showing midsystolic aortic valve notching *(arrow),* from the same patient as in **A.** **C.** M-mode echocardiogram of the aortic valve before (left) and after (right) myectomy in a patient with hypertrophic obstructive CM. Midsystolic aortic notching *(arrowhead)* has disappeared after myectomy.

pertrophy. Systolic anterior motion of the anterior mitral valve can also be seen in other hyperdynamic cardiac conditions. 2D echocardiography is the method of choice to establish the diagnosis of hypertrophic CM. Furthermore, detailed morphologic characterization is also provided by 2D echo imaging [8,14]. The most frequent morphologic variety of hypertrophic CM consists of diffuse hypertrophy of the entire ventricular septum and anterolateral free wall (70–75%), basal septum (10–15%), concentric hypertrophy (5%), apical hypertrophic CM (< 5%), and hypertrophy of the lateral wall (1–2%). *Apical hypertrophic CM* may be missed by 2D echocardiography unless an apical examination is done carefully. Parasternal examination may not show any evidence of LV hypertrophy since the hypertrophy is usually confined to the apex (Fig. 10-6). Due to massive apical hypertrophy, epicardial motion may

Fig. 10-6. 2D echocardiogram of apical hypertrophic CM. **A.** The parasternal long-axis view is unremarkable. Wall thickness of the ventricular septum (VS) and posterior wall (PW) is normal. **B.** Apical four-chamber view during diastole (left) and systole (right). The apical wall thickness during diastole is markedly increased (18 mm, *arrow*) and the apical cavity is nearly obliterated except for a small slit during systole *(arrow)*. **C.** Apical short-axis view during diastole (left) and systole (right), demonstrating apical hypertrophy and apical cavity obliteration. **D.** Typical electrocardiogram of apical hypertrophic CM with a marked increase in QRS voltage and giant negative T-waves in the precordial (V_2–V_5), I, and aVL leads.

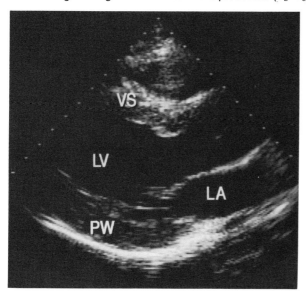

A

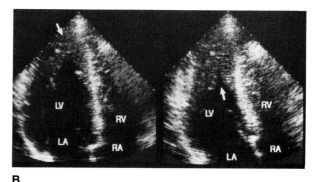

B

C

D

suggest a dyskinetic apex but endocardial motion shows near-complete apical cavity obliteration. This condition is typically associated with giant T-wave inversion in the precordial leads [9] (see Fig. 10-6D).

Doppler (Pulsed-Wave, Continuous-Wave) and Color-Flow Imaging

Left Ventricular Outflow Tract Obstruction

The degree of LV obstruction is readily assessed by continuous-wave Doppler echocardiography. Increased flow velocity across the LVOT is typically detected from the apical transducer position, but other transducer positions should also be tried. The resulting Doppler spectrum has a characteristic late-peaking "dagger-shaped" appearance (Fig. 10-7). Using the simplified Bernoulli equation, the peak velocity can be readily converted to the LVOT pressure gradient. Good correlation exists between Doppler-derived and catheter-derived pressure gradients [15–17] (Fig. 10-8). The dynamic nature of LVOT obstruction can be documented by continuous-wave Doppler during the Valsalva maneuver and during amyl nitrite inhalation (Fig. 10-9).

Mitral Regurgitation

Mitral regurgitation is a frequent accompaniment of the obstructive form of hypertrophic CM. The typical jet is posterolaterally directed and temporally occurs after the onset of LVOT obstruction: ejection→obstruction→leak [18]. It produces a high-velocity jet away from the apex, which may be confused with the LVOT gradient. Flow duration and Doppler spectral

Fig. 10-7. Continuous-wave Doppler spectra obtained from the apex (APX) and high left parasternal (LPS) transducer position, demonstrating severe LVOT obstruction. Note the typical late-peaking configuration resembling a dagger or ski slope. The maximum velocity is 4.2 m/sec, corresponding to the peak LVOT gradient of 70 mm Hg ($= 4 \times 4.2^2$).

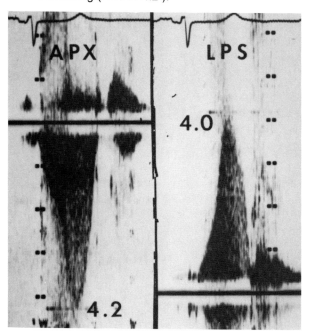

Fig. 10-8. Simultaneous continuous-wave Doppler and cardiac catheterization study. LV apex and outflow pressures are recorded to determine the severity of outflow obstruction. Doppler velocities are converted to pressure gradients, using the simplified Bernoulli equation, which correlate well with maximum (max) catheter-derived gradients. The resting gradient is 15 to 20 mm Hg and it is markedly accentuated in the post-extrasystolic contractions (second and fifth beats), with resultant gradients derived by catheter of 88 and 94 mm Hg and by Doppler of 89 and 94 mm Hg, respectively. It should also be noted that the LV pressure tracing has a late-peaking appearance corresponding to the late-peaking Doppler profile.

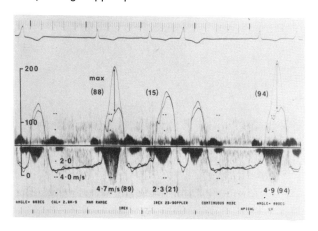

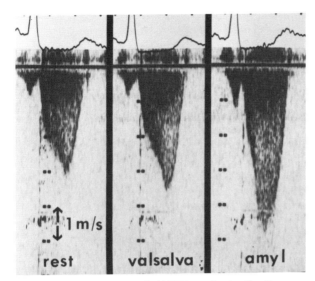

Fig. 10-9. Dynamic LVOT gradients. Continuous-wave Doppler from the apex shows a jet velocity of 3.0 m/sec at rest (gradient = 36 mm Hg). During the Valsalva maneuver, the velocity increased to 3.5 m/sec (gradient = 50 mm Hg) and after inhalation of amyl nitrite, the velocity increased to 4.8 m/sec (gradient = 92 mm Hg).

configuration help to differentiate mitral regurgitation from LVOT obstruction (Fig. 10-10). Color-flow imaging helps to separate the mitral regurgitation from LVOT flow and guide the continuous-wave Doppler beam. Color-flow imaging is also the best means to assess the severity of mitral regurgitation [18] (Fig. 10-11). The peak velocity of the mitral regurgitant jet can also be utilized to determine the magnitude of LVOT obstruction, for example,

Mitral regurgitant jet velocity = 7 m/sec

LV–left atrial gradient = 4×7^2 = 196 mm Hg

LV pressure = 196 + 20 (left atrial pressure)
                      = 216 mm Hg

If the blood pressure is 120/80 mm Hg,

LVOT gradient = 216 − 120 = 96 mm Hg

Diastolic Filling Pattern
Pulsed-wave Doppler is useful in locating the site of maximum obstruction, especially in

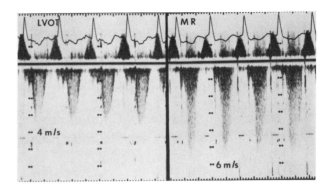

A

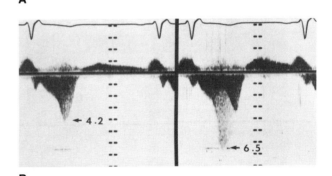

B

Fig. 10-10.   A. Continuous-wave Doppler spectra from LVOT obstruction and mitral regurgitation (MR) obtained from the apex. They may be difficult to differentiate from each other. Mitral regurgitation in hypertrophic CM usually begins at midsystole when there is systolic anterior motion of the mitral valve. Therefore, the Doppler spectrum of mitral regurgitation may superficially resemble LVOT flow velocity spectra. However, the rising slope at midsystole is usually perpendicular to the baseline in mitral regurgitation, whereas it is curvilinear until it reaches the highest velocity in the LVOT signal. Furthermore, the MR velocity signal extends beyond ejection and culminates into mitral forward flow during onset of diastole. Remember that MR velocity will always be higher than LVOT jet velocity. **B.** It is possible to have multiple intracavitary obstruction sites. There are two distinct late-peaking continuous-wave Doppler spectra (right): one with a velocity of 4.2 m/sec and another with a velocity of 6.5 m/sec. The higher velocity is not a mitral regurgitant jet as the rising slope is curvilinear.

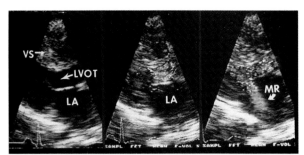

Fig. 10-11. 2D and color-flow imaging demonstrating the beginning of systolic anterior motion (SAM) during early systole (left), which narrows the LVOT and results in obstruction. During midsystole (center), the obstruction becomes most marked, resulting in turbulent flow in the LVOT. Mitral regurgitation (MR) becomes most prominent in mid to late systole (right) after the onset of LVOT obstruction. The sequence of events consists of early rapid ejection followed by development of LVOT obstruction secondary to systolic anterior motion, which leads to mitral regurgitation (ejection → obstruction → leak).

Fig. 10-12. Doppler pattern of abnormal relaxation in a patient with hypertrophic CM. The typical features include reduced E velocity (0.5 m/sec), increased A velocity (1.0 m/sec), decreased E/A ratio (0.5), and prolonged DT (320 msec).

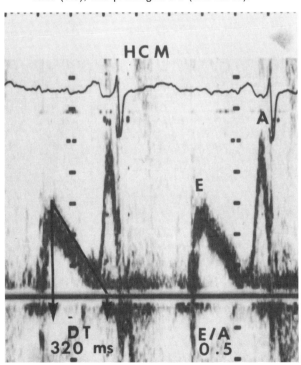

midcavity or apical hypertrophic CM. It is, however, most useful in the evaluation of LV diastolic filling in hypertrophic CM [19, 20]. Predominant diastolic abnormality in hypertrophic CM is slow and prolonged relaxation of the massively hypertrophied myocardium. The LV pressure decay during isovolumic relaxation is slow and, consequently, IVRT is prolonged, early rapid filling (E) is retarded, and the DT is prolonged (Fig. 10-12). However, not all patients with hypertrophic CM have this pattern. The diastolic filling pattern may become pseudonormalized, or a restrictive pattern may develop when the left atrial pressure becomes elevated. The therapeutic and prognostic implications of various filling patterns in hypertrophic obstructive CM remain to be further investigated.

Isovolumic Relaxation Flow

Due to asynchronous relaxation of the hypertrophied myocardium, transient intracavitary pressure gradient develops in the LV during the isovolumic relaxation period. Early relaxation and outward movement of the apical segment when the LVOT is obstructed result in transient LV flow redistribution from the base to the apex of the heart. Due to the apically directed flow, its Doppler velocity signals appear above the baseline similar to mitral inflow velocity (Fig. 10-13). Its peak flow velocity may be higher than the E velocity. It is clinically important to recognize isovolumic relaxation flow since it can be mistaken for E velocity, especially in patients with atrial fibrillation or fused E and A velocities during tachycardia. In patients with midcavity or, particularly, apical hypertrophy, the basal portion of the LV may relax first while the LV apical pressure remains higher than that at the basal portion during the isovolumic relaxation period. Therefore, the blood flow redistributes from the apical portion of the LV to the basal portion and its Doppler velocity signal appears below the baseline (Fig. 10-14). Occasionally, a midcavity pressure gradient continues through a part of diastole, and flow from the apex to the base continues through the early period of diastole.

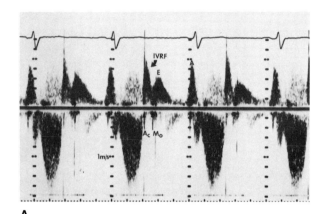

A

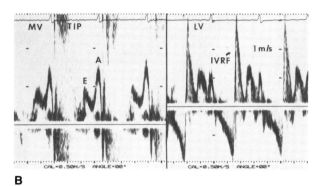

B

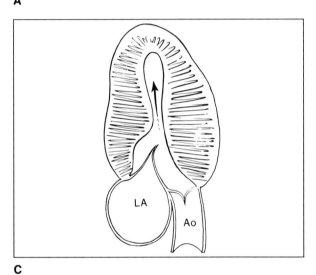

C

Fig. 10-13. **A.** Continuous-wave Doppler from the apex demonstrating isovolumic relaxation flow (IVRF), the velocity of which can be higher than the E velocity. **B.** Pulsed-wave Doppler from the apex with the sample volume at the mitral valve (MV) tip (left) and in the LV midcavity (right). IVRF is recorded best at the midcavity since the flow is directed from the base of the heart to the apex across the narrowest portion of the LV at the papillary muscle level. Note the peak IVRF velocity is 1.5 m/sec, markedly exceeding the mitral E velocity of 0.5 m/sec. **C.** Schematic diagram of IVRF *(arrow)* toward the apex due to an intracavitary gradient produced by the early relaxation of the apex in hypertrophic CM. The aortic and mitral valves are closed.

Dynamic Left Ventricular Outflow Tract Obstruction in the Elderly

Not all dynamic LVOT obstruction is due to hypertrophic CM. If ventricular systolic function becomes hyperdynamic (due to medication or other factors) in the setting of basal septal hypertrophy, the LVOT becomes obstructed in dynamic fashion and it behaves hemodynamically exactly the same as hypertrophic obstructive CM. This tends to happen in elderly patients with a history of hypertension, although hypertension is not a prerequisite [21]. They can be quite symptomatic with dyspnea, chest pain, and/or hypotension, which are exacerbated by vasodilator, diuretic, or digoxin therapy. Although this has been called "hypertensive hypertrophic cardiomyopathy," it is clearly a different entity from true hypertrophic CM. Another frequent clinical setting associated with dynamic LVOT obstruction is the postoperative period when intravascular volume is depleted and the patient is treated with inotropic agent(s).

Transesophageal Echocardiography

There are two clinical situations where TEE is useful in patients with hypertrophic obstructive CM: firstly, to assist and evaluate intraoperatively the result of myectomy (see Chap. 17) and secondly, to evaluate the mitral leaflets and chordal apparatus in a patient with hypertrophic obstructive CM who develops sudden hemodynamic deterioration. A subgroup of patients with hypertrophic obstructive CM develops chordal rupture, resulting in severe mitral regurgitation [22] (Fig. 10-15). These patients require mitral valve repair or replacement in addition to myectomy. TEE is also indicated to delineate the LVOT anatomy and assess hemodynamics in a patient with suboptimal surface (transthoracic) study.

Limitations and Pitfalls

2D echo features of hypertrophic CM can be mimicked by chronic hypertension, especially in combination with renal failure, cardiac amyloidosis, pheochromatosis, and Friedreich's ataxia. Therefore, echo findings of markedly increased LV wall thickness should be interpreted in their clinical context. Even dynamic LVOT obstruction can be present in these clinical conditions. Apical hypertrophic CM occasionally escapes echocardiographic detection since LV wall thickness is not significantly increased at the basal and papillary muscle levels so that parasternal long- and short-axis views may appear normal (see Fig. 10-6). It is best identified by apical short-axis and four-chamber views with good endocardial visualization, demonstrating thickened apical walls and systolic cavity obliteration. Due to the massive apical hypertrophy, the epicardial motion of the apex may appear to be dyskinetic. Apical hypertrophy should be differentiated from apical cavity obliteration due to hypereosinophilic syndrome (see Chap. 11). There is a small apical cavity during diastole in apical hypertrophic CM whereas no apical cavity is present in the eosinophilic thrombotic obliteration of the apex. Not infrequently, false-positive diagnosis of asymmetric septal hypertrophy is made due to right ventricular papillary muscle and prominent trabeculations overlying the interventricular septum (Fig. 10-16).

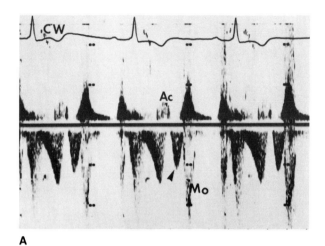

A

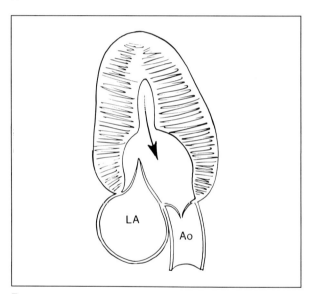

B

Fig. 10-14. **A.** IVRF *(arrowhead)* in a patient with apical hypertrophy and midcavity or apical obliteration. The flow is directed away from the apex because the LV apical pressure remains higher than that at the basal portion of the LV during the isovolumic relaxation period. **B.** Schematic drawing of IVRF *(arrow)* away from the apex in midcavitary or apical obstruction. LV pressure at the apex is higher than at the basal area, and there is a transient intracavitary gradient from the apex to the base during the isovolumic relaxation time. The aortic and mitral valves are closed. Ac = aortic valve closure.

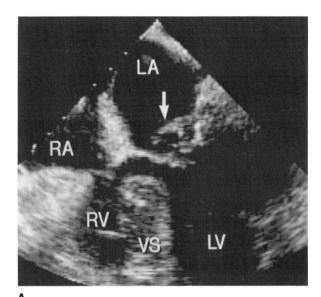

A

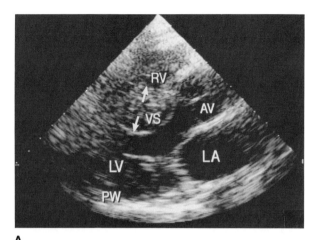

A

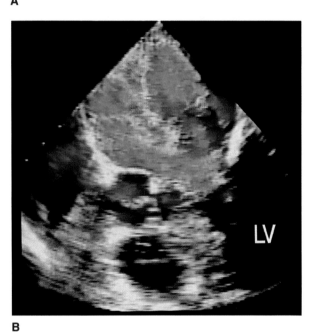

B

Fig. 10-15. **A.** TEE shows rupture of chordae tendineae *(arrow)* of the mitral valve, resulting in a flail segment in a patient with hypertrophic obstructive CM. The ventricular septum (VS) is markedly thickened. **B.** Color-flow imaging shows severe mitral regurgitation with the jet occupying the entire left atrial cavity.

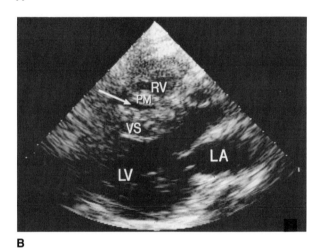

B

Fig. 10-16. **A.** The ventricular septum (VS) appears markedly thickened *(arrows),* consistent with hypertrophic CM. **B.** However, the asymmetric septal hypertrophy was mimicked by right ventricular muscle bands and papillary muscle (PM) overlying the ventricular septum. With slight tilt and rotation, an echo-free space *(arrow)* between these two structures could be demonstrated, hence avoiding misdiagnosis.

Restrictive Cardiomyopathy

Primary restrictive CM is characterized by impaired LV filling due to intrinsic myocardial stiffening without an identifiable cause [23]. This can occur with or without apical cavity obliteration. LV systolic function is frequently well preserved in the initial stages, but LV diastolic pressure rises rapidly due to the reduced compliance. This in turn results in increased atrial pressures and in marked biatrial enlargement. Therefore, characteristic 2D echo features of primary restrictive CM include normal LV and right ventricle cavity size and normal wall thickness with normal or reduced global systolic function. The right ventricle may eventually become mildly enlarged depending on the presence and magnitude of pulmonary hypertension. The atria are characteristically moderately to markedly dilated (Fig. 10-17). Restrictive CM is accompanied by restrictive diastolic filling (the reverse is *not* true). The characteristic hemodynamic profile is a "dip and plateau" or "square root sign" in the LV diastolic pressure tracing, corresponding to a shortened DT of the early rapid filling wave (E) on Doppler spectrum (Fig. 10-18). The mitral

inflow velocity pattern in restrictive CM is typically as follows:

Increased E velocity ($\geq$ 1.0 m/sec)

Decreased A velocity ($\leq$ 0.5 m/sec)

Increased E/A ratio ($\geq$ 2.0)

Decreased DT ($\leq$ 150 msec)

Decreased IVRT ($\leq$ 70 msec)

Pulmonary or hepatic vein flow in restrictive CM is as follows:

Systolic forward flow is less than diastolic forward flow

Increased diastolic (atrial) flow reversals with inspiration in the hepatic vein

Restrictive CM should be distinguished from *restrictive hemodynamics* or *physiology* [24]. The latter indicates a hemodynamic abnormality of impaired LV filling and a rapid rise in ventricular diastolic pressure from decreased compliance and/or increased left atrial pressure

Fig. 10-17. Characteristic 2D echo images of primary restrictive CM from parasternal long-axis (left) and apical four-chamber (right) views. The ventricular size and systolic function are normal, but compliance is decreased. The reduced compliance interferes with diastolic filling and results in atrial dilatation. Both the left and right atria are moderately dilated.

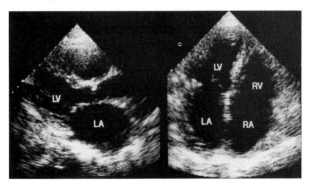

Fig. 10-18. Pulsed-wave Doppler recording of mitral inflow, typical of restrictive diastolic filling. DT is shortened (100 msec) and the E/A ratio is also markedly increased (3.0) mainly due to decreased mitral flow velocity with atrial contraction (A).

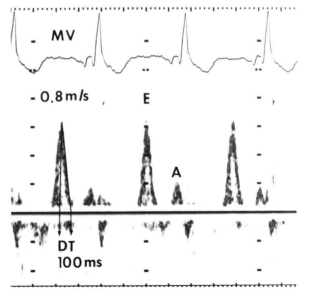

regardless of the underlying pathology, whereas the former indicates an inherent myocardial process producing the typical morphologic and hemodynamic conditions.

Secondary restrictive CM shares the same LV and/or right ventricular filling abnormality and hemodynamics, but with an identifiable underlying myocardial pathology. This includes some of the infiltrative cardiomyopathies (amyloidosis, glycogen storage disease), hypereosinophilic syndrome, endomyocardial fibrosis, and myocardial tumor. Although hemodynamics are similar, hence diastolic filling patterns, 2D echocardiography is able to differentiate various forms of secondary restrictive cardiomyopathy. These entities are discussed separately in Chapter 12.

It is often difficult to differentiate restrictive CM from constrictive pericarditis on the basis of clinical findings, laboratory tests, and hemodynamic assessment. Recently, Hatle and colleagues [25] observed that Doppler evaluation of diastolic filling pattern could separate restriction from constriction. In restriction, diastolic filling is characteristic, with increased early rapid filling flow velocity (E), shortened DT, and decreased late filling from atrial contraction (A). There is no respiratory variation in the diastolic flow, but in constriction there is significant respiratory variation in ventricular filling, which is the distinguishing feature. This is discussed in detail in Chapter 13.

References

1. Corya BC, et al. Echocardiographic features of congestive cardiomyopathy compared with normal subjects and patients with coronary artery disease. *Circulation* 1974;49:1153–1159.

2. Lavine SJ, Arends D. Importance of the left ventricular filling pressure on diastolic filling in idiopathic dilated cardiomyopathy. *Am J Cardiol* 1989;64:61–65.

3. St. Goar FG, et al. Left ventricular diastolic dysfunction in end-stage dilated cardiomyopathy: simultaneous Doppler echocardiography and hemodynamic evaluation. *J Am Soc Echocardiogr* 1991;4:349–360.

4. Abramson SV, et al. Pulmonary hypertension predicts mortality and morbidity in patients with dilated cardiomyopathy. *Ann Intern Med* 1992;116:888–895.

5. Sugrue DD, et al. The clinical course of idiopathic dilated cardiomyopathy: a population-based study. *Ann Intern Med* 1992;117:117–123.

6. Michels VV, et al. The frequency of familial dilated cardiomyopathy in a series of patients with idiopathic dilated cardiomyopathy. *N Engl J Med* 1992;326:77–82.

7. Wigle ED, et al. Hypertrophic cardiomyopathy: the importance of the site and extent of hypertrophy. A review. *Prog Cardiovasc Dis* 1985;28:1–83.

8. Maron BJ, Gottdiener JS, Epstein SE. Patterns and significance of distribution of left ventricular hypertrophy in hypertrophic cardiomyopathy. *Am J Cardiol* 1981;48:418–428.

9. Yamaguchi H, et al. Hypertrophic non-obstructive cardiomyopathy with giant negative T waves (apical hypertrophy): ventriculographic and echocardiographic features in 30 patients. *Am J Cardiol* 1979;44:401–412.

10. Keren G, et al. Apical hypertrophic cardiomyopathy: evaluation by noninvasive and invasive techniques in 23 patients. *Circulation* 1985;71:45–56.

11. Shah PM, Gramiak R, Kramer DH. Ultrasound localization of left ventricular outflow obstruction in hypertrophic obstructive cardiomyopathy. *Circulation* 1969;40:3–11.

12. Tajik AJ, Giuliani ER. Echocardiographic observations in idiopathic hypertrophic subaortic stenosis. *Mayo Clin Proc* 1974;49:89–97.

13. Popp RL, Harrison DC. Ultrasound in the diagnosis and evaluation of therapy in idiopathic hypertrophic subaortic stenosis. *Circulation* 1969;40:905–914.

14. Tajik AJ, Seward JB, Hagler DJ. Detailed analysis of hypertrophic obstructive cardiomyopathy by wide angle two dimensional sector echocardiography (Abstract). *Am J Cardiol* 1979;43:348.

15. Steward WJ, et al. Intraoperative Doppler echocardiography in hypertrophic cardiomy-

opathy: correlations with the obstructive pressure gradient. *J Am Coll Cardiol* 1987; 10:327–335.

16. Sasson Z, et al. Doppler echocardiographic determination of the pressure gradient in hypertrophic cardiomyopathy. *J Am Coll Cardiol* 1988;11:752–756.

17. Grigg LE, et al. Transesophageal Doppler echocardiography in obstructive hypertrophic cardiomyopathy: clarification of pathophysiology and importance in intraoperative decision making. *J Am Coll Cardiol* 1992;20:42–52.

18. Nishimura RA, et al. Evaluation of hypertrophic cardiomyopathy by Doppler color flow imaging: initial observations. *Mayo Clin Proc* 1986;61:631–639.

19. Yock PG, Hatle L, Popp RL. Patterns and timing of Doppler detected intracavitary and aortic flow in hypertrophic cardiomyopathy. *J Am Coll Cardiol* 1986;9:1047–1058.

20. Maron BH, et al. Noninvasive assessment of left ventricular diastolic function by pulsed Doppler echocardiography in patients with hypertrophic cardiomyopathy. *J Am Coll Cardiol* 1987;10:733–742.

21. Topol EJ, Traill TA, Fortuin NJ. Hypertensive hypertrophic cardiomyopathy of the elderly. *N Engl J Med* 1985;312:277–283.

22. Zhu WX, et al. Mitral regurgitation due to ruptured chordae tendineae in patients with hypertrophic obstructive cardiomyopathy. *J Am Coll Cardiol* 1992;20:242–247.

23. Seward J, Tajik AJ. Restrictive cardiomyopathy. *Curr Opin Cardiol* 1987;2:499–501.

24. Appleton CP, Hatle LK, Popp RL. Demonstration of restrictive ventricular physiology by Doppler echocardiography. *J Am Coll Cardiol* 1988;11:757–768.

25. Hatle LK, Appleton CP, Popp RL. Differentiation of constrictive pericarditis and restrictive cardiomyopathy by Doppler echocardiography. *Circulation* 1989;79(2):1–13.

11

Cardiac Diseases due to Systemic Illness

The heart is frequently affected by various systemic illnesses, causing morphologic, functional, and hemodynamic abnormalities. Cardiac involvement is usually predictable for a particular systemic illness and frequently represents a poor prognosis. Cardiac involvement due to systemic diseases includes secondary forms of cardiomyopathies (dilated, infiltrative, or restrictive), the valvular diseases, pericardial diseases (pericardial effusion, tamponade, or constriction), intracardiac mass, and marantic or Libman-Sacks endocarditis. Echocardiography is the method of choice for the detection and evaluation of these cardiac abnormalities. 2D echo studies provide morphologic and functional information; Doppler and color-flow studies provide information regarding intracardiac pressures, the severity of valvular stenosis and regurgitation, and diastolic filling pattern. Not uncommonly, echocardiographic detection of a particular cardiac abnormality may be the first diagnostic clue, for example, typical tricuspid and pulmonary valve involvement and appearance in carcinoid, or increased ventricular wall thicknesses and granular appearance in cardiac amyloidosis. Table 11-1 lists various cardiac manifestations of systemic illnesses frequently seen in the echocardiography laboratory, and their cardiac abnormalities are discussed in more detail, along with illustrative examples, in this chapter.

Table 11-1. Echocardiographic features of systemic illnesses

Amyloidosis
  Increased LV and RV wall thickness (moderate–marked)
  Normal LV cavity size
  Gradual deterioration of ventricular systolic function
  Granular appearance of myocardium (abnormal texture)
  Pericardial effusion
  Spectrum of diastolic dysfunction
  Thickening of the valves and multivalvular regurgitation
Ankylosing spondylitis
  Dilatation of the aortic annulus
  Dilatation of sinuses of Valsalva
  Thickened aortic valve with aortic regurgitation
Carcinoid
  Thickening and retraction of tricuspid valve with severe
    tricuspid regurgitation
  Tricuspid stenosis, usually mild
  Pulmonary valve thickening and retraction with
    pulmonic stenosis
  Right ventricular volume overload
  Thickening of left-side valves (< 15%)
Friedreich's ataxia
  LV hypertrophy, usually concentric (68%), resembling
    hypertrophic cardiomyopathy
  Dilated LV with systolic dysfunction (7%)
Hemochromatosis
  Appearance of dilated cardiomyopathy, dilated LV with
    decreased systolic function
  Normal ventricular wall thickness
  Restrictive diastolic filling characteristic at the advanced
    stage
Hypereosinophilic syndrome
  Posterior mitral leaflet thickening and tethering
  Ventricular apical thrombus with cavity obliteration
  Rarely, diffuse myocarditis with LV cavity increased in
    size with systolic dysfunction

Marfan's syndrome
  Dilatation of the ascending aorta
  Dilatation of the aortic annulus and the sinus of
    Valsalva
  Aortic dissection
  Mitral valve prolapse
Muscular dystrophy (Duchenne's)
  Posterior basal and lateral wall fibrosis
Pheochromocytoma
  Concentric LV hypertrophy (20%)
  Myocarditis (acute) with catecholamine crisis
Rheumatoid arthritis
  Pericardial effusion
  Constrictive pericarditis
  Cardiac granuloma
Sarcoidosis
  Regional wall motion abnormalities
  Thinning of the basal and posterolateral walls
  Posterobasal aneurysm
  Restrictive morphology
Systemic lupus erythematosus (SLE)
  Pericarditis
  Tamponade
  Myocarditis
  Endocarditis, Libman-Sacks
Tuberous sclerosis
  Rhabdomyoma
  Cardiomyopathy

Amyloidosis

This systemic disease due to deposition of amyloid fibrils in various organs may involve the myocardium, resulting in infiltrative cardiomyopathy. Contrary to the general perception, not all infiltrative cardiomyopathies produce restrictive cardiac morphology or hemodynamics. When myocardial infiltration is primarily interstitial as in amyloidosis, the predominant morphologic feature is an increase in myocardial wall thickness without a dilated left ventricular (LV) cavity [1, 2] (Fig.

11-1). Ventricular systolic function is not significantly reduced until it reaches the advanced stage with a marked increase in the wall thickness (15 mm). The LV wall thickness determined by 2D echocardiography is one of the important prognostic variables in patients with cardiac amyloidosis. Amyloid deposits in the heart are diffuse, involving the valves, myocardium, interatrial septum, and pericardium. It is common to detect multivalvular regurgitation due to diffuse amyloid deposits in the cardiac valves. Amyloid deposits make myocardial texture sparkle on 2D echocardiog-

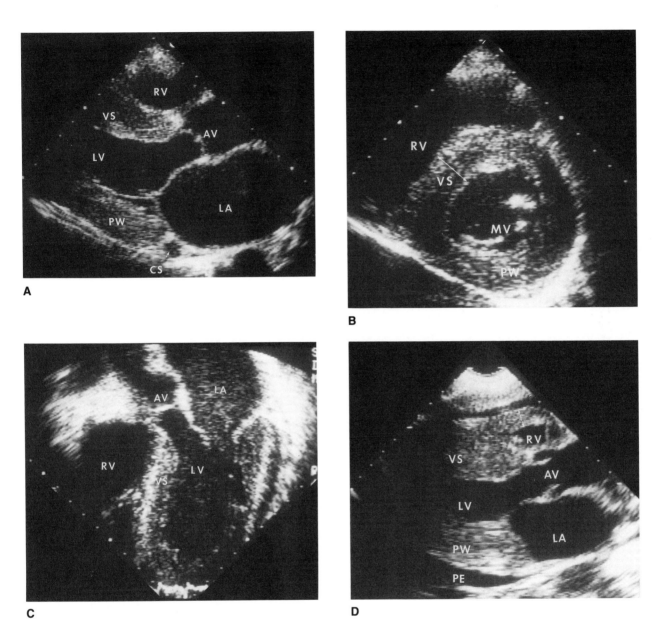

Fig. 11-1. Typical 2D echocardiograms of cardiac amyloidosis. Typical findings include (1) diffuse ventricular wall thickness, (2) pericardial effusion, (3) sparkling granular appearance of the myocardium, (4) thickened valves (due to amyloid infiltrates), and (5) deteriorating ventricular systolic function as wall thickness increases. **A.** The parasternal long-axis view shows the typical findings of cardiac amyloidosis, described above. The coronary sinus (CS, *arrow*) is enlarged due to right atrial pressure increased. **B.** The parasternal short-axis view shows marked concentric increase in LV wall thickness. The arrows indicate the thickness (= 18 mm) of the ventricular septum (VS). **C.** The apical long-axis view with the apex-down format. There is spontaneous echo contrast in the left atrium (LA) due to sluggish blood flow and left atrial enlargement. **D.** The subcostal view shows pericardial effusion (PE) and increased right ventricular (RV) wall thickness of 10 mm *(arrows)*.

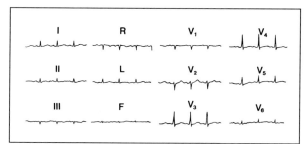

Fig. 11-2. Typical electrocardiogram of cardiac amyloidosis showing low QRS voltage despite increased LV wall thickness. (From JK Oh et al. Dynamic left ventricular outflow tract obstruction in cardiac amyloidosis detected by continuous-wave Doppler echocardiography. *Am J Cardiol* 1987;59:1009–1010.)

raphy, which produces a beautiful image, but the sparkling appearance alone is not diagnostic of cardiac amyloidosis. Other conditions may produce similar echocardiographic features, for example, hypertensive disease (especially in patients with renal failure), glycogen storage disease [3], and hypertrophic cardiomyopathy. However, the patients with cardiac amyloidosis usually do have a low QRS voltage on the electrocardiogram (Fig. 11-2), whereas patients with LV hypertrophy, hypertrophic cardiomyopathy, or glycogen storage disease have increased QRS voltages of the LV hypertrophy pattern. At an early stage of cardiac amyloidosis, systolic function can be hyperdynamic and it is not uncommon to see hemodynamic features of systolic anterior motion of the mitral valve and intracavitary obstruction as in hypertrophic cardiomyopathy [4]. As the disease progresses, however, the systolic function gradually deteriorates. Pulsed-wave Doppler echocardiography has been helpful in the evaluation of the diastolic abnormalities of cardiac amyloidosis. The initial diastolic abnormality of cardiac amyloidosis is abnormal relaxation due to increased ventricular wall thickness; the pattern becomes restrictive when progressive amyloid cardiac infiltration decreases LV compliance and increases left atrial pressure [5, 6] (Fig. 11-3). The filling pattern may even normalize temporarily ("pseudonormalized") as a result of combined relaxation abnormality and increased left atrial filling

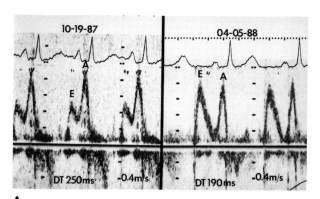

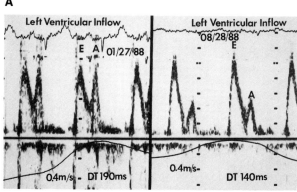

Fig. 11-3. Serial mitral inflow Doppler velocities from two patients with cardiac amyloidosis. **A.** The initial Doppler (left) showed a relaxation abnormality with decreased E, increased A, and prolonged deceleration time (DT). Six months later (right), it became pseudonormalized with progressive cardiac amyloidosis. **B.** In another patient, the initial study (left) showed a DT of 190 msec with normal E and A. Seven months later (right), the mitral inflow became typical of a restrictive pattern (increased E, decreased A, and decreased DT), which indicates that the initial Doppler pattern was of a "pseudonormalized" inflow. (From AL Klein et al. Serial Doppler echocardiographic follow-up of left ventricular diastolic function in cardiac amyloidosis. *J Am Coll Cardiol* 1990;16:1135–1141.)

pressure before becoming frankly restrictive. It has been demonstrated that deceleration time (DT) is one of the most important prognostic variables in cardiac amyloidosis [7]. The shorter the DT, the poorer the prognosis. The average survival for patients with a DT of 150 msec or shorter was less than 1 year, compared to 3 years when the DT was longer than 150 msec (Fig. 11-4). Therefore, echocardiographic eval-

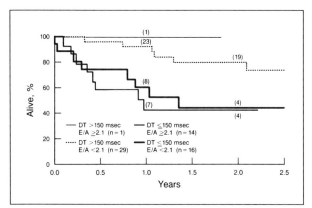

Fig. 11-4. Survival curve of patients with cardiac amyloidosis. The patients with a DT of 150 msec or lower had a 1-year mortality rate of 50%, whereas it was 90% when the DT was above 150 msec. (From AL Klein et al. Prognostic significance of Doppler measures of diastolic function in cardiac amyloidosis. *Circulation* 1991;83:808–816.)

uation of cardiac amyloidosis provides comprehensive morphologic, functional (systolic and diastolic), and prognostic information.

Carcinoid

Carcinoid heart disease is caused by a slow-growing metastatic carcinoid tumor, usually originating in the ileum. Cardiac involvement occurs almost exclusively with hepatic metastases and is caused by substances released by the tumor such as serotonin and bradykinin. Since the tumor substances are inactivated by the lung, the predominant cardiac involvement is on the right side, but it may involve the left side (7% of cases) most likely due to the patent foramen ovale which allows the passage of tumor substances from the right to the left atrium or due to pulmonary metastasis [9]. The predominant pathology of cardiac carcinoid is fibrosis of the cardiac valves and endocardium, especially the tricuspid and pulmonary valves [8, 9]. These valvular abnormalities produce characteristic thickening (fibrosis) and restricted motion of the valves that are responsible for severe tricuspid regurgitation, usually mild tricuspid stenosis, and varying degrees of pulmonary stenosis (Figs. 11-5 and 11-6). These morphologic changes

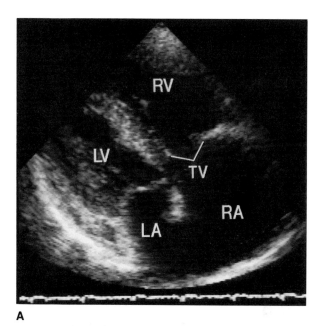

A

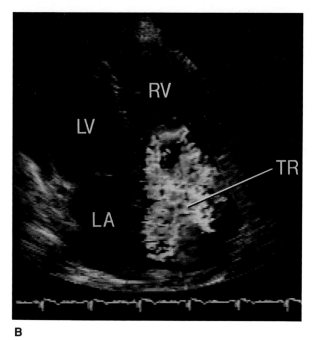

B

Fig. 11-5. 2D systolic frame of right ventricular inflow view showing carcinoid involvement of the tricuspid valve (TV). **A.** Anterior and septal tricuspid leaflets do not coapt due to retraction and thickening resulting in severe tricuspid regurgitation (TR). **B.** Color-flow imaging shows a severe tricuspid regurgitation jet filling the entire right atrial cavity, which is dilated. (From PA Pellikka et al. Carcinoid heart disease: clinical and echocardiographic spectrum in 74 patients. *Circulation* 1993;87:1188–1196.)

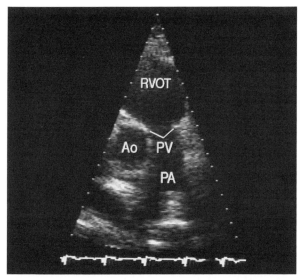

A

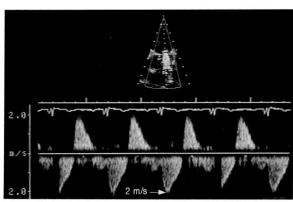

B

of carcinoid valvular involvement are readily detected by 2D echocardiography. The tricuspid valve is thickened and retracted with limited mobility, and coaptation is incomplete, resulting in severe tricuspid regurgitation. The severe tricuspid regurgitation produces a right ventricular volume overload pattern with an enlarged right ventricle and ventricular septal motion abnormalities. The pulmonary valve, also thickened and retracted, resulting in pulmonic stenosis, is occasionally difficult to image by the transthoracic approach. The transesophageal longitudinal-axis view of the right ventricular outflow tract may be needed to visualize the pulmonary valve. Characteristically, the wall thickness of the ventricles is normal in carcinoid heart disease, and carcinoid plaque over the endocardial walls in the right cardiac chambers may be seen by transesophageal echocardiographic (TEE) examination. Carcinoid may also produce a metastatic

Fig. 11-6.   A. Parasternal short-axis view at the pulmonary valve (PV) level showing carcinoid involvement of the pulmonary valve. The pulmonary valve annulus is narrowed and the valve is diminutive to the extent of being poorly visualized. **B.** Continuous-wave Doppler spectrum from the pulmonary valve shows mild pulmonary stenosis with a peak velocity of 2 m/sec and regurgitation signal with a short DT, consistent with severe pulmonary regurgitation. (From PA Pellikka et al. Carcinoid heart disease: clinical and echocardiographic spectrum in 74 patients. *Circulation* 1993;87:1188–1196.)

Fig. 11-7.   Myocardial metastasis (M) in the LV wall of a 61-year-old man who also had carcinoid involvement of the tricuspid and pulmonary valves. This was confirmed pathologically after removal. (From PA Pellikka et al. Carcinoid heart disease: clinical and echocardiographic spectrum in 74 patients. *Circulation* 1993;87:1188–1196.)

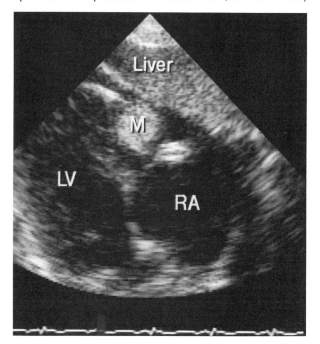

tumor embedded in the myocardium [8] (Fig. 11-7). 2D echocardiographic features of carcinoid heart disease are distinctive and readily distinguishable from other lesions producing right heart failure, such as Epstein's anomaly, right ventricular contusion, right ventricular infarct, tricuspid valve dysplasia, and severe tricuspid regurgitation due to intrinsic valvular abnormalities. Rarely, patients with excessive use of ergot may develop cardiac valvular lesions resembling carcinoid involvement [10].

Hemochromatosis

Idiopathic hemochromatosis is an autosomal recessive disease with an incidence of 2 to 3 per 1,000 population. It is characterized by large deposits of iron in the various organs including the heart, liver, testes, and pancreas. When the

heart is involved with hemochromatosis, the disease is usually in the advanced stage with multiorgan involvement. The severity of myocardial dysfunction is proportional to the amount of iron deposited in the myocardium. Myocardial deposit of excessive iron interferes with myocardial cellular function, resulting in LV dilatation and systolic dysfunction as seen in dilated cardiomyopathy, and progressive congestive heart failure is the most frequent cause of death in patients with hemochromatosis. Therefore, in patients who present with heart failure and features of dilated cardiomyopathy of unknown etiology, iron level, iron-binding capacity, and serum ferritin level should be determined. Typical 2D echocardiographic findings of cardiac hemochromatosis include mild LV dilatation, LV systolic dysfunction, normal wall thicknesses and cardiac valves, and biatrial enlargement [11] (Fig. 11-8). Cardiac chamber

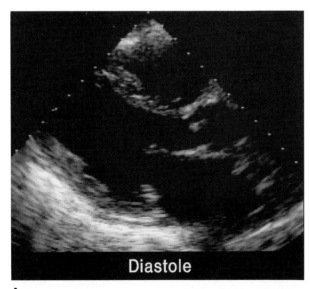

A

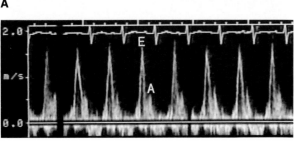

C

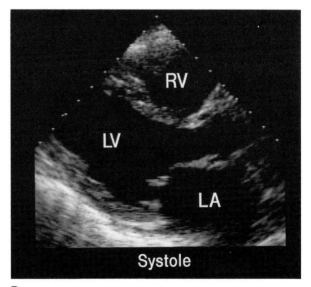

B

Fig. 11-8. 2D echocardiogram (parasternal long-axis view) of severe hemochromatosis of the heart. The features are similar to those of dilated cardiomyopathy. The LV cavity is mildly dilated and there is severe global systolic dysfunction with ejection fraction of 15% **(A, B).** Mitral diastolic filling demonstrates restrictive hemodynamics (increased E, decreased A, and DT of 90 msec) indicative of decreased compliance and increased left atrial pressure **(C).**

dilatation produces varying degrees of mitral and tricuspid valve regurgitation. When a patient presents with congestive heart failure, the LV diastolic filling pattern is usually restrictive (Fig. 11-8C) while the morphologic features are of dilated cardiomyopathy. These typical echocardiographic findings were found in 37% of patients with hemochromatosis seen at the Mayo Clinic [11] and most of the patients with the above echocardiographic findings of cardiac involvement died in 6 months. However, LV dysfunction can be reversed, sometimes completely, by chronic phlebotomies; therefore, serial echocardiographic examination is useful to monitor the response of LV function.

Hypereosinophilic Syndrome

Hypereosinophilic syndrome is defined as a persistent eosinophilia with more than 1500 eosinophils/mm^3 and evidence of organ involvement. Cardiac involvement is very common in hypereosinophilic syndrome and it involves both the right and left sides with endocardial thickening of the inflow areas and thrombotic-fibrotic obliteration of the ventricular apices. Typical echocardiographic features

include limited motion of the posterior mitral leaflet (resulting in mitral regurgitation of varying severity) along with thickening of the inferobasal LV wall, endocardial thrombotic-fibrotic lesion, and biapical obliteration by thrombus [12] (Fig. 11-9). The apical cavity obliteration and eosinophilic involvement of the endocardium decrease the ventricular compliance and limit ventricular diastolic filling, producing restrictive physiology on pulsed-wave Doppler echocardiography. Rarely, acute hypereosinophilic crisis produces diffuse myocarditis with ventricular cavity dilatation with a marked decrease in systolic function, and patients usually die from severe heart failure or uncontrollable ventricular arrhythmias.

Sarcoidosis

Sarcoidosis is a granulomatous disease of unknown etiology involving multiple organs. The most important manifestation of sarcoidosis is caused by pulmonary involvement, resulting in diffuse pulmonary fibrosis, right-side heart failure, and pulmonary hypertension. Cardiac involvement is uncommon, occurring in less than 20% of patients. Myocardium is involved by noncaseating granulomas, producing myo-

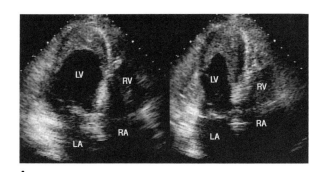
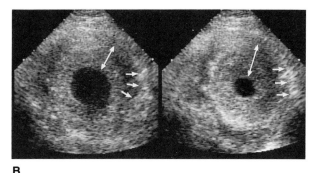

A   **B**

Fig. 11-9. Apical four-chamber **(A)** and short-axis **(B)** views in a patient with hypereosinophilic syndrome, showing apical obliteration due to deposits of thrombus and eosinophils. Underlying myocardial contractility is not impaired. Between diastolic (left) and systolic (right) frames, there is significant wall thickening with systole. In the short-axis view **(B)**, obliterative thrombus material is shown (←—→), and the endocardial segment is indicated by three arrows. This condition should be differentiated from apical hypertrophic cardiomyopathy in which the apical cavity is obliterated by the hypertrophied myocardium, whereas in the hypereosinophilic heart the apex is obliterated by thrombus-eosinophilic material.

cardial fibrosis and regional wall motion abnormalities. The fibrosis occurs predominantly at the mid and basal levels of the LV, although global involvement may occur. Thinning and aneurysmal formation do occur mainly at the basal inferior and lateral portions of the LV. Therefore, 2D echocardiographic features include a dilated LV with regional wall motion abnormalities, especially at the mid and basal levels of the LV [13]. Posterior basal aneurysm may be seen. These echocardiographic features were seen in 14% of the patients with sarcoidosis examined at the Mayo Clinic, and the symptoms of congestive heart failure were more common in the patients with the above-mentioned echocardiographic features [13]. Although angiotensin-converting enzyme (ACE) level is commonly used to diagnose sarcoidosis, most of the patients with echocardiographic features of cardiac involvement had a normal ACE level and noncaseating granulomas in the endomyocardial biopsy specimen. Therefore, a normal ACE level does not exclude active cardiac sarcoidosis and should not deter one from obtaining endomyocardial biopsy specimens to make the diagnosis.

Systemic Lupus Erythematosus

Lupus is a systemic disease characterized by the presence of antinuclear antibodies (ANAs). These antibodies produce immune complexes that cause inflammation of various organs. The most common cardiac involvement is pericarditis, found in more than two-thirds of patients, and detection of pericardial effusion by echocardiography is one of the diagnostic criteria for systemic lupus erythematosus (SLE). Despite the frequent presence of pericardial effusion, tamponade and constrictive pericarditis are uncommon. The myocardium may be involved by vasculitis, resulting in myocarditis, but significant LV systolic dysfunction is again rare. Another characteristic cardiac lesion of SLE is Libman-Sacks endocarditis with verrucous valvular lesion usually involving the mitral valve [14]. It is most commonly found on the basal portion of the mitral valve but can extend to the chordal structure or papillary muscles (Fig. 11-10). Aortic valve involvement with *Libman-Sacks endocarditis* is uncommon. These lesions are difficult to see on transtho-

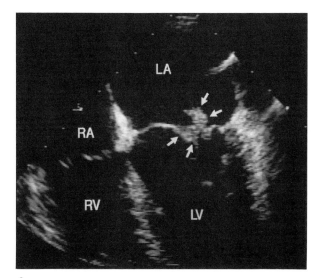
A

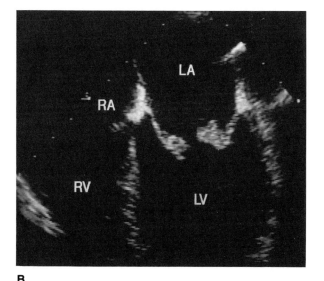
B

Fig. 11-10. Libman-Sacks endocarditis in a 36-year-old woman with SLE and no clinical evidence of bacterial endocarditis. Systolic **(A)** and diastolic **(B)** frames of the horizontal TEE view of the mitral valve show large verrucous vegetations *(arrows)*.

racic echocardiograms, but detection is enhanced by TEE. Metastatic tumors also involve cardiac valves, producing lesions similar to those seen in Libman-Sacks endocarditis. This is called *marantic endocarditis* and occurs most commonly with Hodgkin's disease and adenocarcinoma of the lung, pancreas, stomach, and colon.

Other Conditions

The heart is affected by many other systemic, rheumatic, endocrine, genetic, and infectious diseases. Pheochromocytoma and Friedreich's ataxia produce a concentric increase in LV wall thickness [15, 16]. *Friedreich's ataxia* is an autosomal recessive disease producing spinal cerebellar ataxia and 90% of the patients with this entity have cardiac involvement. For the most part they have 2D echocardiographic findings similar to hypertrophic cardiomyopathy although LV hypertrophy is more often concentric. Asymmetric septal hypertrophy is unusual and LV outflow tract obstruction is not common. In a minority of patients (7%), the LV may be dilated with decreased systolic function due to a diffuse interstitial fibrosis [16]. Most of the patients with *pheochromocytoma* have normal echocardiographic findings except for hyperdynamic systolic function but occasionally one does see concentric LV hypertrophy (20%) [15]. When a patient with pheochromocytoma develops catecholamine crisis, acute myocarditis may result with LV dilatation with decreased systolic function, which may be reversible on treatment of the pheochromocytoma.

Certain neuromuscular diseases also involve the myocardial segment, especially *Duchenne's dystrophy* involving the inferobasal area due to myocardial fibrosis. 2D echocardiographic findings of Duchenne's dystrophy are similar to those of inferior myocardial infarction. Patients with hypothyroidism or rarely hyperthyroidism may develop dilated cardiomyopathy, which resolves when the underlying endocrine abnormalities are corrected. Certain

chemicals have direct toxic effects on the myocardium, resulting in secondary dilated cardiomyopathy. These chemicals include alcohol, doxorubicin, and ipecac syrup (Emetin). The myocardial dysfunction may not be reversible when the chemical insult is withdrawn.

Cardiac involvement is frequent in patients with acquired immunodeficiency syndrome (AIDS) and manifests as dilated cardiomyopathy, pericardial effusion/tamponade, endocarditis due to opportunistic organisms, myocarditis, and/or metastatic cardiac neoplasm [17].

References

1. Siqueira-Filho AG, et al. M-mode and two-dimensional echocardiographic features in cardiac amyloidosis. *Circulation* 1981; 63:188–196.

2. Cueto-Garcia L, et al. Serial echocardiographic observations in patients with primary systemic amyloidosis: an introduction to the concept of early (asymptomatic) amyloid infiltration of the heart. *Mayo Clin Proc* 1984;59:589–597.

3. Olson LJ, et al. Cardiac involvement in glycogen storage disease III: morphologic and biochemical characterization with endomyocardial biopsy. *Am J Cardiol* 1984;53:980–981.

4. Oh JK, et al. Dynamic left ventricular outflow tract obstruction in cardiac amyloidosis detected by continuous-wave Doppler echocardiography. *Am J Cardiol* 1987;59:1009–1010.

5. Klein AL, et al. Serial Doppler echocardiographic follow-up of left ventricular diastolic function in cardiac amyloidosis. *J Am Coll Cardiol* 1990;16:1135–1141.

6. Klein AL, et al. Doppler characterization of left ventricular diastolic function in cardiac amyloidosis. *J Am Coll Cardiol* 1989;13: 1017–1026.

7. Klein AL, et al. Prognostic significance of Doppler measurements of diastolic function in cardiac amyloidosis: a Doppler echocardiography study. *Circulation* 1991;83:808–816.

8. Pellikka PA, et al. Carcinoid heart disease: clinical and echocardiographic spectrum in 74 patients. *Circulation* 1993;87:1188–1196.

9. Callahan JA, et al. Echocardiographic features

of carcinoid heart disease. *Am J Cardiol* 1982;50:762–768.

10. Redfield MM, et al. Valve disease associated with ergot alkaloid use: Echocardiographic and pathologic correlations. *Ann Intern Med* 1992;117:50–52.

11. Olson LJ, Baldus WP, Tajik AJ. Echocardiographic features of idiopathic hemochromatosis. *Am J Cardiol* 1987;60:885–889.

12. Gottdiener JS, et al. Two-dimensional echocardiographic assessment of the idiopathic hypereosinophilic syndrome: anatomic basis of mitral regurgitation and peripheral embolization. *Circulation* 1983;67:572–578.

13. Burstow D, et al. Two-dimensional echocardi-ographic findings in systemic sarcoidosis. *Am J Cardiol* 1989;63:478–482.

14. Libman E, Sacks B. A hitherto undescribed form of valvular and mitral endocarditis. *Arch Intern Med* 1924;33:701–737.

15. Shub C, et al. Dynamic left ventricular outflow tract obstruction associated with pheochromocytoma. *Am Heart J* 1981;102:286–290.

16. Alboliras ET, et al. Spectrum of cardiac involvement in Friedreich's ataxia: clinical, electrocardiographic and echocardiographic observations. *Am J Cardiol* 1986;58:518–524.

17. Francis CK. Cardiac involvement in AIDS. *Curr Probl Cardiol* 1990;15:571–632.

12

Pericardial Diseases

Detection of pericardial effusion was one of the most exciting initial clinical applications of cardiac ultrasound. Today echocardiography continues to play a significant role in the diagnosis and management of pericardial disease [1–4]: With M-mode, 2D sector images, and Doppler, it is the gold standard in detecting pericardial effusion and determining its hemodynamic significance. When pericardial effusion needs to be drained, pericardiocentesis can be performed safely under the guidance of 2D echocardiography. Although it is often difficult to establish a definite diagnosis of constrictive pericarditis with 2D echocardiography alone, the characteristic respiratory variations in Doppler flow velocities are present in most patients with constriction. Furthermore, congenitally absent pericardium and pericardial cyst are reliably diagnosed by 2D echocardiography. Transesophageal imaging may be required to provide better assessment of pericardial thickness and other structural abnormalities of the pericardium.

Pericardial Effusion/ Tamponade

When the potential pericardial space is filled with fluid or blood, it is detected as an "echo-free" space. When the amount of effusion is greater than 25 ml, echo-free space persists throughout the cardiac cycle. A smaller amount of pericardial effusion may be detected as a posterior echo-free space present only during the systolic phase. As pericardial effusion increases, movement of the parietal pericardium decreases. When there is a massive amount of pericardial effusion, the heart may have a "swinging" motion in the pericardial cavity (Fig. 12-1), which is responsible for the electrocardiographic manifestation of cardiac tamponade, *electrical alternans.* However, the swinging motion is not always present in cardiac tamponade. Various M-mode and 2D echocardiographic signs in this life-threatening condition have been reported [5–7]: decreased excursion and E-F slope of the mitral valve, exaggerated late diastolic posterior motion of the right ventricular wall at end-expiration, early diastolic collapse of the right ventricle (Fig. 12-2A, B), late diastolic right atrial inversion (Fig. 12-2C), and the plethora of the inferior vena cava with blunted respiratory changes. In the case of acute myocardial rupture, one may see clotted blood in the pericardial sac, highly suggestive of hemopericardium (Fig. 12-3). When there is air in the pericardial sac (pneumopericardium) due to esophageal perforation, cardiac imaging (both transthoracic and transesophageal) is very difficult since ultrasound does not penetrate air well.

Recently, Doppler echocardiography features were reported to be more sensitive than the aforementioned signs [8, 9]. The Doppler findings of cardiac tamponade are based on the following characteristic respiratory variations in intrathoracic and intracardiac hemodynamics (Fig. 12-4). Normally, intrapericardial pressure (hence, left ventricular [LV] diastolic

pressure) and intrathoracic pressure decrease by the same degree during inspiration, but in cardiac tamponade, intrapericardial pressure decreases substantially less than the intrathoracic pressure. Therefore, the LV filling pressure gradient (from pulmonary wedge pressure to the LV diastolic pressure, depicted as the shaded area in Fig. 12-4) decreases with inspiration. With the decreased LV filling, the mitral valve opening is delayed, lengthening the isovolumic relaxation time (IVRT) and decreasing mitral E velocity. Due to the ventricular coupling in cardiac tamponade with relatively fixed cardiac volume, reciprocal changes occur in the right side of the cardiac chambers (Fig. 12-5).

Pulmonary and hepatic venous flow velocities reflect similar respiratory flow changes of the mitral and tricuspid valves, respectively: inspiratory decrease and expiratory increase in the pulmonary vein diastolic forward flow, and increase in expiratory reversal of hepatic venous flow [10] (Fig. 12-6).

Echo-guided Pericardiocentesis

The most effective treatment for cardiac tamponade is removal of pericardial fluid. Although pericardiocentesis is "lifesaving," blind percutaneous attempt carries a high complication rate including pneumothorax and puncture of the cardiac walls. 2D echocardiography can guide pericardiocentesis by locating the optimal site of puncture, determining the depth of the pericardial effusion and the distance from the puncture site to the effusion, and monitoring the results of the pericardiocentesis [10–13] (Fig. 12-7). At the Mayo Clinic, most pericardiocentesis procedures are performed by an echocardiographer with 2D echocardiographic guidance. More than 500 2D echo-guided pericardiocentesis procedures have been performed without any mortality.

Constrictive Pericarditis

M-mode and 2D echocardiographic features of constrictive pericarditis include thickened

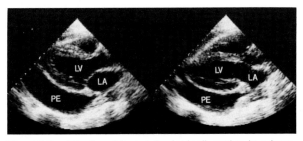

Fig. 12-1. The heart has a "swinging" motion in a large amount of pericardial effusion (PE), which is an ominous sign of cardiac tamponade. When the left ventricular (LV) cavity is close to the surface (left), the QRS voltage increases on the electrocardiogram, whereas it decreases when the LV swings away from the surface (right), producing total electrical alternans.

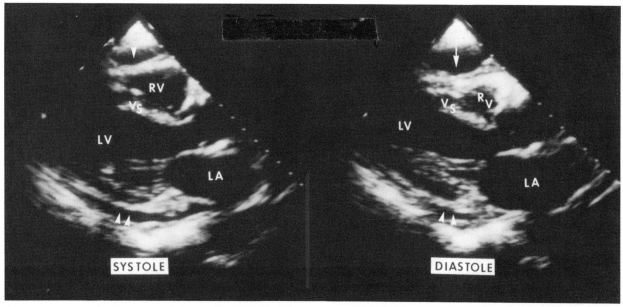

A

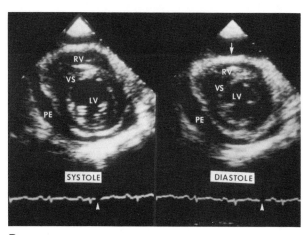

B

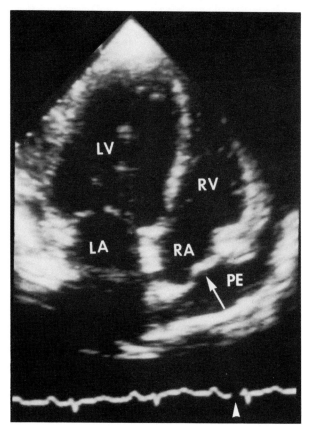

C

Fig. 12-2. Parasternal long- **(A)** and short-axis **(B)** views of a patient with tamponade during systole and diastole. The pericardial effusion *(double arrowhead;* PE) appears small in the long axis and moderate in the short axis during systole. But during early diastole, the right ventricular (RV) free wall collapses *(arrow).* Apical four-chamber view **(C)** demonstrating late diastolic *(arrowhead* on the ECG) collapse of the right atrial wall *(arrow).* This sign is sensitive, but not specific for tamponade. When right atrial inversion is longer than a third of the R-R interval, it is specific for hemodynamically significant pericardial effusion.

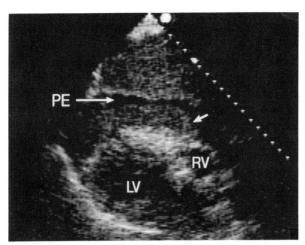

Fig. 12-3. Subcostal echocardiogram of a patient with cardiogenic shock after acute myocardial infarction. In addition to pericardial effusion (PE), there is an echodense structure *(small arrow)* along the ventricular walls, which indicates clot formation. Urgent pericardiocentesis was performed to temporize the clinical situation, then the patient underwent an emergency operation and survived. (Courtesy of S. Hayes, M.D.)

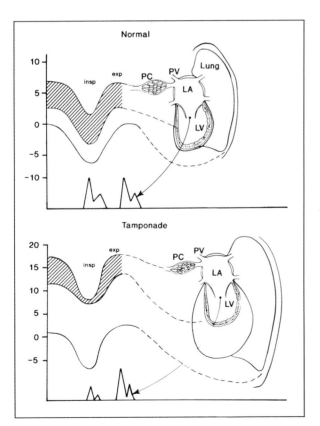

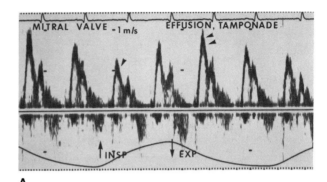

Fig. 12-5. Typical pulsed-wave Doppler pattern of tamponade recorded with nasal respirometer.
A. Mitral inflow velocity decreases *(arrowhead)* after inspiration (INSP) and increases *(double arrowhead)* after expiration (EXP).
B. Tricuspid inflow velocity has the opposite changes. E velocity increases *(double arrowhead)* after inspiration and decreases *(arrowhead)* after expiration. (From JK Oh et al. Transient constrictive pericarditis. *Mayo Clin Proc* [in press].)

◀ **Fig. 12-4.** Schematic drawing of intrathoracic and intracardiac pressure changes with respiration in normal and tamponade physiology. The shaded area indicates LV filling pressure gradients (difference between pulmonary capillary wedge pressure and LV diastolic pressure). At the bottom of each drawing, a schematic mitral inflow Doppler velocity profile is shown to reflect LV diastolic filling. In tamponade, there is a reduction in LV filling after inspiration (insp) due to a smaller pressure decrease in the pericardium and LV compared to pressure change in the pulmonary capillaries (PC). LV filling is restored after expiration (exp). (Modified from JT Sharp et al. Hemodynamics during induced cardiac tamponade in man. *Am J Med* 1960;29:640–646.)

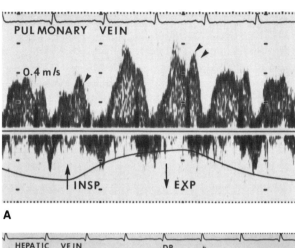

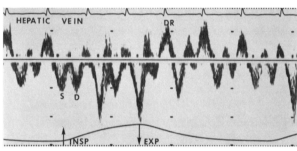

Fig. 12-6. Pulmonary vein and hepatic vein Doppler patterns of tamponade. **A.** Diastolic forward pulmonary venous flow decreases *(arrowhead)* after inspiration (INSP) and increases *(double arrowhead)* after expiration (EXP) **B.** The hepatic vein has a significant reduction in diastolic forward flow and an increase in diastolic reversals (DR) after expiration. (From JK Oh et al. Transient constrictive pericarditis. *Mayo Clin Proc* [in press].)

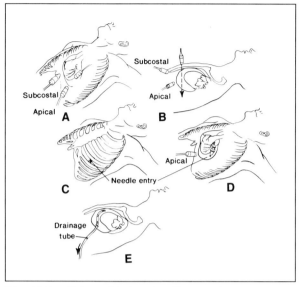

Fig. 12-7. Echo-guided pericardiocentesis.

Step 1. Locate an area on the chest or subcostal region from where the largest amount of pericardial effusion could be visualized, and mark (A–C).

Step 2. Determine the depth of effusion from the marked position and the optimal angulation.

Step 3. After sterile preparation and local anesthesia, perform pericardiocentesis (D).

Step 4. When in doubt about the location of the needle, inject saline solution through the needle and image from a remote site to locate the bubbles.

Step 5. Monitor the completeness of the pericardiocentesis by repeated echocardiography.

Step 6. Place a 6F or 7F pigtail catheter in the pericardial space to minimize reaccumulation (E).

Step 7. Drain any residual or reaccumulated fluid and flush the pigtail catheter with 5 to 10 ml of heparinized saline solution every 4 to 6 hours. If there is no reaccumulation of pericardial fluid in 2 to 3 days by repeated echocardiographic examination, the pigtail catheter can be removed. Always send pericardial fluid for cell counts, glucose and protein measurements, culture, and cytology. (From JA Callahan et al. Pericardiocentesis assisted by two-dimensional echocardiography. *J Thorac Cardiovasc Surg* 1983;85:877–879.)

pericardium, abnormal ventricular septal motion, flattening of LV posterior wall during diastole, respiratory variation in ventricular size, and dilated inferior vena cava [14–18] (Fig. 12-8), but these findings are not sensitive or specific. Recently, Doppler features of constriction, quite distinct from the Doppler features of restrictive hemodynamics, were reported by Hatle and coauthors [19]. Although the underlying pathologic mechanism is different from that of cardiac tamponade, hemodynamic events in constriction in terms of respiratory variation during left and right ventricular filling are similar to those of tamponade. The thickened pericardial barrier prevents full transmission of intrathoracic pressure changes with respiration to the pericardial and intracardiac cavity, creating respiratory variations in the left-side filling pressure gradient (pressure difference between pulmonary vein and left atrium). Therefore, the mitral inflow and the pulmonary venous flow velocities decrease im-

mediately after the onset of inspiration and increase with expiration [19–21] (Fig. 12-9). Reciprocal changes occur in the tricuspid valve and the hepatic venous flow velocities due to the relatively fixed cardiac volume in constriction. With decreased filling to the right cardiac chambers on expiration, there are exaggerated diastolic flow reversals and decreased diastolic forward flow in the hepatic vein with the onset

Fig. 12-8. Typical M-mode echocardiogram of constrictive pericarditis with the following characteristic findings: (1) Pericardial (P) thickness is increased. (2) Septal motion is abnormal; septum moves toward the LV with inspiration and toward the RV with expiration. (3) LV posterior wall is flattened during diastole. (4) During respiration there is variation in the ventricular size: LV end-diastolic dimension is smaller with inspiration (INSP; ED$_i$) than with expiration (EXP; ED$_e$). (From JK Oh et al. Transient constrictive pericarditis. *Mayo Clin Proc* [in press].)

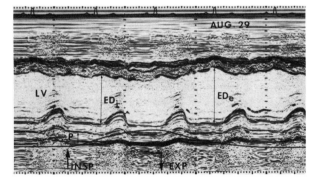

Fig. 12-9. Recording of simultaneous pulmonary vein (PV) Doppler via transesophageal study and intracardiac pressures from the LV and pulmonary capillary wedge (PCWP). Respirometer recording is also displayed with upward deflection for inspiration (INSP) and downward deflection for expiration (EXP). The PCWP is 35 mm Hg at end-diastole. At early diastole, pulmonary capillary wedge pressure is much higher after expiration than after inspiration, whereas respiratory variation in LV diastolic pressure (LVDP) is only slight. Hence, the pressure gradient between the pulmonary capillary wedge and LV diastolic pressures is reduced after inspiration and increased after expiration. The respiratory variation in LV filling gradient is reflected in diastolic pulmonary vein forward flow Doppler velocity (0.2 m/sec with inspiration and 0.6 m/sec with expiration). The marked increase in pulmonary vein diastolic foward flow velocity is indicated by an arrow. The variation in pulmonary vein systolic forward flow velocities is not as marked. (Modified from JK Oh et al. Diagnostic accuracy of Doppler echocardiography in constrictive pericarditis. *J Am Coll Cardiol* [in press].)

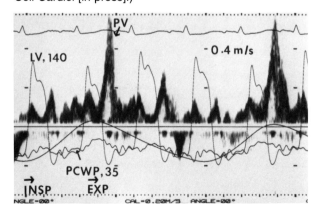

of expiration. In contrast, hepatic vein flow reversals are more prominent with inspiration in restrictive hemodynamics. It is, however, not unusual to see significant diastolic flow reversals in hepatic vein Doppler during both inspiration and expiration in patients with advanced constriction or combined constriction and restriction. The deceleration time (DT) of the early filling wave (E) of the mitral and tricuspid valves may or may not be shortened in constriction but is always shortened in restriction. The Doppler features of constriction and restriction are summarized in Figure 12-10, and representative Doppler spectra of constrictive pericarditis are shown in Figure 12-11. Table 12-1 shows Doppler velocity values obtained from 25 patients with constrictive pericarditis.

Fig. 12-10. Schematic drawing of Doppler velocities from mitral inflow (MV), tricuspid inflow valve (TV), and hepatic vein (HV) along with electrocardiographic (ECG) and respirometer recordings (Resp) indicating inspiration (i) and expiration (e).

Normal
Mitral inflow
  a. No (≤ 10%) respiratory variation in E
  b. DT of 160 msec or more
Tricuspid inflow
  a. Mild (≤ 15%) respiratory variation in E
  b. DT of 160 msec or more
Hepatic vein
  a. Systolic forward (S) flow greater than diastolic forward (D) flow (in sinus rhythm)
  b. Systolic forward flow less than diastolic forward flow (in atrial fibrillation)
  c. Slight increase in systolic (SR) and diastolic reversals (DR) with expiration

Constriction
Mitral inflow
  a. Inspiratory E less than expiratory E (≥ 25% change)
  b. DT, not always, but usually shortened (≤ 160 msec)
Tricuspid inflow
  a. Inspiratory E greater than expiratory E (≥ 40% change)
  b. DT usually shortened (≤ 160 msec)
Hepatic vein
  a. Decreased diastolic forward flow with expiration
  b. Marked decrease in diastolic forward flow and increase in diastolic flow reversals with expiration

Constriction is usually diagnosed on the basis of changes in mitral inflow and hepatic vein flow velocity with respiration. When mitral inflow is difficult to obtain, pulmonary vein diastolic forward flow velocity changes of 25% or more with respiration are used to represent respiratory variation in LV filling. Pulmonary vein Doppler may be obtained by transesophageal echocardiography (see Fig. 12-9).

Restriction
Mitral inflow
  a. No respiratory variation of E velocity
  b. Increased E velocity (usually ≥ 1.0 m/sec)
  c. Decreased A velocity (usually ≤ 0.5 m/sec)
  d. Increased E/A ratio (≥ 2.0)
  e. Shortened DT of E (≤ 160 msec)
Tricuspid inflow
  a. Mild respiratory variation (≤ 15%) in E velocity
  b. Increased E/A ratio (≥ 2.0)
  c. Shortened DT of E (≤ 160 msec)
Hepatic vein
  a. Systolic forward flow (S) less than diastolic forward flow (D)
  b. Increase in systolic and diastolic flow reversals with inspiration

(Modified from JK Oh et al. Diagnostic accuracy of Doppler echocardiography in constrictive pericarditis. *J Am Coll Cardiol* [in press].)

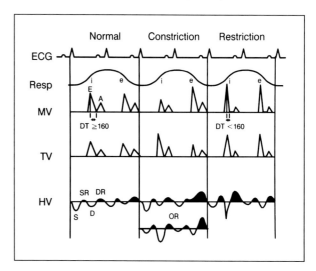

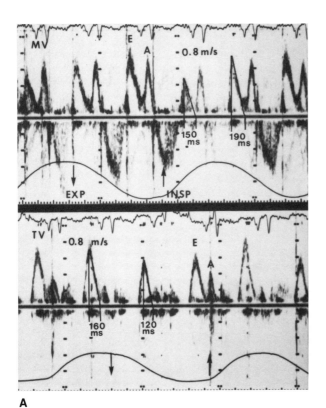

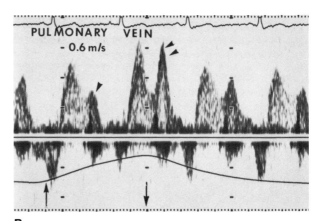

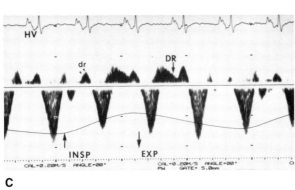

Fig. 12-11. Representative Doppler pattern of constrictive pericarditis. **A.** Mitral (MV) and tricuspid (TV) inflow Doppler velocities. Mitral E velocity is decreased after the onset of inspiration (INSP, 0.5 m/sec) and is increased after expiration (EXP, 0.8 m/sec). DT is shorter with inspiration (150 msec) than after expiration (190 msec). Opposite changes are present in tricuspid inflow Doppler velocities. **B.** Pulmonary venous Doppler velocities demonstrating decreased diastolic forward flow *(arrowhead)* after inspiration (↑) and increased diastolic forward flow *(double arrowhead)* after expiration (↓). **C.** Hepatic vein (HV) flow velocities demonstrating increased diastolic reversal flow (DR) after expiration (EXP) compared to inspiratory diastolic reversals (dr). However, diastolic flow reversals appear prominent even at end-inspiration due to slight time lag between the actual onset of expiration and its recording by respirometer. It is preferable to analyze cardiac cycles with the entire diastole immediately after the onset of inspiration or expiration. (From JK Oh et al. Diagnostic accuracy of Doppler echocardiography in constrictive pericarditis. *J Am Coll Cardiol* [in press]; and from JK Oh et al. Transient constrictive pericarditis. *Mayo Clin Proc* [in press].)

Congenitally Absent Pericardium

This defect usually involves the left side of the pericardium and is more frequent in males. Due to the marked shift of the cardiac chambers to the left (Fig. 12-12), the congenitally absent pericardium mimics the right ventricular volume overload pattern [22, 23]. Due to the pericardial defect, cardiac motion is exag-

gerated, especially the posterior wall of the LV, and also the entire cardiac structure is shifted to the left; hence, the right ventricular cavity is more prominent and the ventricular septal motion becomes abnormal. This entity should be kept in mind as a differential diagnosis of right ventricular volume overload. This condition is also associated with a high incidence of atrial septal defect, bicuspid aortic valve, and bronchogenic cysts.

Pericardial Cyst

Pericardial cyst is typically a benign structural abnormality of the pericardium that is usually detected as an incidental mass lesion on chest x-ray films. Its most frequent location is at the right costophrenic angle, but it is also found at the left costophrenic angle, hilum, and superior mediastinum. It needs to be differentiated from malignant tumors, cardiac chamber enlargement, and diaphragmatic hernia. 2D echocardiography is useful in differentiating pericardial cyst from other solid structures since cyst, filled with clear fluid, is shown as an echo-free structure (Fig. 12-13).

Pericardial Effusion Versus Pleural Effusion

Pericardial effusion is usually circumferentially located. If there is an echo-free space anteriorly alone, it is more likely an epicardial fat pad than pericardial effusion. Posteriorly, pericardial effusion is located anterior to the descending thoracic aorta, whereas pleural effusion is present posterior to the aorta (Fig. 12-14). 2D ultrasound imaging is also helpful in thoracentesis to locate an optimal puncture site (Fig. 12-15).

Transesophageal Echocardiography

When transthoracic echocardiography is not adequate to obtain satisfactory imaging of the pericardium and hemodynamic assessment of ventricular filling, transesophageal echocardiography should be considered. Hemodynamically compromising loculated pericardial

Table 12-1. Data from 25 patients with constriction

	Inspiration	Expiration	% Change
Mitral valve Doppler velocities			
E (m/sec)	0.55 ± 0.19	0.85 ± 0.26	55
A (m/sec)	0.41 ± 0.16	0.53 ± 0.18	29
E/A ratio	1.46 ± 0.71	1.62 ± 0.52	—
DT (msec)	146 ± 34	155 ± 41	—
Tricuspid valve Doppler velocities			
E (m/sec)	0.65 ± 0.15	0.42 ± 0.13	55
A (m/sec)	0.40 ± 0.15	0.31 ± 0.11	29
E/A ratio	2.03 ± 0.97	1.60 ± 0.80	—
DT (msec)	142 ± 31	142 ± 34	—
Hepatic vein Doppler velocities (m/sec)			
S	0.29	0.21	—
D	0.35	0.20	—
SR	−0.05	−0.14	—
DR	−0.14	−0.31	—

DT = deceleration time; S = systolic forward flow; D = diastolic forward flow; SR = systolic reversals; DR = diastolic reversals. Source: From JK Oh et al. Diagnostic accuracy of Doppler echocardiography in constrictive pericarditis. *J Am Coll Cardiol* [in press].

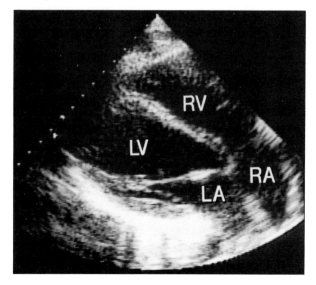

Fig. 12-12. 2D still-frame obtained from the normal apical position (left fifth intercostal space at the midclavicular line) in a patient with a congenitally absent pericardium. Due to leftward shift of the heart, the right ventricle (RV) is at the center of the apical image, rather than the LV apex; this is often confused with right ventricular volume overload. This patient underwent cardiac catheterization elsewhere to evaluate an atrial septal defect, which showed no shunt prior to this evaluation.

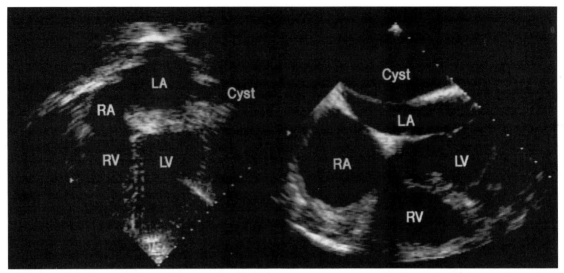

Fig. 12-13. Transthoracic and transesophageal echocardiographic images of a pericardial cyst. Apex-down apical four-chamber view (left) showing a large echo-free cystic structure next to the left atrium (LA) and LV. Transverse transesophageal four-chamber view (right) showing a large pericardial cyst compressing the left atrial posterior wall.

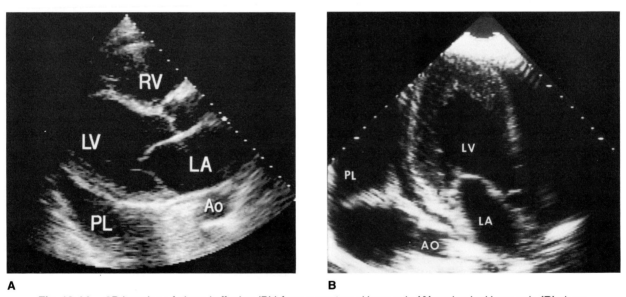

A   B

Fig. 12-14. 2D imaging of pleural effusion (PL) from parasternal long-axis **(A)** and apical long-axis **(B)** views. While pericardial effusion is present between the descending thoracic aorta (Ao, AO) and the posterior cardiac walls, pleural effusion (PL) is present behind the descending thoracic aorta.

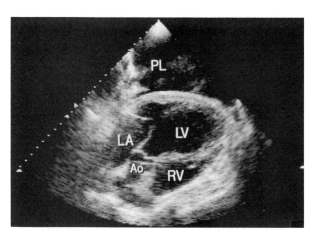

Fig. 12-15. 2D echocardiographic examination from the back, through pleural effusion (PL). This unique view may be the only available ultrasound window to the heart in some patients.

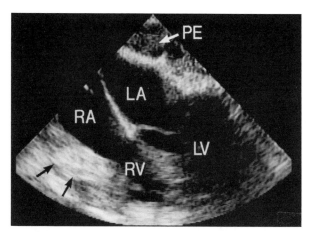

Fig. 12-16. Horizontal TEE four-chamber view showing loculated pericardial effusion (PE) and hematoma behind the left atrium (LA) in a hypotensive patient after coronary artery bypass surgery. Right cardiac chambers are also compressed by hematoma *(black arrows)*.

effusion may escape detection by transthoracic echo, and transesophageal echo has been especially helpful in postoperative patients with tamponade due to loculated hemopericardium (Fig. 12-16). It is also useful to obtain pulmonary venous flow pulsed-wave Doppler velocity with simultaneous respirometer in the evaluation of constrictive pericarditis (see Fig. 12-9). Transesophageal echocardiography may prove to be helpful in measuring the thickness of the pericardium and evaluating abnormal structures near the pericardium (e.g., pericardial cyst, metastatic tumor).

Clinical Impact

Echocardiography is usually one of the first diagnostic procedures in patients suspected to have a pericardial problem. It should be able to provide complete assessment of a pericardial effusion (how much and how significant), the best site for pericardiocentesis if necessary, and the diagnosis of constrictive pericarditis. In some patients, constrictive pericarditis is transient, usually following acute pericarditis [24]. Development and resolution of transient constrictive hemodynamics are readily assessed by serial 2D Doppler echocardiography [25]. Detection of respiratory filling and central venous flow velocities may provide the initial diagnostic clue to constrictive pericarditis, even in patients with no clinical suspicion of pericardial abnormality.

References

1. Feigenbaum H, Waldhausen JA, Hyde LP. Ultrasound diagnosis of pericardial effusion. *JAMA* 1965;191:711–714.

2. Feigenbaum H, Zaky A, Waldhausen JA. Use of ultrasound in the diagnosis of pericardial effusion. *Ann Intern Med* 1966;65:443–452.

3. Tajik AJ. Echocardiography in pericardial effusion. *Am J Med* 1977;63:29–39.

4. Lemire F, et al. Further echocardiographic observations in pericardial effusion. *Mayo Clin Proc* 1976;51:13–18.

5. Schiller NB, Botvinick EH. Right ventricular compression as a sign of cardiac tamponade: an analysis of echocardiographic ventricular dimensions and their clinical implications. *Circulation* 1977;56:774–779.

6. Armstrong WF, et al. Diastolic collapse of the right ventricle with cardiac tamponade: an

echocardiographic study. *Circulation* 1982; 65:1491–1496.

7. Gillam LD, et al. Hydrodynamic compression of the right atrium: a new echocardiographic sign of cardiac tamponade. *Circulation* 1983; 68:294–301.

8. Appleton CP, Hatle LK, Popp RL. Cardiac tamponade and pericardial effusion: respiratory variation in transvalvular flow velocities studied by Doppler echocardiography. *J Am Coll Cardiol* 1988;11:1020–1030.

9. Burstow DJ, et al. Cardiac tamponade: characteristic Doppler observations. *Mayo Clin Proc* 1989;64:312–324.

10. Callahan JA, Seward JB, Tajik AJ. Cardiac tamponade; pericardiocentesis directed by two-dimensional echocardiography. *Mayo Clin Proc* 1985;60:344–347.

11. Callahan JA, et al. Pericardiocentesis assisted by two-dimensional echocardiography. *J Thorac Cardiovasc Surg* 1983;85:877–879.

12. Callahan JA, et al. Two-dimensional echocardiographically guided pericardiocentesis: experience in 117 consecutive patients. *Am J Cardiol* 1985;55:476–479.

13. Kopecky SL, et al. Percutaneous pericardial catheter drainage: report of 42 consecutive cases. *Am J Cardiol* 1986;58:633–635.

14. Tei C, et al. Atrial systolic notch on the interventricular septal echogram: an echocardiographic sign of constrictive pericarditis. *J Am Coll Cardiol* 1983;1:907–912.

15. Engel PJ, et al. M-mode echocardiography in constrictive pericarditis. *J Am Coll Cardiol* 1985;6:471–474.

16. Gibson TC, et al. An echocardiographic study of the interventricular septum in constrictive pericarditis. *Br Heart J* 1978;38:738–743.

17. Pandian NG, et al. Diagnosis of constrictive pericarditis by two-dimensional echocardiography: studies in a new experimental model and in patients. *J Am Coll Cardiol* 1984; 4:1164–1173.

18. Candell-Riera J, et al. Echocardiographic features of the interventricular septum in chronic constrictive pericarditis. *Circulation* 1978;57:1154–1161.

19. Hatle LK, Appleton CP, Popp RL. Differentiation of constrictive pericarditis and restrictive cardiomyopathy by Doppler echocardiography. *Circulation* 1989;79:1–13.

20. Schiavone WA, Calafiore PA, Salcedo EE. Transesophageal Doppler echocardiographic demonstration of pulmonary venous flow velocity in restrictive cardiomyopathy and constrictive pericarditis. *Am J Cardiol* 1989; 63:1286–1288.

21. Oh JK, et al. Diagnostic accuracy of Doppler echocardiography in constrictive pericarditis. *J Am Coll Cardiol* [in press].

22. Nasser WK, et al. Congenital absence of the left pericardium. *Circulation* 1970;41:469–478.

23. Kansal S, Roitman D, Sheffield LT. Two-dimensional echocardiography of congenital absence of pericardium. *Am Heart J* 1985;109:912–915.

24. Sagrista-Sauleda J, et al. Transient cardiac constriction: An unrecognized pattern of evolution in effusive acute idiopathic pericarditis. *Am J Cardiol* 1987;59:961–966.

25. Oh JK, et al. Transient constrictive pericarditis: Diagnosis by two-dimensional Doppler echocardiography. *Mayo Clin Proc* [in press].

13

Pulmonary Hypertension

Determination of pulmonary artery pressure is a routine part of the echocardiographic examination since it reflects the severity of left-side heart diseases (e.g., mitral regurgitation, mitral stenosis, left ventricular [LV] systolic dysfunction), provides a prognosis, and is a measure of pulmonary hypertension. Although certain 2D echocardiographic features suggest pulmonary hypertension, Doppler echocardiography is the primary means to determine actual pulmonary pressures. Systolic and diastolic pulmonary artery pressures are determined from tricuspid and pulmonary regurgitation velocities, respectively. Transesophageal echocardiography (TEE) provides superb visualization of the main, right, and proximal portion of the left pulmonary arteries and hence is useful in the detection of pulmonary artery thromboembolism.

2D Echocardiography

Pulmonary hypertension is easily recognized when the following M-mode and 2D echocardiographic features are present [1–4] (Figs. 13-1 and 13-2):

1. Diminished or absent "a" (atrial) wave of the pulmonary valve
2. Midsystolic closure or notching of the pulmonary valve
3. Enlarged right cardiac chambers
4. D-shaped LV cavity due to the flattened ventricular septum

However, these features are not sensitive for pulmonary hypertension. They are qualitative and do not provide actual hemodynamic data.

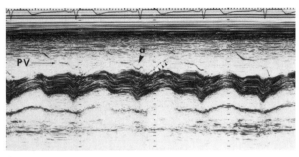

A

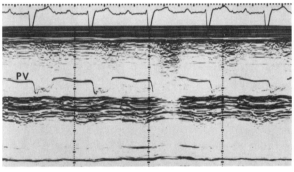

B

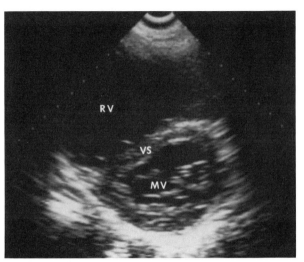

Fig. 13-2. Parasternal short-axis view demonstrating the D-shaped left ventricular cavity and enlarged right ventricular (RV) cavity in pulmonary hypertension. Similar appearances are present in right ventricular volume overload. However, flattening of the ventricular septum (VS) persists during the entire cardiac cycle in right ventricular and pulmonary artery pressure overload whereas it disappears during systole in right ventricular volume overload.

Fig. 13-1. **A.** Normal M-mode echocardiogram of the pulmonary valve (PV) with atrial wave (a) deflection. **B.** M-mode of the pulmonary valve in pulmonary hypertension. The atrial wave is absent and there is midsystolic closure of the valve, giving the shape of "W" during systole.

Doppler Echocardiography

Doppler echocardiography allows estimation of pulmonary artery pressure by measuring tricuspid regurgitation velocity, right ventricular outflow tract flow acceleration time, and pulmonary regurgitation velocity.

Tricuspid Regurgitation Velocity

Tricuspid regurgitation velocity reflects the pressure difference between the right ventricle and the right atrium [5–7] (Fig. 13-3). Therefore, systolic right ventricular pressure can be estimated by adding the right atrial pressure to the transtricuspid gradient derived from the tricuspid regurgitation velocity (i.e., transtricuspid pressure gradient = 4 × tricuspid regurgitation velocity^2). The right atrial pressure

can be estimated clinically by measuring jugular venous pressure or by the respiratory motion of the inferior vena cava (IVC) seen on 2D echocardiograms. When the diameter of the IVC decreases by 50% or more with inspiration (Fig. 13-3C), the right atrial pressure is usually less than 10 mm Hg, and those with less than 50% inspiratory collapse tend to have right atrial pressures of 10 mm Hg or higher [8]. However, correlation with cardiac catheterization values demonstrated that addition of an empiric constant (as right atrial pressure) yields a satisfactory value: 14 when jugular venous pressure is normal and 20 when jugular venous pressure is elevated [6]. In the absence of pulmonic stenosis, right ventricular systolic pressure is equal to pulmonary artery systolic pressure. The normal tricuspid regurgitation velocity is 2.0 to 2.5 m/sec. A higher velocity indicates either pulmonary hypertension or pulmonic stenosis (Fig. 13-4). Tricuspid

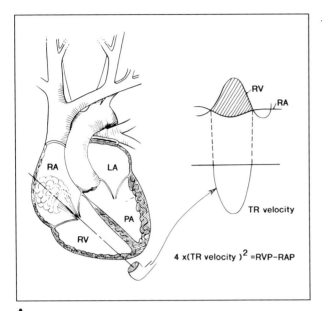

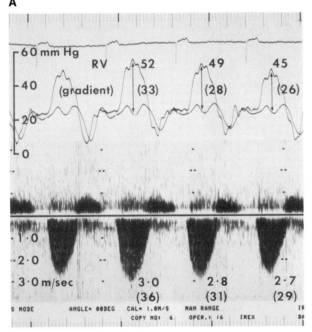

A

B

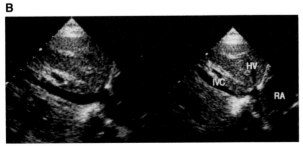

C

◀ **Fig. 13-3.** **A.** Schematic drawing of the right cardiac chambers to demonstrate how to measure systolic right ventricular (RV) pressure from tricuspid regurgitation (TR) velocity. 4 × (peak TR velocity)^2 represents the peak systolic transtricuspid pressure gradient from the right ventricle to the right atrium (RA). Therefore, systolic right ventricular pressure is estimated by adding right atrial pressure to the pressure gradient derived from tricuspid regurgitation velocity. RAP = right atrial pressure; RVP = right ventricular pressure. **B.** Simultaneous right ventricular–right atrial pressure tracings and tricuspid regurgitation velocity recording by continuous-wave Doppler. Pressure gradients (36, 31, and 29 mm Hg) derived from the peak Doppler velocities of the second, third, and fourth beats (3.0, 2.8, and 2.7 m/sec, respectively) are close to the catheter-derived right ventricular–right atrial gradients (33, 28, and 26 mm Hg). **C.** Subcostal view of the inferior vena cava (IVC), hepatic vein (HV), and right atrium (RA) during expiration (left) and inspiration (right) in a patient with normal right atrial pressure. The IVC collapses more than 50% with inspiration.

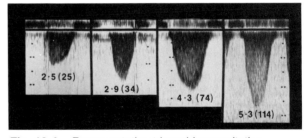

Fig. 13-4. Representative tricuspid regurgitation velocities. The numbers in parentheses are derived from peak velocities using the simplified Bernoulli equation.

regurgitation velocity may be lower than 2.0 m/sec when there is near equalization of pressures between the right atrium and the right ventricle with severe tricuspid regurgitation.

Tricuspid regurgitation is present in more than 75% of the normal adult population. When the tricuspid regurgitation jet is trivial and its continuous-wave Doppler spectrum is suboptimal, injection of agitated saline solution into an arm vein enhances the tricuspid regurgitation velocity signal.

Technical Caveat

Doppler velocity recordings from aortic stenosis and mitral regurgitation can mimic the tricuspid regurgitant jet. All three Doppler jets move away from the apex but they can be differentiated by angulation of the transducer, Doppler peak velocity, flow duration, and accompanying diastolic signal. Tricuspid regurgitation is most medially directed and tricuspid inflow (diastole) velocity is usually lower than 0.5 m/sec unless the tricuspid regurgitation is severe. Flow duration is shortest in aortic stenosis. Mitral regurgitant jet peak velocity is usually, but not always, higher than 4 m/sec and always higher than that of aortic stenosis in the same patient (see Chap. 7, Fig. 7-12).

Right Ventricular Outflow Tract Flow Acceleration Time

It has been demonstrated that the right ventricular outflow tract flow has a characteristic pattern as pulmonary artery pressure increases

Fig. 13-5. Right ventricular outflow tract flow velocity recordings by pulsed-wave Doppler. The sample volume is placed in the region of the pulmonary valve annulus. Normal flow pattern (left). Acceleration time (Ac T) is the time interval between the beginning of the flow and its peak velocity (between two arrows). It is 130 msec. Normal is 120 msec or higher. Flow velocity in pulmonary hypertension (right). The acceleration time is shortened to 40 msec.

Mean PA pressure = 79 − (0.45 × 40)
= 61 mm Hg

using Mahan's regression equation (where PA = pulmonary artery) [9].

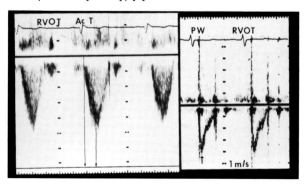

(Fig. 13-5). The acceleration phase becomes shorter with increased pulmonary artery pressure. Several investigators derived regression equations to estimate the mean pulmonary artery pressure (MPAP) from the right ventricular outflow tract acceleration time (AcT) [9, 10]:

Log_{10} (MPAP) = −0.0068 (AcT) + 2.1
(Kitabatake et al. [10])

MPAP = 79 − 0.45 (AcT)
(Mahan et al. [9])

Mahan's equation is simpler and preferred for estimating mean pulmonary artery pressure. It should be noted, however, that acceleration time is dependent on cardiac output and heart rate [11]. With increased cardiac output through the right cardiac chambers (as in atrial septal defect), acceleration time may be normal even when pulmonary artery pressure is elevated. If the heart rate is less than 60 or more than 100 beats/min, the acceleration time needs to be corrected for heart rate.

Pulmonary Regurgitation Velocity

The end-diastolic velocity of pulmonary regurgitation (PR) reflects the end-diastolic pressure gradient between the pulmonary artery and right ventricle (Figs. 13-6 and 13-7). At end-diastole, right ventricular pressure should be equal to right atrial pressure (RAP). Therefore,

PAEDP = 4 × PR EDV^2 + RAP

where PAEDP = pulmonary artery end-diastolic pressure, and
EDV = end-diastolic velocity.

The peak Doppler-determined pulmonary artery and right ventricular pressure gradient from the peak early diastolic pulmonary regurgitation is useful in estimating *mean* pulmonary artery pressure. According to Masuyama and colleagues [12] this pressure gradient approximates mean pulmonary artery pressure (PAP). Therefore,

Mean PAP = 4 × peak PR $velocity^2$

Utilizing the above multiple Doppler parameters, one can estimate systolic, diastolic, and

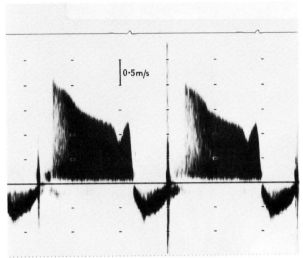

Fig. 13-6. Continuous-wave Doppler spectrum of pulmonary regurgitation velocity in a patient with normal pulmonary artery pressure. Since the pressure difference between the pulmonary artery (PA) and right ventricle (RV) is small during diastole, contraction of the right atrium (hence, increase in right atrial and RV pressures) decreases the PA-RV pressure gradient, resulting in a dip in pulmonary regurgitation velocity. When pulmonary pressure is high, usually right atrial contraction does not make a significant change in PA-RV pressure gradients; hence, there is no dip in the continuous-wave Doppler signal of pulmonary regurgitation.

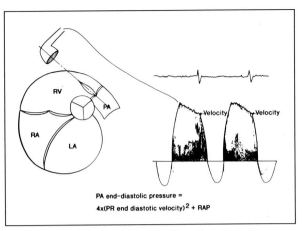

Fig. 13-7. Schematic drawing of continuous-wave Doppler interrogation of pulmonary regurgitation (PR) from the left parasternal window and the pulmonary regurgitation Doppler spectrum. If end-diastolic pulmonary regurgitation velocity is 3 m/sec, end-diastolic pulmonary artery pressure = 4×3^2 + 20 = 56 mm Hg, assuming a right atrial pressure (RAP) of 20 mm Hg.

mean pulmonary artery pressures (Fig. 13-8). Fortunately, tricuspid and pulmonary regurgitation are present in more than 85% of normal patients. The incidence is higher in patients with pulmonary hypertension. Tricuspid regurgitation velocity signal is enhanced by the injection of a contrast agent into the right atrium via a right-arm vein. Once echocardiography establishes that pulmonary artery pressure is elevated, its potential causes should be evaluated thoroughly by 2D Doppler and color-flow imaging to look for left-side failure (LV failure, mitral stenosis, mitral regurgitation, etc.), left-to-right shunt, atrial septal defect, ventricular septal defect, cor pulmonale, or pulmonary embolism.

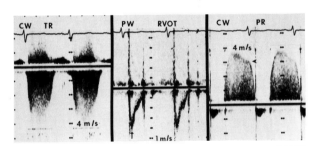

Fig. 13-8. Estimation of pulmonary artery pressure (PAP) from tricuspid regurgitation (TR) velocity, right ventricular outflow tract (RVOT) flow velocity acceleration time, and pulmonary regurgitation (PR) velocity.

Systolic PAP = $4 \times TR^2$ + RAP
$= 4 \times 4^2 + 20$
= 84 mm Hg,

where RAP = right atrial pressure.

Mean PAP = $79 - 0.45 \times 60$
= 52 mm Hg (Mahan)

Mean PAP = $4 \times$ peak PR^2
$= 4 \times 3.5^2$
= 49 mm Hg (Masuyama)

Cor Pulmonale and Pulmonary Embolism

Transthoracic Echocardiography

It may be difficult to distinguish acute cor pulmonale (i.e., pulmonary embolism) from chronic obstructive lung disease. Right ventricular hypertrophy is common in the chronic form. In both forms, the right chambers are dilated and there is 2D and Doppler evidence of right ventricular pressure overload as described above. The LV cavity is relatively small and hyperdynamic unless left-side cardiac pathology is also present. Figure 13-9 shows a still-frame from the subcostal 2D echocardiographic image in a patient who had hemodynamic collapse after orthopedic surgery. The right chambers are dilated and the ventricular septum is deviated to the left due to the increased right ventricular pressure from acute pulmonary embolism.

Occasionally, *thrombi in transit* are detected in the right cardiac chambers [13]. They are highly mobile and have the appearance of popcorn or a

Fig. 13-9. Subcostal 2D echocardiogram demonstrates dilated right ventricle (RV) and atrium (RA) with the ventricular septum (VS) deviated to the left in a patient who had cardiac arrest. When the dilated right chambers are detected in the setting of an acute hemodynamic event, pulmonary embolus should be considered. Right ventricular infarct is almost always associated with infarction of LV inferoseptal region.

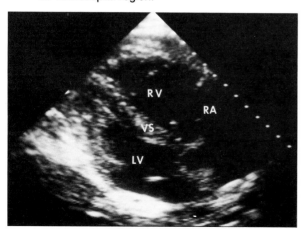

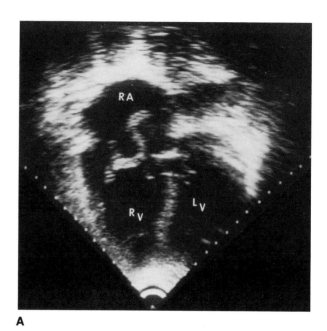

A

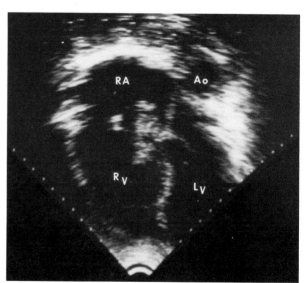

B

Fig. 13-10. Apex-down apical view demonstrating mobile thrombi in the right chamber. The shape of the mass changes due to its highly mobile nature. **A.** During systole, it has the shape of a snake. **B.** During diastole, it traverses the tricuspid valve, in the shape of popcorn.

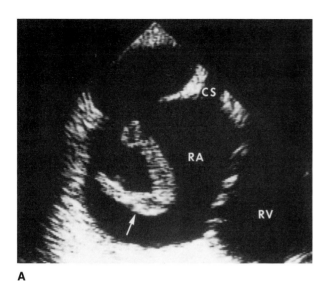

A

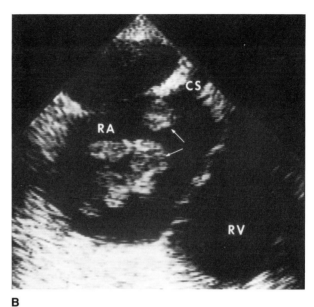

B

Fig. 13-11. Two separate frames **(A, B)** from horizontal TEE imaging of mobile right atrial (RA) thrombi in transit *(arrow in* **A;** *arrows* in **B**). The configuration of the thrombi is dynamic. In all patients with pulmonary embolism, varying degrees of this phenomenon probably exist. When the thrombi are large, the duration of their presence in the right chambers is longer than for smaller thrombi.

snake (Figs. 13-10 and 13-11). The mobile mass comes from en bloc embolization of venous thrombicast. Patients inevitably have pulmonary embolism and should be treated vigorously with anticoagulation agents, thrombolytic therapy, or even surgical removal. The same kind of thrombus material is responsible for paradoxical embolus when the foramen ovale is patent (see Chap. 14). At the Mayo Clinic, we have successfully treated mobile right atrial thrombi with the following thrombolytic regimen: streptokinase, 250,000 units by bolus, followed by 100,000 units/hour by continuous infusion. Right atrial thrombi usually dissolve within 24 to 48 hours. Therapeutic results are monitored by repeated echocardiographic examinations. When there are left atrial thrombi due to paradoxical emboli, thrombolytic therapy is contraindicated and surgical removal is the most effective treatment.

Transesophageal Echocardiography

The main pulmonary artery and its bifurcation to the right and the left branches are well seen by TEE. Thrombus in the proximal part of the pulmonary artery can be detected easily by

Fig. 13-12. TEE of pulmonary artery thrombus. Longitudinal-plane view (left) showing the right pulmonary artery (RPA) with a large thrombus *(arrow).* Horizontal-plane basal view (right) showing the right pulmonary artery with thrombus *(arrows).*

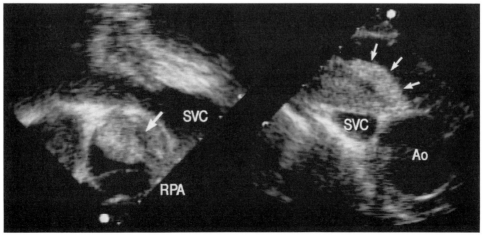

183

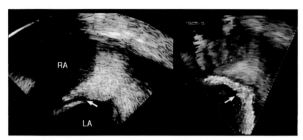

Fig. 13-13. Longitudinal TEE view of the patent foramen ovale *(arrow)* in a patient with right ventricular infarct and hypoxemia. Color-flow imaging shows a large right-to-left shunt *(arrow)* via the patent foramen ovale. It was surgically closed and oxygen saturation was normalized (from 60 to 96%).

TEE (Fig. 13-12). As shown in Figure 13-11, thrombi in transit in the right chambers are also seen easily by TEE. When transthoracic echocardiography is not able to characterize a right-side intracardiac mass, TEE should be considered. A recent study demonstrated that TEE detected central pulmonary thromboemboli in 35 (58%) of 60 patients with severe pulmonary embolism, mostly in the right pulmonary artery [14]. Although it is more difficult to visualize the left pulmonary artery by TEE, even with the longitudinal plane, the sensitivity of TEE in the detection of pulmonary thrombi is 97%, using pulmonary angiography, computed tomography, autopsy, or surgery as a reference standard.

When right atrial pressure is elevated, there may be significant right-to-left shunt via the patent foramen ovale, resulting in severe hypoxemia. Since the entire atrial septum is clearly seen by TEE, the patients with refractory hypoxemia in the setting of elevated right atrial pressure should undergo transesophageal contrast and color-flow echocardiographic examination (Fig. 13-13).

References

1. Weyman AE, et al. Echocardiographic patterns of pulmonic valve motion with pulmonary hypertension. *Circulation* 1974;50:905–910.

2. Goodman DJ, Harrison DC, Popp RL. Echocardiographic features of primary pulmonary hypertension. *Am J Cardiol* 1974;33:438–443.

3. Nanda NC, et al. Echocardiographic evaluation of pulmonary hypertension. *Circulation* 1974; 50:575–581.

4. Lew W, Karliner JS. Assessment of pulmonary valve echogram in normal subjects and in patients with pulmonary arterial hypertension. *Br Heart J* 1979;42:147–161.

5. Yock PG, Popp RL. Noninvasive estimation of right ventricular systolic pressure by Doppler ultrasound in patients with tricuspid regurgitation. *Circulation* 1984;70:657–662.

6. Currie, PJ, et al. Continuous wave Doppler determination of right ventricular pressure. A simultaneous Doppler catheterization study in 127 patients. *J Am Coll Cardiol* 1985;6:750–756.

7. Hatle L, Angelsen BAJ, Tromsdal A. Noninvasive estimation of pulmonary artery systolic pressure with Doppler ultrasound. *Br Heart J* 1981;45:157.

8. Kircher BJ, Himelman RB, Schiller NB. Noninvasive estimation of right atrial pressure from the inspiratory collapse of the inferior vena cava. *Am J Cardiol* 1990;66:493–496.

9. Mahan G, et al. Estimation of pulmonary artery pressure by pulsed Doppler echocardiography (Abstract). *Circulation* 1983;68(suppl III):367.

10. Kitabatake A, et al. Noninvasive evaluation of pulmonary hypertension by a pulsed Doppler technique. *Circulation* 1983;68:302–309.

11. Chan KL, et al. Comparison of three Doppler ultrasound methods in the prediction of pulmonary artery pressure. *J Am Coll Cardiol* 1987;9:549–554.

12. Masuyama T, et al. Continuous-wave Doppler echocardiographic detection of pulmonary regurgitation and its application to non-invasive estimation of pulmonary artery pressure. *Circulation* 1986;74:484.

13. Proano M, et al. Successful treatment of pulmonary embolism and associated mobile right atrial thrombus with use of a central thrombolytic infusion. *Mayo Clin Proc* 1988;63:1181–1185.

14. Wittlich N, et al. Detection of central pulmonary artery thromboemboli by transesophageal echocardiography in patients with severe pulmonary embolism. *J Am Soc Echocardiogr* 1992;5:515–524.

14

Tumors and Masses

Echocardiography is the diagnostic procedure of choice to evaluate an intracardiac mass or thrombus. Although incidence of intracardiac mass is relatively low, its detection has a direct therapeutic implication. By its appearance, location, and attachment site shown on 2D echocardiography, it is usually possible to differentiate various intracardiac masses with satisfactory confidence [1–8].

Primary Tumor

The most common primary cardiac tumor is a myxoma. It is usually located in the left atrium and attached to the atrial septum by a stalk. During diastole, it frequently protrudes through the mitral orifice, resulting in hemodynamic compromise similar to that of mitral stenosis (Figs. 14-1 and 14-2). A metastatic tumor to the lung and the pulmonary vein may give rise to a left atrial mass similar to a left atrial myxoma. This is occasionally seen with osteogenic sarcoma (chondrosarcoma) or melanoma (Fig. 14-3). The second most frequent location for myxoma is the right atrium (Fig. 14-4). However, the most common right atrial tumor is a rhabdomyoma in children with tuberous sclerosis (Fig. 14-5). It is usually multiple and also present in the right ventricle or right ventricular outflow tract and even in the pulmonary artery. The presence of rhabdomyoma can be diagnosed even before birth by fetal echocardiography. This tumor may regress spontaneously after birth. The most common tumor in the ventricle is fibroma. It is usually located in the ventricular free wall and well demarcated (Fig. 14-6). Occasionally, it

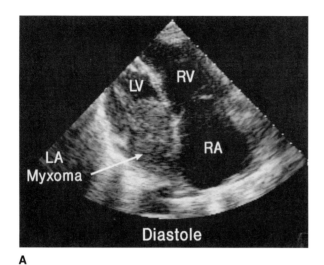
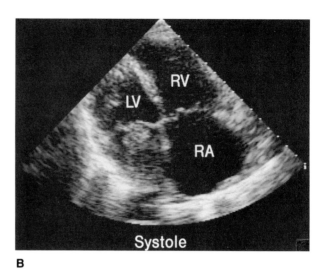

A   **B**

Fig. 14-1. Still-frames **(A, B)** from a transthoracic 2D echocardiogram of a typical left atrial (LA) myxoma. A large mass occupies most of the left atrial cavity and protrudes across the mitral valve during diastole. Attachment is difficult to see from this transthoracic examination.

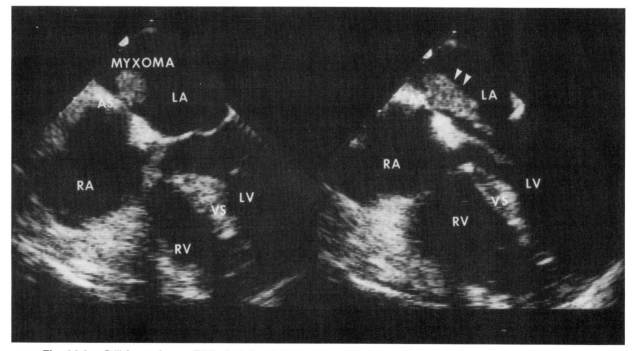

Fig. 14-2. Still-frame from a TEE of a left atrial myxoma, which is usually attached to the atrial septum (AS). During diastole (right), the tumor *(arrowheads)* protrudes across the mitral valve.

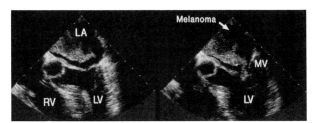

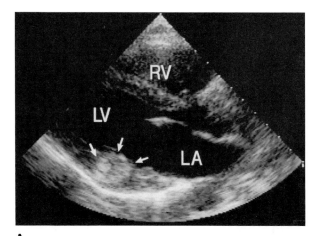

A

Fig. 14-3. TEE showing a large left atrial (LA) mass in a patient with metastatic melanoma. The mass protrudes across the mitral valve (MV) during diastole and could be traced back to the pulmonary vein.

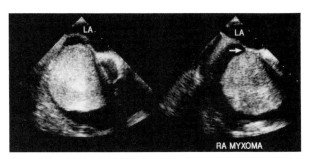

Fig. 14-4. TEE horizontal-plane view (left, systole; right, diastole) of a right atrial myxoma attached to the atrial septum *(arrow).* The myxoma occupies most of the right atrial cavity.

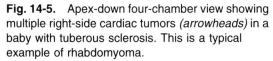

Fig. 14-5. Apex-down four-chamber view showing multiple right-side cardiac tumors *(arrowheads)* in a baby with tuberous sclerosis. This is a typical example of rhabdomyoma.

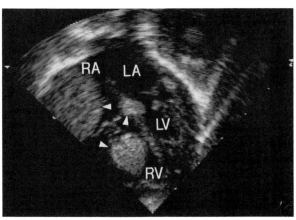

B

Fig. 14-6. Parasternal long- **(A)** and short-axis **(B)** views of a left ventricle (LV) fibroma *(arrows).* It is well circumscribed in the posterior free wall. It may cause ventricular arrhythmia but does not produce any hemodynamic abnormality.

grows into the ventricular cavity and interferes with ventricular filling (Fig. 14-7). The most frequent malignant primary cardiac tumors are hemangiosarcoma, rhabdomyosarcoma, and fibrosarcoma. Angiosarcoma occurs most commonly in the right atrium whereas rhabdomyosarcoma and fibrosarcoma can occur anywhere in the heart. The prognosis of malignant primary cardiac tumor is grim. The types of primary cardiac tumors observed at the Mayo Clinic from 1977 to 1983 are listed in Table 14-1.

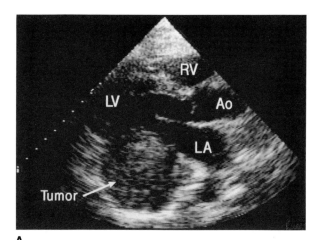

A

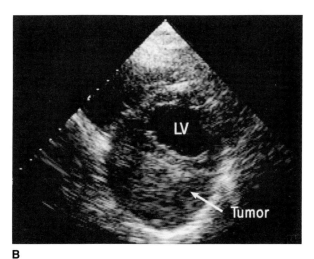

B

Fig. 14-7. A, B. A large LV fibroma (tumor) occupying a significant portion of the LV cavity. It interferes with LV filling at the mitral valve level.

Metastatic Tumor and Other Masses

Malignant tumors can metastasize to the heart. They are most frequently from the lung, breast, kidney, liver, lymphoma, melanoma (see Fig. 14-3), and osteogenic sarcoma. Hypernephroma and hepatoma tend to metastasize to the inferior vena cava and the right atrium contiguously. Whenever a right atrial mass is detected, the inferior vena cava should be care-

Table 14-1. Types of primary cardiac tumors (January 1977–June 1983)

Tumor type	No.
Myxoma	27 (72%)
Left atrium	23 (62%)
Right atrium	4 (10%)
Myxosarcoma (left atrium)	1 (3%)
Hemangiosarcoma (right atrium)	1 (3%)
Ventricular fibroma	3 (8%)
Papillary fibroelastoma	5 (14%)
All tumors	37

Source: Modified from FE Fyke III et al. Primary cardiac tumors: experience with 30 consecutive patients since the introduction of two-dimensional echocardiography. *J Am Coll Cardiol* 1985;5:1465–1473.

fully scanned. The right atrium also harbors various normal and abnormal structures that appear as a mass on 2D echocardiography. Among them are the eustachian valve, a pacemaker wire, a balloon or central-line catheter, and thrombus. Each structure, however, has characteristic features, and careful examination should be able to differentiate one entity from the others. Thrombi from the lower-extremity deep veins have to go through the right atrium en route to the pulmonary circulation. They are mobile, have a characteristic popcorn or snake-like appearance, and are always associated with pulmonary embolism (see Chap. 13) [9]. In patients with mobile right atrial thrombi, the mortality is high with heparin therapy alone. Although surgical removal has been advocated, these patients can be treated successfully with continuous infusion of a thrombolytic agent. Left atrial thrombus is most common in patients with mitral stenosis or atrial fibrillation, and infrequently occurs as paradoxical embolus from a right atrial thrombus passing through the patent foramen ovale (Fig. 14-8). However, even in the most ideal patient, transthoracic echocardiography has its limitations in detecting left atrial appendage thrombus. The left atrial appendage is visualized in all patients from a transesophageal window (Fig. 14-9). Ventricular thrombus is easily differentiated from a tumor since the former

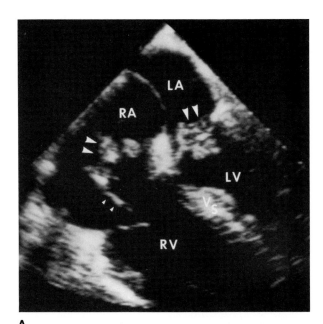

A

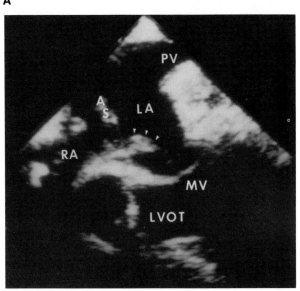

B

Fig. 14-8. **A.** Horizontal four-chamber TEE view showing biatrial thrombi *(large arrowheads)* in a patient with dyspnea and cold left foot due to a peripheral embolic event. The small arrowheads show the pacemaker wire. The atrial septum bulges toward the left atrium (LA) due to right atrial (RA) pressure. **B.** Horizontal basal TEE view in the same patient demonstrates thrombus *(arrowheads)* traversing the patent foramen ovale: paradoxical embolism.

is almost always associated with akinetic to dyskinetic myocardium underlying the thrombus. An exception is the thrombus formation in hypereosinophilic cardiomyopathy, which obliterates the ventricular apex (Fig. 14-10).

Transesophageal Echocardiography

Transesophageal echocardiography (TEE) is more sensitive in detecting an intracardiac mass or thrombus, with the possible exception of an apical thrombus since the apex may not be seen from an esophageal window. Otherwise, due to superior imaging quality, TEE can characterize an intracardiac mass or thrombus better than the transthoracic approach [10] (Fig. 14-11). The entire left atrium and its appendage are clearly seen by TEE in all patients. Its resolution is so excellent that it is even able to detect prethrombotic sluggish blood flow in the left atrium and the left atrial appendage, which has been described as a "spontaneous echo contrast" (Fig. 14-12). According to Daniel and associates [11], the patients with spontaneous echo contrast have a higher chance of embolic event or left atrial thrombus formation. Therefore, one of the most frequent indications of TEE is to look for a cardiac source of embolic events to the cerebral or peripheral circulation. Another important diagnostic consideration in patients with an embolic event from the heart is to look for the patent foramen ovale. About one-fourth of the normal population have a patent foramen ovale. This may not result in any problems unless right atrial pressure is elevated in patients with pulmonary embolism, right ventricular failure, or right ventricular infarct. The foramen ovale will enlarge further and is conducive to result in paradoxical embolus. TEE is an excellent tool to image the entire atrial septum, and the patent foramen ovale has a characteristic appearance, especially from a longitudinal view. Contrast echocardiography (injecting agitated saline into the right atrium through an arm

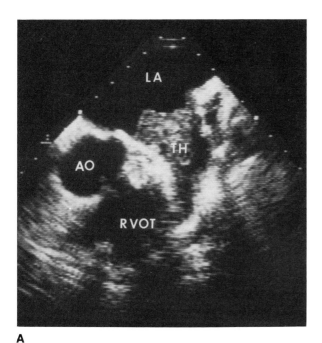

A

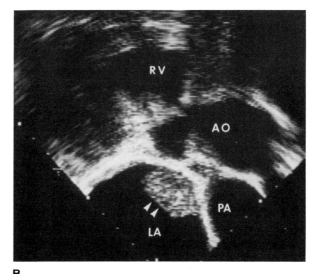

B

Fig. 14-9.   Transesophageal view of the left atrium (LA) and its appendage with thrombus. **A.** On the horizontal basal short-axis view, the left atrial appendage is shown as a crescent moon shape and is filled with thrombus (TH). **B, C.** Longitudinal views of the left atrium and left atrial appendage with thrombus *(arrowheads).*

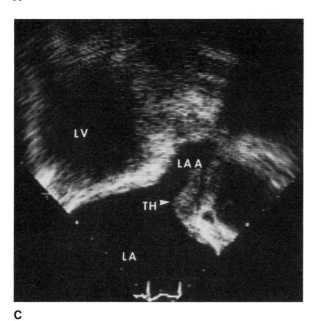

C

Fig. 14-10.   Apical long-axis view by transthoracic ▶ echocardiography demonstrating an apical mass *(arrowheads).* The apical thickness is increased *(large arrow)* compared to that of the posterior wall *(small arrow)* due to the apical accumulation of thrombus and eosinophils.

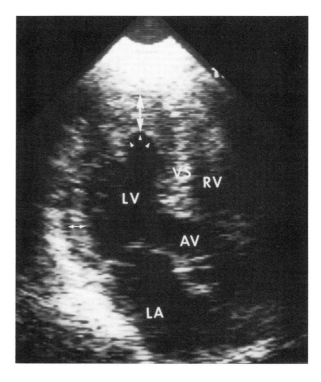

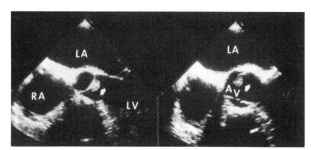

Fig. 14-11. Horizontal TEE detection of aortic valve fibroelastoma during diastole and systole *(arrow)*. This lesion was not detected by transthoracic examination.

Fig. 14-12. Spontaneous echo contrast in the LV shown by horizontal **(A)** and longitudinal **(B)** transesophageal imaging.

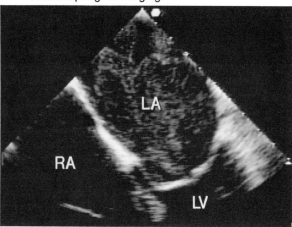

A

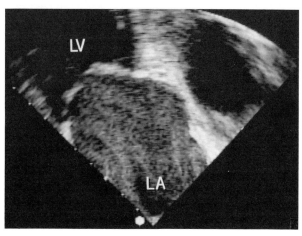

B

vein) allows visualization of the passage of fluid (contrast) through the patent foramen ovale to the left cardiac chambers with and without release of the Valsalva maneuver (Fig. 14-13). However, it is not clear how the finding of the patent foramen ovale should be handled therapeutically in patients with an embolic event. Closure of the patent foramen ovale may be considered in young patients with documented deep-vein thrombosis and recurrent embolic events while on warfarin therapy.

Because TEE is extremely sensitive for detection of left atrial and left atrial appendage thrombus, cardioversion of atrial fibrillation may be attempted safely without prolonged anticoagulation when TEE excludes the presence of left atrial thrombi [12].

Role of Echocardiography in Nonrheumatic Atrial Fibrillation

The clinical trial Stroke Prevention in Atrial Fibrillation [13, 14] has identified clinical and echocardiographic risk factors for stroke in patients with nonrheumatic atrial fibrillation. Three clinical variables—recent congestive heart failure, a history of hypertension, and previous arterial thromboembolism—were independently associated with a higher risk (7.7%/year). In patients with no clinical risk factor, LV systolic dysfunction and left atrial enlargement on echocardiography could separate the extremely low-risk group (1%/year) from the moderate-risk group (7.5%/year). So far, there has been no large clinical study to demonstrate TEE findings to be predictive of subsequent thromboembolism.

Pseudotumor—Pitfalls

Not all "masses" detected by echocardiography are a thrombus or an intracardiac tumor. An aberrant appearance of a normal cardiac or extracardiac structure may be interpreted as

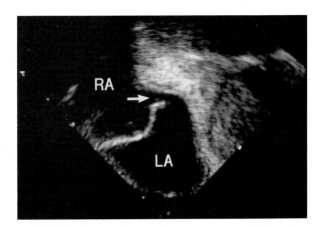

A

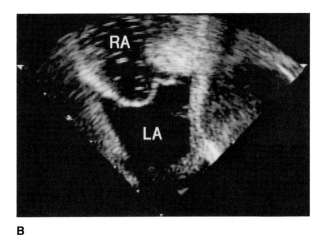

B

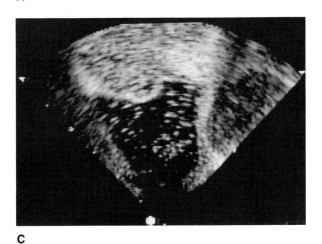

C

Fig. 14-13. Longitudinal TEE view showing contrast echo study to detect right-to-left shunt via the patent foramen ovale (PFO). **A.** Prior to injection of contrast material, TEE suggests a patent foramen ovale *(arrow)*. **B.** Agitated saline was injected into a right-arm vein and initial bolus is seen in the right atrium (RA). **C.** Contrast shunts through the patent foramen ovale and opacifies the left atrium.

Fig. 14-14. Lipomatous hypertrophy of the atrial septum *(double arrows)*. It has the characteristic "dumbbell" appearance. The lipomatous hypertrophy may extend up to the superior vena cava. This patient also has fatty infiltration of the tricuspid annulus *(arrow)*.

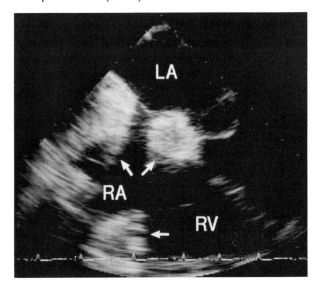

an intracardiac mass. This pitfall is very important to recognize and has become more common after the introduction of TEE [15]. The normal structures frequently interpreted as an intracardiac mass include a large eustachian valve, lipomatous hypertrophy of the atrial septum [16] (Fig. 14-14), fatty tricuspid valve annulus, and diaphragmatic hernia by TTE [17] (Fig. 14-15). In TEE, the "Q-tip" appearance of a globular structure separating the left upper pulmonary vein from the left atrial appendage (Fig. 14-16) and the potential space of the transverse sinus (Fig. 14-17), which may harbor fibrin material in the presence of pericardial effusion, have been interpreted as an intracardiac mass.

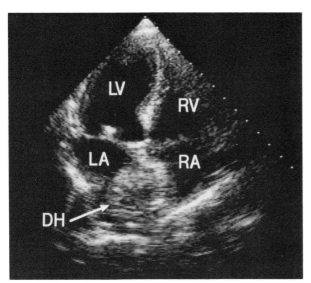

Fig. 14-15. Diaphragmatic hernia (DH) shown as a mass behind the atria. This can be confidently diagnosed by demonstrating liquid bubbles after consumption of a carbonated drink.

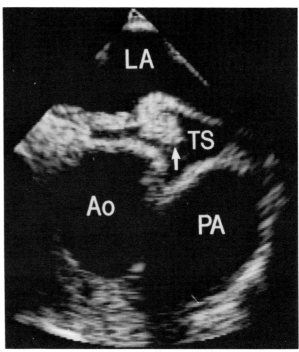

Fig. 14-17. TEE short-axis view of the transverse sinus (TS) with fibrin material *(arrow)* and pericardial effusion.

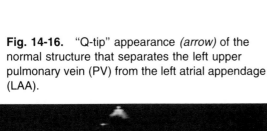

Fig. 14-16. "Q-tip" appearance *(arrow)* of the normal structure that separates the left upper pulmonary vein (PV) from the left atrial appendage (LAA).

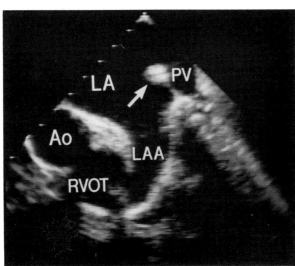

References

1. Schattenberg TT. Echocardiographic diagnosis of left atrial myxoma. *Mayo Clin Proc* 1968;43:620–627.

2. Nasser WK, et al. Atrial myxoma. II. Phonocardiographic, echocardiographic, hemodynamic, and angiographic features in nine cases. *Am Heart J* 1972;83:810–824.

3. Harbold NB Jr, Gau GT. Echocardiographic diagnosis of right atrial myxoma. *Mayo Clin Proc* 1973;48:284–286.

4. Lappe DL, Bulkley BH, Weiss JL. Two-dimensional echocardiographic diagnosis of left atrial myxoma. *Chest* 1978;74:55–58.

5. Come PC, Kurland GS, Vine HS. Two-dimensional echocardiography in differentiating right atrial and tricuspid valve mass lesions. *Am J Cardiol* 1979;44:1207–1212.

6. DePace NL, et al. Two dimensional echocardiographic detection of intraatrial masses. *Am J Cardiol* 1981;48:954–960.

7. Shub C, et al. Cardiac papillary fibroelastomas: two-dimensional echocardiographic recognition. *Mayo Clin Proc* 1981;56:629–633.

8. Fyke FE III, et al. Primary cardiac tumors: experience with 30 consecutive patients since the introduction of two-dimensional echocardiography. *J Am Coll Cardiol* 1985; 5:1465–1473.

9. Proano M, et al. Successful treatment of pulmonary embolism and associated mobile right atrial thrombus with use of a central thrombolytic infusion. *Mayo Clin Proc* 1988; 63:1181–1185.

10. Reeder GS, et al. Transesophageal echocardiography and cardiac masses. *Mayo Clin Proc* 1991;66:1101–1109.

11. Daniel WG, et al. Left atrial spontaneous contrast in mitral valve disease: an indicator for an increased thromboembolic risk. *J Am Coll Cardiol* 1988;11:1204–1211.

12. Manning WJ, et al. Cardioversion from atrial fibrillation without prolonged anticoagulation with use of transesophageal echocardiography to exclude the presence of atrial thrombi. *N Engl J Med* 1993;328:750–755.

13. The Stroke Prevention in Atrial Fibrillation investigators. Predictors of thromboembolism in atrial fibrillation: I. Clinical features of patients at risk. *Ann Intern Med* 1992;116:1–5.

14. The Stroke Prevention in Atrial Fibrillation investigators. Predictors of thromboembolism in atrial fibrillation: II. Echocardiographic features of patients at risk. *Ann Intern Med* 1992;116:6–12.

15. Seward JB, et al. Critical appraisal of transesophageal echocardiography: limitations, pitfalls, and complications. *J Am Soc Echocardiogr* 1992;5:288–305.

16. Fyke FE, et al. Diagnosis of lipomatous hypertrophy of the atrial septum by two-dimensional echocardiography. *J Am Coll Cardiol* 1983;1:1352–1357.

17. Nishimura RA, et al. Diaphragmatic hernia mimicking an atrial mass: a two-dimensional echocardiographic pitfall. *J Am Coll Cardiol* 1985;5:992–995.

15

Diseases of the Aorta

Using the multiple transthoracic and transesophageal imaging windows, the entire thoracic aorta can be visualized by echocardiography [1–7]. The entire arch and the proximal portion of the descending thoracic aorta are well seen on suprasternal notch examination and should be a routine part of the transthoracic examination in all patients (Fig. 15-1A). Diseases involving the aorta include aortic aneurysm, aortic dissection, coronary sinus aneurysm with or without rupture into the surrounding cardiac chambers (most commonly to the right cardiac chambers), aortic ulcer or intramural hematoma, aortic rupture, atheromatous debris, aortic abscess, and coarctation of the aorta. The dimension of the ascending aorta and the arch is best measured from the parasternal long-axis and suprasternal views, respectively. The various measurement sites for the aorta are shown in Figure 15-1B since the dimension of the aorta should be measured from the same locations during repeat echocardiography for follow-up of aortic aneurysm and Marfan's syndrome (Fig. 15-2).

The entire segments of the thoracic aorta and proximal brachiocephalic vessels can be imaged by transesophageal echocardiography (TEE) (Fig. 15-3). The midascending aorta to the proximal portion of the arch may not be visualized by horizontal plane imaging due to the interposed air-filled trachea and bronchi. The longitudinal plane, however, should allow visualization of that segment (see Chap. 3). The location and the extent of aortic pathologies can be confidently identified by biplane TEE examination (Fig. 15-3B).

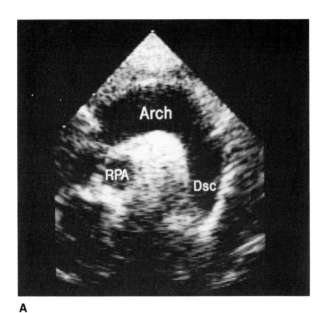

A

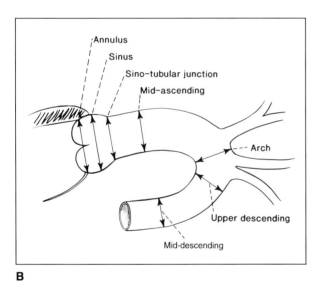

B

Fig. 15-1.   A. Long-axis view of the aorta from the suprasternal notch window. The entire transverse (Arch) and the proximal portion of the descending thoracic (Dsc) aorta are clearly seen. Cross section of the right pulmonary artery (RPA) is visualized in this view. **B.** A schematic drawing of aortic annulus, sinus of Valsalva, ascending aorta, arch, and descending thoracic aorta illustrates various sites to measure aortic dimension. Accurate serial determinations from the same sites are important in the follow-up of patients with aortic aneurysm or Marfan's syndrome.

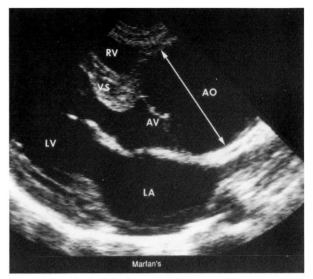

Fig. 15-2.   Typical 2D image of the ascending aorta in Marfan's syndrome (annuloaortic ectasia). The proximal portion of the aorta (aortic annulus and the sinuses of Valsalva) is diffusely enlarged *(arrow)*. Annulus dilatation results in chronic aortic regurgitation. Progressive aortic dilatation predisposes the patients to aortic rupture, and it is advised to perform prophylactic surgery (Bentall procedure) when the aortic diameter reaches 6 cm [8]. Aortic dissection is also frequent. Cardiac complications (heart failure, aortic rupture, and aortic dissection) are the most common cause of death in patients with Marfan's syndrome, accounting for more than 90% of deaths. Mitral valve prolapse is another frequent associate.

Aortic Dissection

Transthoracic Echocardiography

Transthoracic echocardiography is a good imaging modality for screening for proximal aortic dissection (the ascending aorta and the arch). Its positive predictive value is very good, but the dissection may not be excluded due to the suboptimal imaging quality of transthoracic echocardiography. Review of 6-year experience at the Mayo Clinic in 67 patients with aortic dissection demonstrated that the sensitivity of transthoracic echocardiography was

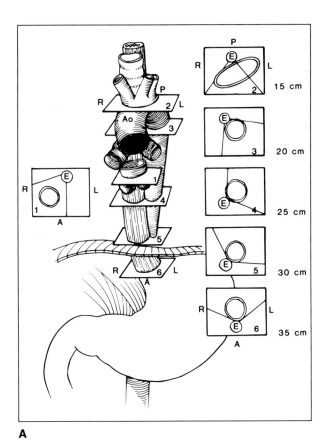

A

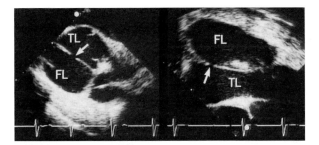

B

Fig. 15-3. **A.** Schematic diagram showing the anatomic relationship of the aorta (Ao), trachea, and esophagus (E). Also shown are various levels of horizontal scan planes of the thoracic aorta (1 = aortic root; 2 = arch; 3 = upper descending aorta; 4–5 = midthoracic aorta; 6 = upper abdominal aorta). Note that the esophagus lies anterior to the aorta at the diaphragm and posterior at the level of the arch. The portion of the distal ascending aorta directly anterior to the trachea is a *blind area* for horizontal TEE. (From JB Seward et al. Transesophageal echocardiography. *Mayo Clin Proc* 1988;63:649–680.) **B.** Biplane TEE images of type II dissection. The horizontal plane (left) shows an intimal flap separating the true lumen (TL) from a false lumen (FL) and a communicating site *(arrow)*. However, the extent of aortic dissection is not determined. The longitudinal plane (right) shows the dissection to be confined to the ascending aorta. The arrow indicates a communicating site in the intimal flap.

Fig. 15-4. Transthoracic parasternal long-axis view showing a dilated ascending aorta (Ao) and an intimal flap *(arrows)* in proximal aortic dissection. A small pericardial effusion (PE) is detected, a worrisome sign for hemopericardium.

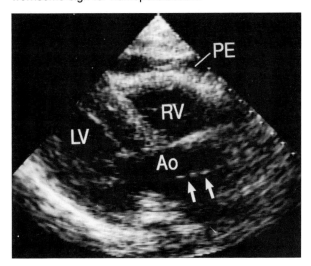

79% and the positive predictive accuracy was 91% [4]. Although all patients with aortic dissection had a dilated aorta by 2D echocardiography, an intimal flap was seen in only 79% of the patients (Fig. 15-4). Five patients (7%) had a false-positive diagnosis, most frequently due to the membranous wall of the thrombus in the lumen of an aneurysmal descending thoracic aorta, which was misinterpreted as an intimal flap. Another limitation of transthoracic echocardiography is the lack of visualization of the entire aorta, especially the descending thoracic aorta. Therefore, transthoracic echocardiography is an inexpensive rapid screening tool for aortic dissection, but negative or suboptimal examination requires further diagnostic evaluation for aortic dissection.

Transesophageal Echocardiography

TEE allows visualization of the entire thoracic aorta from both horizontal and longitudinal views using biplane transducers, due to the intimate anatomic relationship between the esophagus and the entire thoracic aorta (see Fig. 15-3). It should be noted that the esophagus lies anterior to the aorta at the level of the diaphragm, but they are intertwined in the thorax so that the esophagus is located posterior to the aorta at the level of the transverse arch. In the horizontal transesophageal view, the distal portion of the ascending aorta and the proximal portion of the transverse aorta may not be well visualized because of the interposed trachea. Because of this unique anatomic relationship between the esophagus and the aorta, the transesophageal view of the aorta must be interpreted in the context of the location of the transesophageal transducer. The blind area on the horizontal plane can now be visualized by the longitudinal view. With the clearer and more complete view of the entire aorta, TEE has changed the role of echocardiography in the diagnosis and the management strategy of aortic dissection. Illustrative TEE images of aortic dissection are shown in Figures 15-5 through 15-8.

A European cooperative study utilizing only horizontal plane views demonstrated that transthoracic and transesophageal echocardiography were at least equal or even superior to computed tomography or aortography in the diagnosis of aortic dissection [9]. A similar result was reported in the United States [10]. No serious complications were noted during TEE. The diagnostic capability will be made easier by biplane or multiplane imaging. With the increasing experience with this unique imaging modality, surgical repair of aortic dissection may be carried out on the basis of TEE detection of aortic dissection. The mortality of patients with aortic dissection increases 1% for every hour after onset, especially in patients· with dissection of the proximal aorta [11]. Echocardiography has the advantage of being portable and quick to perform (about 10–15 minutes for each examination). Since TEE can produce a mild increase in heart rate and blood

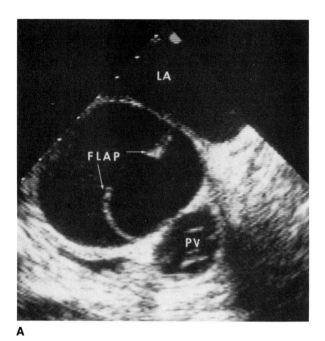

Fig. 15-5. Horizontal TEE of type I aortic dissection. **A.** With the transducer oriented toward the ascending aorta, an undulating flap (in real time) is demonstrated with a large defect, a communication site, in the dilated proximal ascending aorta. **B.** With the transducer oriented toward the descending thoracic aorta, the extent of dissection to the descending aorta is seen. The false lumen (FL) is huge, separated by an intimal flap from the small true lumen (TL).

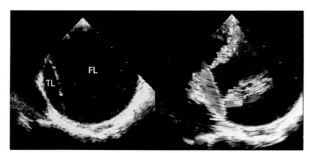

Fig. 15-6. Horizontal TEE of type III dissection. 2D imaging (left) clearly identifies a typical dissection of the descending thoracic aorta. The true lumen (TL) is small compared to the large false lumen (FL). The echo dropout area in the flap indicates a communicating site. Color-flow imaging (right) during systole shows flow from the true to the false lumen via two intimal tear sites.

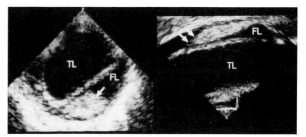

Fig. 15-7. Biplane TEE of type III dissection. The horizontal plane image (left) shows the true (TL) and false lumina (FL). The false lumen is partially thrombosed *(arrow)*. The longitudinal plane image (right) shows the descending thoracic aorta with the transducer located at the bottom of the figure. The false lumen (FL) is partially thrombosed *(arrows)*.

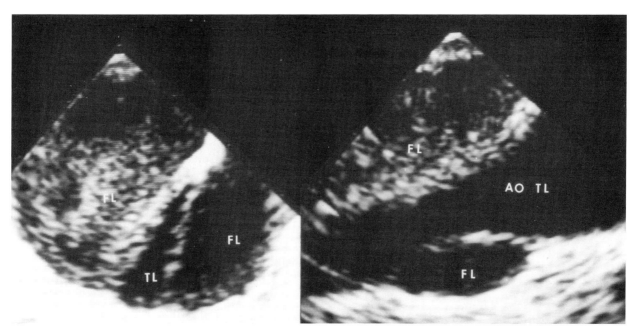

Fig. 15-8. Biplane TEE of a dissection in the descending thoracic aorta. Horizontal view (left). The true lumen (TL) is sandwiched between two false lumina (FL). The false lumen close to the esophagus is almost completely thrombosed, whereas the other false lumen is not. Longitudinal view (right). This is an example of spiral dissection.

pressure, it would be prudent to sedate the patient well prior to the passage of the transesophageal probe when aortic dissection is suspected clinically. Echocardiography also has the advantage of evaluating the potential complications of aortic dissection: hemopericardium, coronary involvement, aortic regurgitation, and left ventricular (LV) systolic dysfunction. Follow-up of patients with aortic dissection is made easier using TEE, after surgical or medical treatment [12]. Morphologic and flow characteristics of aortic dissection during follow-up may be important in their future prognosis.

Clinical presentations of other aortic pathologies can be identical to those of aortic dissection; they are aortic intramural hematoma and aortic penetrating ulcer [13]. Unlike aortic dissection, no undulating intimal flap is present; hence, diagnosis is more difficult. TEE has been shown to be promising in the detection of the subtle, but potentially fatal aortic pathologies such as intramural hematoma (Fig. 15-9) or ulcer. Although resolution of such lesions has been noted with antihypertensive treatment,

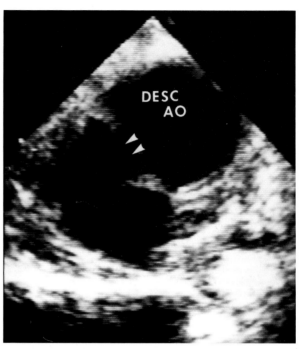

Fig. 15-10. Horizontal TEE view of the descending thoracic aorta in a hypotensive patient after a motor vehicle accident. The aorta has a tear *(arrowheads)* with a large pseudoaneurysm.

Fig. 15-9. Transverse TEE view of the descending thoracic aorta in a hypertensive patient with severe back pain, demonstrating intramural hematoma. The soft tissue mass with a smooth surface appears different from aortic debris. This dissolved over the next 6 months while the patient was on antihypertensive medications including a beta-blocker.

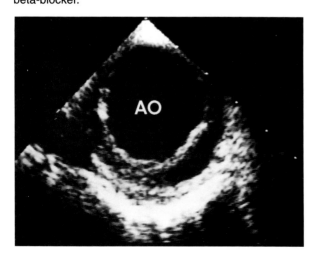

they have a high likelihood of rupture so that surgical repair is usually recommended.

Other Pathologies

Aortic Rupture

Aortic rupture is one of the most feared complications of deceleration injury due to a motor vehicle accident. Figure 15-10 shows an example of such a complication diagnosed by TEE. TEE can be safely performed in patients after a motor vehicle accident unless they have serious cervical spinal injury.

Aortic Debris

Since imaging of the aorta is a routine part of the TEE examination, various morphologic abnormalities of the aorta have been described. Atherosclerotic plaques and debris are common findings in elderly patients [14] and their

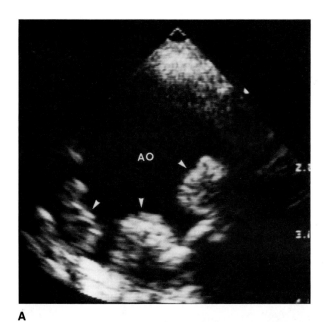

A

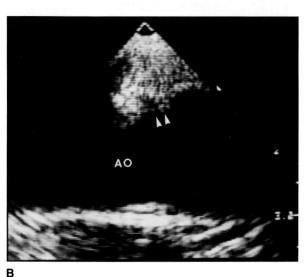

B

Fig. 15-11. Biplane TEE images of aortic debris in the descending thoracic aorta. **A.** Horizontal view showing mobile irregular masses (in real time) *(arrowheads)* attached to the aortic wall. This is a typical appearance of atherosclerotic plaque in the aorta. **B.** Longitudinal view showing aortic debris *(arrowheads)*.

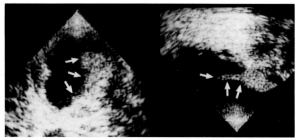

Fig. 15-12. Biplane TEE images of aortic debris *(arrows)* partially obstructing the descending thoracic aorta in a patient with (ischemic) cardiomyopathy and a livedo below the umbilicus. The combination of low cardiac output and significant obstruction of the descending aorta by the aortic debris resulted in a low-flow state in the lower extremities. The livedo disappeared when cardiac output increased with dopamine administration.

clinical significance needs further observation. Unlike intramural hematoma, aortic plaques are usually irregular in shape and frequently mobile (Fig. 15-11). It has been noted that the incidence of aortic debris is higher in patients with systemic embolization. Aortic plaque can be hemodynamically compromising or flow-limiting, especially in the setting of low cardiac output (Fig. 15-12).

Aortic Aneurysm

Since the entire thoracic aorta can be visualized by transthoracic and transesophageal echocardiography, aortic dilatation is easily documented. When aneurysm reaches the diameter of 6 cm, the incidence of rupture increases and smaller aneurysms require serial follow-up studies measuring dimensions at specific locations of the aorta (see Fig. 15-1B). Pseudoaneurysm carries a more ominous prognosis. It is a result of a tear of the aortic wall, and there is leakage of blood from the aorta to the pseudoaneurysm which is contained. Due to its tendency to rupture, repair of the pseudoaneurysm is usually recommended. Pseudoaneurysm has a different appearance from true aneurysm. It is important to demonstrate the rupture point where communication

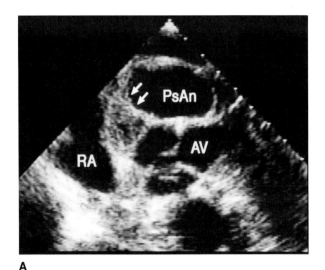

A

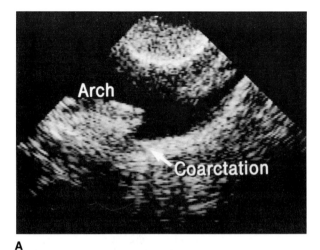

A

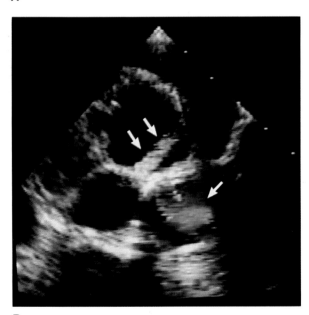

B

Fig. 15-13. Aortic pseudoaneurysm in a 78-year-old man. **A.** Horizontal TEE at the aortic valve (AV) level showing a large aortic pseudoaneurysm (PsAn). It is partially thrombosed *(arrows)*. **B.** Color-flow imaging during diastole demonstrates communicating flow from the aorta to the pseudoaneurysm *(arrows)*. Also, aortic regurgitation *(arrow)* is present. A similar echocardiographic finding is seen in patients with aortic root abscess.

B

Fig. 15-14. Suprasternal 2D and continuous-wave Doppler studies of coarctation of the aorta. **A.** 2D image showing the narrowing of the descending thoracic aorta at the usual location. **B.** Continuous-wave Doppler spectrum of coarctation. Peak velocity is 4 m/sec, corresponding to a peak pressure gradient of 64 mm Hg. Continuous diastolic flow *(upward arrow)* is typical in severe coarctation since aortic pressure to coarctation remains high during diastole.

occurs between the aorta and the pseudoaneurysm (Fig. 15-13).

Coarctation of the Aorta

Coarctation of the aorta is a narrowing of the descending thoracic aorta, usually immediately distal to the left subclavian artery. It is important to consider coarctation in patients with hypertension since it is surgically treatable. Echocardiographically, coarctation is diagnosed by showing narrowing of the descending thoracic aorta and increased Doppler flow velocity across the narrowing (Fig. 15-14). Therefore, suprasternal notch 2D and continuous-wave Doppler examinations should be routinely performed in patients with hypertension.

References

1. Victor MF, et al. Two-dimensional echocardiographic diagnosis of aortic dissection. *Am J Cardiol* 1981;48:1155–1159.

2. Mathew T, Nanda NC. Two-dimensional and Doppler echocardiographic evaluation of aortic aneurysm and dissection. *Am J Cardiol* 1984;54:379–385.

3. Granato JE, Dee P, Gibson RS. Utility of two-dimensional echocardiography in suspected ascending aortic dissection. *Am J Cardiol* 1985;56:123–129.

4. Khandheria BK, et al. Aortic dissection: review of value and limitations of two-dimensional echocardiography in a six-year experience. *J Am Soc Echocardiogr* 1989;2:17–24.

5. Erbel R, et al. Detection of aortic dissection by transesophageal echocardiography. *Br Heart J* 1987;58:45–51.

6. Seward JB, et al. Transesophageal echocardiography: technique, anatomic correlations, implementation, and clinical applications. *Mayo Clin Proc* 1988;63:649–680.

7. Seward JB, et al. Biplanar transesophageal echocardiography: anatomic correlations, image orientation, and clinical applications. *Mayo Clin Proc* 1990;65:1193–1213.

8. Gott VL, et al. Surgical treatment of aneurysms of the ascending aorta in the Marfan syndrome. Results of composite graft repair in 50 patients. *N Engl J Med* 1985;314:1070.

9. Erbel R, et al. The European Cooperative Study Group for Echocardiography. Echocardiography in diagnosis of aortic dissection. *Lancet* 1989;1:457–461.

10. Ballal RS, et al. Usefulness of transesophageal echocardiography in assessment of aortic dissection. *Circulation* 1991;84:1903–1914.

11. Jamieson WRE, et al. Aortic dissections: early diagnosis and surgical management are the keys to survival. *Can J Surg* 1982;25:145–149.

12. Mohr-Kahaly S, et al. Ambulatory follow-up of aortic dissection by transesophageal two-dimensional and color-coded Doppler echocardiography. *Circulation* 1989;80:24–33.

13. Standson AW, et al. Penetrating atherosclerotic ulcers of the thoracic aorta: natural history and clinicopathologic correlations. *Ann Vasc Surg* 1986;1:15–23.

14. Lanza GM, et al. Plaque and structural characteristics of the descending thoracic aorta using transesophageal echocardiography. *J Am Soc Echocardiogr* 1991;4:19–28.

16

Congenital Heart Disease

Echocardiography has markedly changed the evaluation, diagnosis, and management of congenital heart disease. A complete echocardiographic examination can establish a goal-directed management, reduce the need for confirmatory cardiac catheterization, and provide serial evaluation of residua and sequelae of congenital heart disease. Comprehensive echocardiography in congenital heart disease would need a much larger text than this manual. Seward and colleagues [1] from our echocardiography laboratory published a comprehensive 2D echocardiographic atlas of congenital cardiac malformations. Readers who desire more detailed information on this subject are referred to the atlas [1]. This manual presents an abbreviated systematic tomographic 2D approach to congenital heart disease as encountered in an adult cardiology practice.

Systematic Tomographic Approach

The most challenging echocardiographic examination is in patients with complex congenital heart disease in which the cardiac structures and viscera are in unusual positions. In these circumstances, a systematic approach to the 2D echocardiographic examination is necessary. The format for image orientation should be the same for every form of congenital heart disease. The following step-by-step approach can be applied to all cardiac anomalies and conforms to the recommendations of the American Society of Echocardiography (ASE).

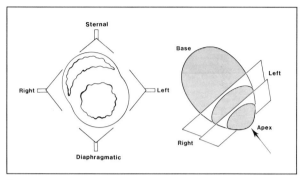

A

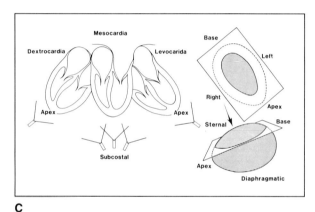

C

B

Fig. 16-1. Schematic orientation to echocardiographic tomographic anatomy in short-axis view **(A)**, long-axis view **(B)**, and four-chamber view **(C)**. (From JB Seward, WD Edwards. *Two-Dimensional Echocardiographic Atlas.* Vol 1. New York: Springer, 1987.)

Short-Axis View

Short-axis views are portrayed as though looking from the apex toward the base of the heart (Fig. 16-1A). From a parasternal or transesophageal transducer position, left-side structures will be to the right of the video screen; right-side structures, to the left; sternal (anterior), to the top; and diaphragmatic (posterior), toward the bottom.

Long-Axis View

The long-axis views of the heart, regardless of transducer position or arrangement of the cardiac chambers, are displayed as though looking from left cardiac structures toward the right (Fig. 16-1B). Parasternal and transesophageal long-axis views are portrayed with the basal (superior) cardiac structures to the viewer's right, sternal (anterior) structures toward the top of the screen, and diaphragmatic (posterior) structures toward the bottom.

Four-Chamber View

Four-chamber views or frontal projections of the heart are by convention more commonly displayed with the apex down (ASE option 1) when imaging congenital anomalies (Fig. 16-1C). Apex down is utilized because it orients cardiac structures in a manner most closely resembling classic anatomic dissections and surgical approach to the heart. The four-chamber view thus orients the heart from its anterior surface to the posterior.

2D Examination

The most important prerequisite to a complete examination is knowing how to position the transducer to obtain the appropriate image orientation. Standard anatomic and transducer references should be utilized to consistently obtain proper display of the image. It is easiest to understand transducer orientation if one begins with examination of the upper abdominal anatomy.

Step 1: Short-Axis Image of the Upper Abdomen

Place the transducer in the epigastrium and direct the beam directly posterior. Orient the ultrasound plane to view the upper abdomen in short axis. To confirm proper short-axis orientation, tilt the transducer from right to left. If the image is properly oriented, tilting the transducer to the patient's right will bring structures on the right side of the screen toward the midline. If the opposite happens, rotate the transducer 180 degrees or do an electronic side-to-side inversion of the image. A proper short-axis transducer orientation is now confirmed. *All* subsequent short-axis views, regardless of the precordial transducer position, are obtained with this same left-to-right orientation of the transducer. If one becomes disoriented, return to the upper abdomen to confirm a consistent transducer image orientation.

Step 2: Long-Axis Image of the Upper Abdomen

Rotate the transducer 90 degrees clockwise from step 1 or orient the transducer into a proper long-axis orientation. To simply confirm a proper orientation, tilt the transducer toward the patient's head. This should bring the structures on the right side of the video screen toward the middle of the picture. If the opposite occurs, reverse the image 180 degrees. The chest, upper abdomen, and cardiac chambers should be displayed toward the right side of the video image and structures toward the feet and lower abdomen to the left side of the image. All long-axis views, regardless of heart position, are obtained with this transducer orientation.

Step 3: Four-Chamber Image

Initially, orient the transducer in a proper short-axis view of the upper abdomen (see above). Tilt the transducer beam toward the chest and the transducer handle toward the feet, parallel with the abdominal wall. The echo of the pulsatile heart will be visible near the bottom of the video screen. Electronically, reorient the image from top to bottom maintaining the same left-right relationship. The ultrasound burst is now at the bottom of the video screen. To confirm the proper left-right image orientation, direct the ultrasonic beam to the patient's right. Right-side structures should move toward the center of the image. If the opposite occurs, either perform electronic side-to-side reversal of the image or rotate the transducer 180 degrees. To confidently determine the position of the heart, alternatively aim the transducer toward the patient's right side, midline, and left side of the chest (Fig. 16-1C). Cardiac pulsations will disclose the cardiac position. This maneuver determines cardiac position to be either dextrocardia (cardiac apex in the right side of the chest), mesocardia (cardiac apex in midline), or levocardia (cardiac apex in the left side of the chest).

Step 4: Precordial Examination

Once the position of the heart in the chest is known, the transducer, in an appropriate short-axis, long-axis, or four-chamber orientation, may be shifted from the abdominal position to the precordium. Use the upper abdomen as an easy point of reference for each transducer reorientation.

Overview of Adult Congenital Heart Disease

The most commonly encountered congenital heart defect of clinical significance after bicuspid valve is atrial septal defect. Presently, with precordial and transesophageal echocardiography (TEE), both anatomic and hemodynamic characteristics of this abnormality can be confidently evaluated in virtually all patients [2–4]. Some anomalies such as the sinus venosus atrial septal defect are difficult to diagnose by precordial echocardiography. However, this anomaly and others can be confidently diagnosed by TEE [5, 6]. Associated anomalous pulmonary venous connections can also be confidently detected. Hemodynamics such as pulmonary artery pressure and flow characteristics can be determined noninvasively. A detailed echo/Doppler examination has eliminated the need for cardiac catheterization in most patients with congenital heart disease. Other congenital cardiac diseases diagnosed in the adult would include small ventricular septal defect, pulmonary stenosis, (residual) coarctation, patent ductus arteriosus, Ebstein's anomaly, left ventricular (LV) outflow tract obstruction including discrete subaortic stenosis, and other acyanotic congenital conditions. A comprehensive echo/Doppler examination is now considered the primary means of diagnosing and characterizing most congenital anomalies.

Patients with cyanotic heart disease are now reaching adulthood in greater numbers because of better medical and surgical management. Tetralogy of Fallot, pulmonary atresia, ventricular septal defect (VSD), and single ventricle are recognized and characterized by echocardiographic morphologic and Doppler hemodynamic observations. Today management of congenital heart disease, including the use of catheterization, is goal-directed and in great part assisted by comprehensive noninvasive ultrasound imaging and hemodynamic examination. Complete or "blind" diagnostic catheterization is no longer a necessary or an acceptable practice. Patients operated on for congenital heart disease are usually left with residua and sequelae that require serial follow-up evaluation, which can be safely obtained using echo/Doppler technology.

Examples of congenital heart disease are provided below.

Atrial Septal Defect

There are four distinct types of atrial septal defects: (1) primum or partial atrioventricular (AV) canal, (2) secundum, (3) sinus venosus, and (4) coronary sinus defect. The secundum defect is most common, followed by the primum, sinus venosus, and coronary sinus defects. The primum defect (partial AV canal) is associated with a cleft mitral valve. Sinus veno-

sus defect is associated with a high incidence of partial anomalous pulmonary venous connection (PAVC). Each form of atrial septal defect is normally associated with a left-to-right shunt, which results in right atrial and ventricular volume overload. Pulmonary hypertension of a magnitude that would preclude surgical repair is rare and can be recognized and quantitated by echo/Doppler studies. Echocardiographic findings of an atrial septal defect usually include right ventricular en-

Fig. 16-2. Two-dimensional and M-mode echo features of atrial septal defect (ASD). (Top) The right ventricle (RV) is dilated and the tricuspid valve (TV) is enlarged due to right ventricular volume overload. Ventricular septal (VS) motion was paradoxical. (Bottom) A wide spectrum of ventricular septal motion abnormalities. The first two M-mode echocardiograms (left) show typical paradoxical motion, and the next two show atypical septal motion. Septal motion may occasionally be normal, as shown in the last column (right). (From JB Seward, WD Edwards. *Two-Dimensional Echocardiographic Atlas.* Vol 1. New York: Springer, 1987.)

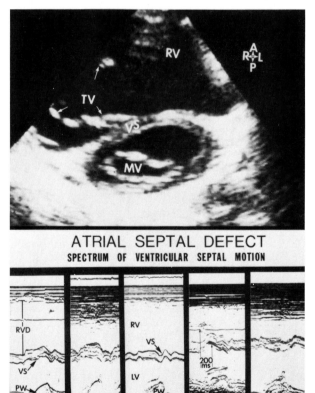

largement and abnormal (paradoxical) ventricular septal motion, which are the signature of volume overload (Fig. 16-2). In addition to visualizing the actual defect by 2D echocardiography, the left-to-right shunt can be visualized by flow imaging [2–4]. A complete transthoracic echocardiographic examination can detect most primum and secundum atrial septal defects; however, the sinus venosus defect, which is normally located near the entry of the superior vena cava, is visualized only in approximately 70% of patients (Fig. 16-3). TEE is exquisitely sensitive for the identifica-tion of all types of atrial septal defects [5, 6] as well as associated anomalous pulmonary venous connection (Figs. 16-4 and 16-5).

Outflow Tract Obstruction

Congenital LV outflow tract obstruction can be classified into subvalvular, valvular, and supra-valvular. A congenitally abnormal aortic valve, usually bicuspid (see Chap. 7), is the most common congenital cardiac anomaly (1–2% incidence) (Fig. 16-6). Bicuspid aortic valves can present with aortic stenosis, regurgitation, or

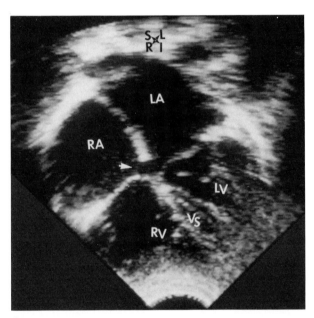

A

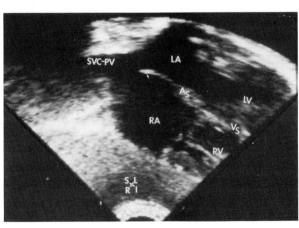

C

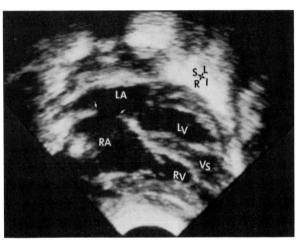

B

Fig. 16-3. Different types of atrial septal defects shown from the subcostal four-chamber transducer position, which allows the best visualization of the atrial septum using surface echocardiography. **A.** Primum atrial septal defect is visualized as an echo dropout *(arrow)* in the lower portion of the atrial septum. Both atrioventricular valves insert at the same level on the crest of the ventricular septum (VS). **B.** The secundum defect is characterized as an echo dropout *(arrows)* in the central portion of the atrial septum. **C.** Sinus venosus defect is shown as an echo dropout in the superior portion of the atrial septum (AS). This defect is usually associated with anomalous pulmonary vein connection. A pulmonary vein is connected to the junction between the superior vena cava and the right atrium. Note that the superior vena cava and an anomalous pulmonary vein (SVC-PV) straddle the defect and the superior portion of the atrial septum *(arrow)*. (From JB Seward et al. *Two-Dimensional Echocardiographic Atlas.* Vol. 1. New York: Springer, 1987.)

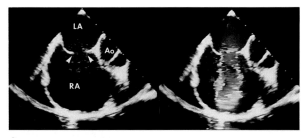

A

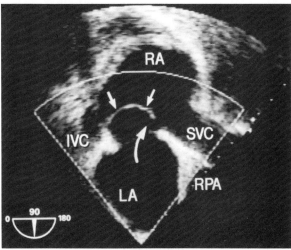

B

Fig. 16-4.   TEE of secundum atrial septal defect. **A.** Horizontal plane in the four-chamber projection. (Left) The transducer is located posterior to the left atrium (LA) within the esophagus. The secundum defect *(arrowheads)* is visualized as a communication between the left and right (RA) atria in the center of the atrial septum. Ao = aortic root. (Right) Color-flow Doppler showing the left-to-right shunt across the defect. **B.** In another patient, longitudinal plane in the axis of the superior (SVC) and inferior (IVC) venae cavae shows a secundum atrial septal defect *(large curved arrow)* in the superior aspect of the aneurysmal membranous atrial septum *(small arrows)*. The posteriorly located left atrium (LA) communicates with the anteriorly located right atrium (RA). This image was obtained by a multiplane probe with the transducer rotated 90 degrees to obtain a longitudinal view.

both. Symptomatic aortic stenosis due to a bicuspid aortic valve usually occurs before the age of 65. Patients with a bicuspid aortic valve also have a higher incidence of proximal aortic dissection and a common association with coarctation of the aorta. 2D/Doppler echocardiographic examination can identify aortic cusp morphology [7] (position of the raphe and commissures) as well as serially determine hemodynamic significance of aortic stenosis [8]. When transthoracic examination is not satisfactory to visualize aortic cusps, TEE should be effective in all patients (Fig. 16-7).

Subvalvular aortic stenosis may be discrete, fibromuscular, diffuse, or dynamic (Fig. 16-8). Congenital dynamic outflow obstruction is commonly encountered with severe pulmonary stenosis, tetralogy of Fallot, and complete transposition of the great arteries.

Supravalvular aortic stenosis most commonly presents as a fibrous thickening of the ascending aortic wall (Fig. 16-9). Doppler hemodynamics in fixed or dynamic outflow obstruction can be noninvasively determined and characterized in nearly all cases (Fig. 16-9).

Internal Cardiac Crux

The internal cardiac crux is a very important echocardiographic anatomic landmark used in the evaluation of many common as well as complex congenital cardiac anomalies. In the four-chamber plane, the components of the internal crux include the atrial septum, ventricular septum, and septal portions of the mitral and tricuspid valves (Fig. 16-10). The tricuspid valve originates from the crest of the ventricular septum whereas the septal portion of the mitral valve inserts at a higher level off the lower atrial septum. The portion of ventricular septum between the two valves represents the atrioventricular septum (i.e., a potential communication between the LV and right atrium). The consistency of the internal cardiac crux anatomy can be used to diagnose both ventricular and atrioventricular valve abnormality. The morphologic mitral valve always inserts higher than the morphologic tricuspid valve. The morphologic mitral valve

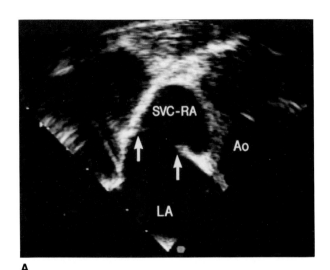

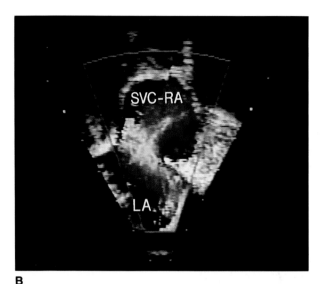

A

B

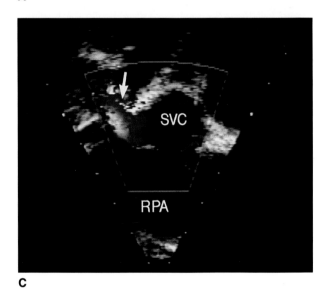

C

Fig. 16-5. TEE of a sinus venosus atrial septal defect. **A.** The defect *(arrows)* is usually located in the posterosuperior atrial septum between the left atrium (LA) and the superior vena cava–right atrial junction (SVC-RA). Ao = aortic root. **B.** Color-flow Doppler shows the left-to-right atrial shunt (color polarity has been reversed). **C.** Withdrawal of the transducer to the level of the right pulmonary artery (RPA) shows the right upper pulmonary vein *(arrow)* anomalously entering the superior vena cava (SVC).

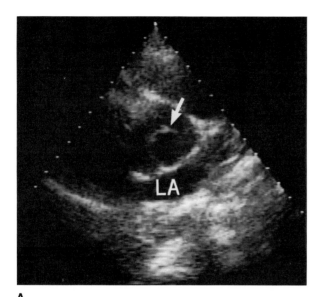

A

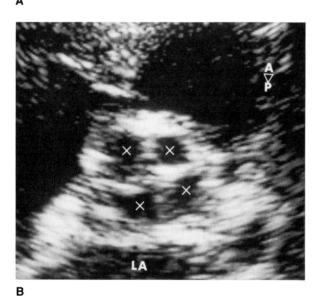

B

Fig. 16-6.   Transthoracic parasternal short-axis view at the aortic valve level showing **(A)** a unicuspid *(arrow)* and **(B)** a quadricuspid (x) aortic valve.

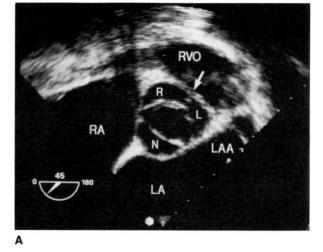

A

B

Fig. 16-7.   TEE in short-axis **(A)** and long-axis **(B)** views of the bicuspid aortic valve (systolic frame). These images were obtained by multiplane probe with the transducer rotated to 45 degrees for the short-axis view and 135 degrees for the long-axis view. In the short-axis view, commissures are seen at 5 and 9 o'clock positions with raphe at the 1 o'clock position *(arrow)*. The anterior cusp is made up of right (R) and left (L) cusps conjoined by a raphe, and the posterior cusp is usual noncoronary (N) cusp. In the long-axis view, the doming of the anterior aortic cusps *(arrow)* is well seen.

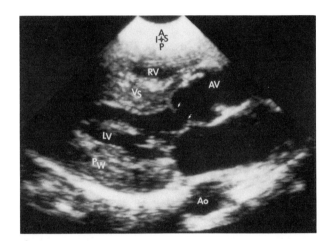

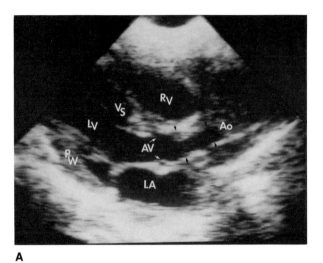

A

A

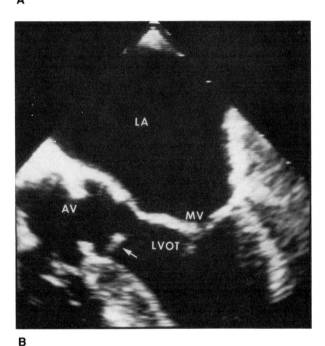

B

Fig. 16-8. **A.** Parasternal long-axis view of discrete membranous subaortic stenosis *(arrows).* A discrete subaortic membrane narrows the LV outflow tract. Note the LV hypertrophy. (From JB Seward et al. *Two-Dimensional Echocardiographic Atlas.* Vol. 1. New York: Springer, 1987.). **B.** TEE four-chamber view of discrete membranous subaortic stenosis *(arrow).*

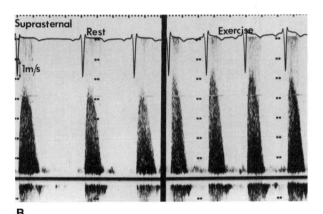

B

Fig. 16-9. **A.** Parasternal long-axis view of supravalvular aortic stenosis, secondary to thickening of the aortic wall *(black arrows)* above the aortic valve (AV). This would result in the typical appearance of an "hourglass" deformity on aortic root angiography. **B.** Continuous-wave Doppler across supravalvular aortic stenosis, from the suprasternal transducer position. At rest, the peak velocity reaches 4.5 m/sec, corresponding to a maximum gradient of 81 mm Hg. With exercise, the peak velocity increases to 5.5 m/sec, which is equal to a maximum gradient of 121 mm Hg.

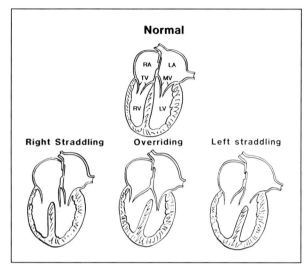

Fig. 16-10. Schematic drawing to illustrate the normal internal cardiac crux, and malalignment of the atrioventricular valve—straddling (i.e., chordal malalignment) and overriding (i.e., annulus malalignment).

is committed to the morphologic LV, and the lower inserting morphologic tricuspid valve to the morphologic right ventricle.

The crux anatomy is best imaged from a precordial, apical, subcostal, or transesophageal four-chamber view. Many complex anomalies of the heart are most confidently diagnosed by their alteration of the crux anatomy (Ebstein's anomaly, tricuspid atresia, corrected transposition, double inlet) [9, 10] (Fig. 16-11 through 16-14). When atrioventricular valve is malaligned with respect to the ventricular septum, the terms *straddling* and *overriding* are used to describe this malalignment (see Fig. 16-10). *Straddling* is used to describe the atrioventricular valve whose chordae insert into two ventricular chambers and *overriding* is used when the annulus is committed into both ventricles. Overriding is considered minor when less than 50% of the annulus is committed to the contralateral ventricle, and major when approximately 50% or more of the annulus is committed to the contralateral ventricle. In the extreme when both atrioventricular valves are committed to a single ventricular chamber, the abnormality is called double-inlet ventricle. All patients with atrioventricular valve straddling have complex congenital heart disease [10].

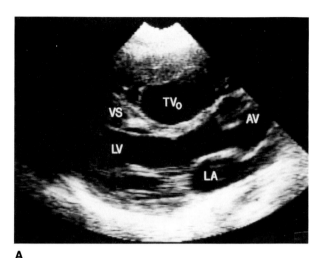

A

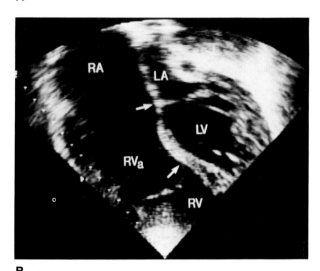

B

Fig. 16-11. Ebstein's anomaly. **A.** Transthoracic parasternal long-axis view. Anteriorly the orifice of the tricuspid valve (TVo) is reoriented toward the right ventricular outflow. **B.** Four-chamber view. The septal leaflet of the tricuspid valve is inserted *(arrows)* downward from its expected position. This downward displacement of the tricuspid valve atrializes (RVa) a portion of the right ventricle (RV).

Ventricular Septal Defect

In the adult, a VSD may be found as an isolated defect or associated with other anomalies such as tetralogy of Fallot or pulmonary atresia. Depending on the location, a VSD is classified as (1) membranous/perimembranous (i.e., the

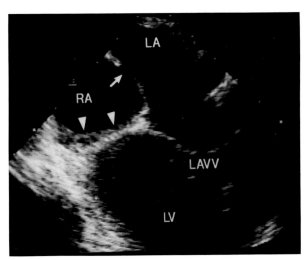

Fig. 16-12. Tricuspid atresia on TEE. In the floor of the right atrium (RA), a fibrous band *(arrowheads)* replaces the tricuspid valve (i.e., tricuspid valve atresia). An atrial septal defect *(arrow)* connects the right and left (LA) atria. A large left atrioventricular valve (LAVV) empties blood from the left atrium into the left ventricle (LV).

▼ **Fig. 16-14.** Double-inlet LV during systole **(A)** and diastole **(B)**. All of the left-side and more than 50% of the right-side atrioventricular valve are committed to the LV. The orifice of the right atrioventricular valve overrides the ventricular septum (VS). The right ventricle (RV) is small. The septal portion of the straddling valve inserts far into the left ventricular cavity *(arrows)*. The left atrioventricular valve is committed entirely to the LV.

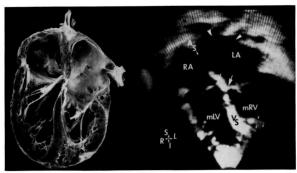

Fig. 16-13. Corrected transposition of the great arteries. The right atrium communicates with a right-side morphologic LV, which connects to the pulmonary artery, and the left atrium communicates with a left-side morphologic right ventricle, which connects to the aorta. Cardiac specimen cut in the four-chamber plane (left). Note that the right atrium communicates with the mitral valve (inserts higher on the ventricular septum), and the left atrium communicates with the lower inserting tricuspid valve and right ventricle. Four-chamber echo image (right) showing the reversed relationship of the cardiac crux (i.e., the right-side mitral valve inserts higher than the left-side tricuspid valve). The morphologic LV (mLV) is to the left below the right atrium (RA), and the morphologic right ventricle (mRV) is below the left atrium (LA). The right ventricle is trabeculated *(small arrows)*. The pulmonary veins *(arrowheads)* enter the left atrium. (From JB Seward et al. *Two-Dimensional Echocardiographic Atlas.* Vol. 1. New York: Springer, 1987.)

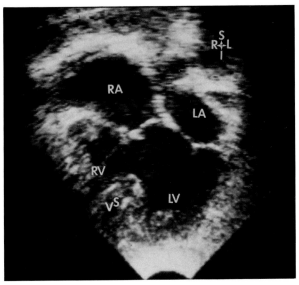

A

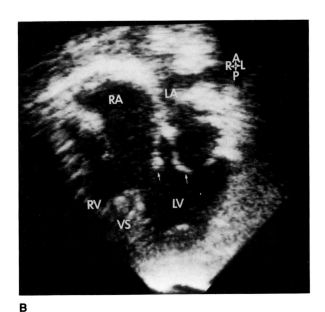

B

most common type; Fig. 16-15), (2) outflow (infundibular/supracrystal), (3) inflow (atrioventricular canal), and (4) muscular (trabecular). Color Doppler echocardiographic examination can identify VSD in more than 90% of cases. Continuous-wave Doppler can measure blood flow velocity and gradient across the VSD, which can then be used to calculate the right ventricular pressure. The right ventricular systolic pressure is calculated by subtracting VSD gradient from the assumed or measured LV systolic pressure (Fig. 16-16). A large VSD would have a smaller pressure difference between the ventricles, and conversely a small VSD would have a large gradient (i.e., velocity) between the ventricles. A membranous or infundibular VSD can be associated with increasing aortic valve regurgitation secondary to variable aortic valve prolapse. Even in the presence of modest aortic valve regurgitation and small VSD flow, this particular defect usually should be closed and the aortic valve repaired to prevent worsening aortic valve regurgitation.

Fig. 16-15. Membranous ventricular septal defect (VSD). (Top left) Subcostal view. The VSD *(large arrow)* is located just below the aortic valve (AV). (Top right) Parasternal short-axis view. The VSD *(small arrows)* is located on the medial aspect of the LV outflow (LVO). (Bottom) Parasternal long-axis view with medial tilt of the image plane. The VSD *(small arrows)* is located in the upper ventricular septum (VS) just beneath the aortic valve (AV). P = papillary muscle.

Patent Ductus Arteriosus

In the adult, patent ductus arteriosus is usually found as an isolated defect since more complex congenital heart diseases associated with it are usually discovered early in infancy. In the fetus, the ductus carries blood from the proximal portion of the left pulmonary artery to the descending thoracic aorta. After birth, if the ductus remains patent, the pulmonary pressures will fall and result in varying degrees of left-to-right shunt (i.e., aorta to pulmonary artery). If the shunt is significant, it may ultimately result in increasing pulmonary hypertension, shunt reversal, and cyanosis. Echocardiographic diagnosis is based on demonstrating persistent anatomic connection and flow between the descending aorta and pulmonary artery. The best imaging view is a high left parasternal long-axis scan of the right ventricular outflow tract and main pulmonary artery [1].

Fig. 16-16. Continuous-wave Doppler recordings from VSD (left), pulmonary regurgitation (center), and tricuspid regurgitation (right) in a patient with VSD. Since peak velocity across the VSD is 4 m/sec, the left ventricular–right ventricular systolic pressure gradient is 64 mm Hg (4×4^2). The systolic blood pressure was 130 mm Hg; thus, the right ventricular systolic pressure is 66 mm Hg (i.e., 130 − 64). A tricuspid regurgitation velocity of 3.7 m/sec equals a gradient of 55 mm Hg (4×3.7^2) from the right ventricle to the right atrium. Assuming a right atrial pressure of 10, the right ventricular systolic pressure equals 65 mm Hg (i.e., 55 + 10), which is nearly identical to the right ventricular systolic pressure estimated from VSD Doppler velocity (66 mm Hg).

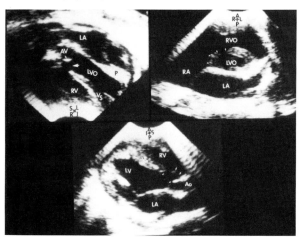

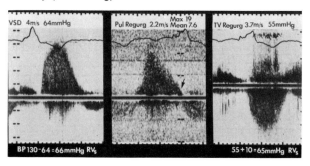

Coarctation

Coarctation of the aorta (see also Chap. 14) represents aortic luminal narrowing typically just distal to the left subclavian artery. Bicuspid aortic valve is a common association. It is also the most common cardiac anomaly seen in patients with Turner's syndrome. The area of aortic narrowing can often be seen from the suprasternal or the high left parasternal transducer position. However, continuous-wave Doppler is the best means to recognize the presence of coarctation as well as to quantitate the magnitude of stenosis. Doppler recording of hemodynamically significant coarctation is characterized by a continuous abnormal flow velocity throughout diastole. In the older patient and any patient with a repaired coarctation, exercise with continuous Doppler assessment is very helpful for recognizing hemodynamically significant (re)coarctation.

Overriding Aorta

Overriding aorta (i.e., aortic valve overriding the ventricular septum; Fig. 16-17) is associated with (1) tetralogy of Fallot, (2) pulmonary atresia with VSD, and (3) truncus arteriosus. Truncus arteriosus is rarely seen in the adult because of the unprotected pulmonary vascular bed. The distinguishing characteristics of these entities include (1) varying degrees of infundibular and pulmonary valvular stenosis in tetralogy; (2) atretic pulmonary valve, hypoplastic pulmonary arteries, systemic-to-pulmonary collateral arteries in pulmonary atresia with VSD; and (3) origin of the pulmonary arteries from the ascending aorta in truncus arteriosus.

Pediatric Congenital Heart Disease

Echocardiography has markedly impacted the indication for cardiac catheterization in children with congenital heart disease. Echocardiography allows early recognition, goal-directed management, and serial hemodynamic assessment of all forms. Cardiac catheterization is predominantly performed to assess pulmonary resistance and extracardiac anatomy (i.e., abnormalities of pulmonary arborization and coarctation and collateral vessels). When utilized in children below the approximate age of 9 or 10 years, TEE requires general anesthesia. Thus TEE is primarily used in the operating room to confirm surgical result or in the catheterization laboratory to assist with therapeutic intervention.

Fetal Congenital Heart Disease

High-resolution echocardiography can now be confidently used to diagnose congenital heart disease in the fetus. This has allowed for prenatal counseling and planning of pregnancy, delivery, and neonatal care. Echocardiography is most effectively utilized to anticipate fetal or neonatal problems and to logically plan treatment strategies.

Fig. 16-17. Parasternal long-axis view of an overriding aortic valve in a patient with pulmonary atresia with VSD. The aortic valve *(arrow)* and aortic root (Ao) override the ventricular septum (VS). Ao = aortic root and thoracic aorta.

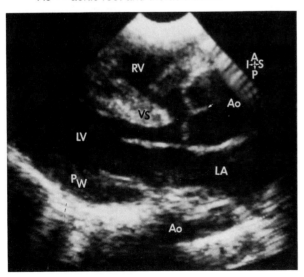

Heart Disease in Pregnancy

Congenital heart disease in the mother or in the fetus is most logically managed with the help of noninvasive echocardiography. Because there are no known harmful effects of ultrasound, it can be safely repeated. Hemodynamic and morphologic characterization as well as serial evaluation for planning of pregnancy can be done noninvasively.

Transesophageal Echocardiography

Due to the superb visualization of the cardiovascular structures, TEE is increasingly utilized in the diagnosis of congenital heart disease [11]. With a smaller probe, it is also possible to perform TEE in infants and small children, although compared to adult patients with congenital heart disease, the need for TEE is less common. This examination is particularly useful in evaluating the atrial septum, cardiac crux, atrial cavities, great arteries and veins of the thorax, and ventricular outflow tracts (Figs. 16-18 and 16-19; see also Figs. 16-4, 16-5, 16-7, and 16-8).

Wide-Field and 3D Imaging

Because most congenital anomalies lie in more than one anatomic plane, wide planes of view are anticipated to be particularly helpful in the understanding of these anomalies. By rotating the transducer in the esophagus, wide-field imaging is feasible and allows better appreciation of cardiovascular structural relationships, especially in congenital heart disease (Fig. 16-20). Closely aligned sets of two-dimensional images can also be interpreted to produce three-dimensional images. It is believed that the next era of echocardiography will occur with the advent of true three-dimensional imaging.

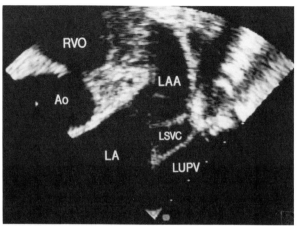

A

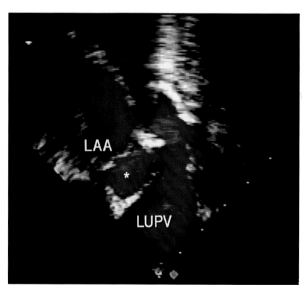

B

Fig. 16-18.   A. Left superior vena cava on TEE (horizontal scan plane in a basal short-axis view). The transducer is posterior to the left atrium (LA). In the partition between the orifice of the left upper pulmonary vein (LUPV) and the left atrial appendage (LAA) courses the persistent left superior vena cava (LSVC). Anteriorly and medially, the aortic root (Ao) and right ventricular outflow (RVO) are also visualized. **B.** Color-flow Doppler confirms flow in the left upper pulmonary vein and left superior vena cava *(asterisk).*

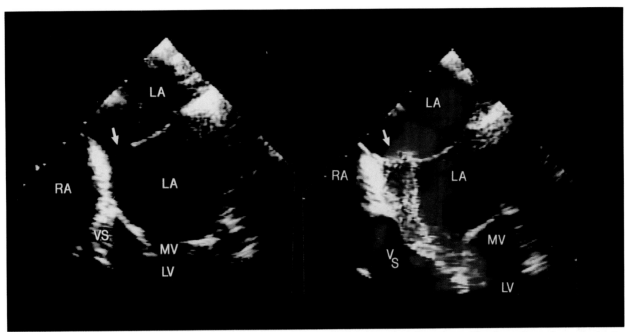

Fig. 16-19. Cor triatriatum on TEE with horizontal transducer in the four-chamber plane. The transducer is posterior to the left atrium (LA) within the esophagus. Within the left atrial cavity is a membrane that divides the left atrium into two cavities. The posterior cavity contains the pulmonary veins and the anterior cavity contains the left atrial appendage (not shown) and mitral valve (MV). The two cavities communicate through a stenotic orifice *(arrow)* in the membrane. Color-flow Doppler (right) shows a turbulent jet across the stenotic membrane.

Fig. 16-20. Wide-field long-axis view of sinus venosus atrial septal defect on TEE. The transducer is posterior in the esophagus and adjacent to the left atrium (LA). The atrial septum (AS) and superior vena cava (SVC) are shown in the long axis. In the superior fatty limbus of the atrial septum is a large sinus venosus atrial septal defect *(arrowhead)*. The wall of the right pulmonary artery (RPA) forms the superior margin of the defect. The membrane of the fossa ovalis (FO), the typical position of a secundum atrial septal defect, remains intact. The right atrium (RA) is located anteriorly.

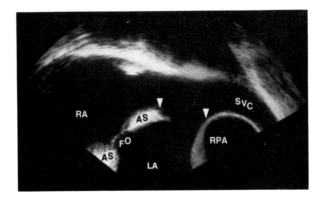

Intraoperative Echocardiography

Echocardiography is increasingly being utilized intraoperatively. No longer is mortality or morbidity an acceptable barometer of surgical success. Instead, successful complete repair with minimal number of residua is the gold standard of care, and this has been accomplished primarily as a result of intraoperative confirmation of anatomy, function, hemodynamics, and blood flow utilizing echocardiography.

References

1. Seward JB, Edwards WD. *Two-Dimensional Echocardiographic Atlas: Congenital Heart Disease,* Vol. 1. New York:Springer, 1987.
2. Shub, C et al. Sensitivity of two-dimensional echocardiography in the direct visualization of atrial septal defect utilizing the subcostal approach: experience with 154 patients. *J Am Coll Cardiol* 1983;2(1):127–135.
3. Khandheria BK, et al. Utility of color flow imaging for visualizing shunt flow in ASD. *Int J Cardiol* 1989;23:91–98.
4. Morimoto K, et al. Diagnosis and quantitative evaluation of secundum-type atrial septal defect by transesophageal Doppler echocardiography. *Am J Cardiol* 1990;66(1):85–91.
5. Oh JK, et al. Visualization of sinus venosus atrial septal defect by transesophageal echocardiography. *J Am Soc Echocardiogr* 1988; 1:275–277.
6. Nanda NC, et al. TEE of the pulmonary veins. *Echocardiography* 1991;8:741–748.
7. Brandenberg RO, et al. Accuracy of two-dimensional echocardiographic diagnosis of congenitally bicuspid aortic valve: Echocardiographic-anatomic correlation in 115 patients. *Am J Cardiol* 1983;51:1469.
8. Oh JK, et al. Prediction of the severity of aortic stenosis by Doppler aortic valve area determination: prospective Doppler-catheterization correlation in 100 patients. *J Am Coll Cardiol* 1988;11:1227–1234.
9. Seward JB, et al. Internal cardiac crux: two-dimensional echocardiography of normal and congenitally abnormal hearts. *Ultrasound Med Biol* 1984;10:735–745.
10. Rice MJ, et al. Straddling atrioventricular valve: two-dimensional echocardiographic diagnosis, classification and surgical implications. *Am J Cardiol* 1985;55:505–513.
11. Seward JB, et al. Transesophageal echocardiography in congenital heart disease. *Am J Cardiac Imag* 1990;4:1–8.

17

Intraoperative Echocardiography

Although epicardial M-mode echocardiography was used in the operating room as early as 1972 to evaluate the result of open mitral commissurotomy [1], it was not until the late 1980s that intraoperative echocardiography became a routine procedure with the widespread use of transesophageal echocardiography (TEE) and incorporation of color-flow imaging. Currently, at the Mayo Clinic, intraoperative TEE represents 25% of all TEE procedures (Fig. 17-1). The purpose of intraoperative echocardiography is threefold: (1) to ensure the optimal result of reconstructive cardiac surgery such as mitral valve repair or congenital defect repair, (2) to minimize cardiovascular complications during surgical procedures (cardiac and noncardiac) in

Fig. 17-1. Number of TEE examinations at the Mayo Clinic in 1991 and 1992. Intraoperative use of TEE accounts for about 25% of all TEE studies. Due to the patients with congenital heart defects, the mean age of patients is relatively young (48 years). OR = operating room.

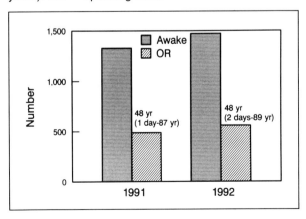

high-risk patients; and (3) to troubleshoot when a patient becomes hemodynamically unstable in the operating room.

Mode

There are two approaches to performing intraoperative echocardiography [2]: (1) epicardial and (2) transesophageal. The advantages and the limitations of each approach are as follows:

Epicardial	Transesophageal
Multiple windows	Limited window
Disturbs surgical field	No interference with surgical field
Intermittent monitoring	Continuous monitoring

At the Mayo Clinic, intraoperative echocardiography is performed mostly by TEE except when

1. the TEE probe cannot be introduced into the esophagus.
2. anterior cardiac structures are obscured by prosthetic material.

Implementation

Intraoperative echocardiography is a multidisciplinary approach and requires cooperation among anesthesiologists, cardiologists, and surgeons. Since the anesthesiologist is in charge of the patient's hemodynamics and airways, it is logical that the transesophageal probe be inserted by the anesthesiologist. If he or she is comfortable with performing TEE, the baseline TEE can be obtained and reviewed with a cardiologist-echocardiographer. Routine monitoring of air embolism or regional wall motion abnormalities is mostly done by the anesthesiologist. In the case of a valve or shunt repair, usually the cardiologist-echocardiographer is actively involved from the beginning of the operation. The TEE findings are discussed with the cardiac surgeon and the anesthesiologist. The identification of the location and extent of morphologic abnormalities of the heart helps the surgeon to direct neces-

sary attention to the particular areas and also helps him or her formulate surgical plans. Echocardiography is repeated soon after the patient comes off the bypass pump, to assess the results of repair. The postoperative echocardiographic findings are discussed with the surgeon. When the structural and hemodynamic results are deemed inadequate, the second pump-run is initiated to revise the repair, after which its results are again evaluated by echocardiography. However, it is not realistic to attempt *perfect* repair in all surgical cases. If a mild hemodynamically insignificant lesion remains, it is better to leave it alone rather than go back to revise the repair. It may be sometimes difficult to determine the long-term outcome of apparently abnormal structures or functions shown on intraoperative echocardiography that are not causing immediate hemodynamic abnormalities. Depending on the surgical procedure, 5 to 10% of cases require a second pump-run [2–6].

Indications and Mitral Valve Repair

The indications for intraoperative echocardiography in 508 patients at the Mayo Clinic in 1992 are shown in Figure 17-2. In adult patients, mitral valve repair is the most common cardiac surgical procedure done using intraoperative echocardiography. Currently at the Mayo Clinic, the mitral valve is repaired, rather than replaced, in more than 95% of patients with various regurgitant mitral valve lesions. Myxomatous degeneration (prolapse, flail, and/or ruptured chordae tendineae) is responsible for mitral regurgitation in 70% of the patients undergoing mitral valve repair [3]. Other etiologies include myocardial ischemia, annulus dilatation, papillary muscle dysfunction, cleft mitral leaflet, and less commonly, rheumatic disease or endocarditis. Valve repair is not recommended for an active endocarditic lesion or in a hemodynamically unstable patient (i.e., shock patient with papillary muscle dysfunction or rupture). Compared with mitral valve replacement, repair is associated with

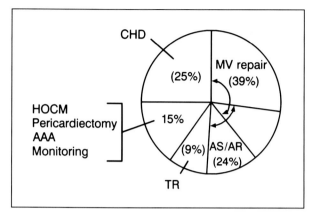

Fig. 17-2. A pie diagram demonstrating indications of intraoperative TEE at the Mayo Clinic in 1992. The most frequent indication of intraoperative TEE was during mitral valve (MV) repair or to evaluate mitral regurgitation with or without concomitant aortic valvular disease or coronary artery disease. Left ventricular monitoring by TEE was done in selected high-risk patients during vascular or major thoracoabdominal surgery. AAA = abdominal aortic aneurysm repair; AS/AR = aortic stenosis/ regurgitation; CHD = congenital heart disease; HOCM = hypertrophic obstructive cardiomyopathy; MV = mitral valve; TH = tricuspid regurgitation.

lower short- and long-term mortality [7–9]. In addition, there is no need for long-term anticoagulation and less risk for infective endocarditis.

Reconstructive cardiac surgery is an individualized procedure and its outcome is less predictable than valve replacement. After the patient is anesthetized, the TEE probe is inserted to obtain the baseline data regarding mitral valve morphology, severity of mitral regurgitation, global systolic function, and other cardiovascular abnormalities (e.g., patent foramen ovale, intracardiac mass, and tricuspid regurgitation). The posterior mitral leaflet is more frequently involved than the anterior leaflet in patients with myxomatous degeneration. The success rate for satisfactory mitral valve repair is much higher for posterior leaflet prolapse or flail segment than for anterior or bileaflet involvement (98.3 versus 77.5%) [3]. Intraoperative TEE examples of posterior, an-

terior, and bileaflet involvement of myxomatous mitral valve are shown in Figures 17-3 through 17-5. For severe mitral regurgitation due to myxomatous degeneration (usually with ruptured chordae), repair consists of (1) quadrangular excision or plication of redundant and/or flail tissue; (2) reconstruction of competent mitral leaflet; (3) shortening of chordae, if elongated; and (4) ring (usually flexible Duran ring) annuloplasty. If the mitral valve has different morphologic mechanisms for severe mitral regurgitation, for example, perforation (Fig. 17-6), cleft mitral valve, endocarditis, and annulus dilatation, the repair procedure is altered accordingly.

The echocardiographer responsible for the intraoperative evaluation should be well familiar with the repair procedure to assess postoperative results. Immediate feedback regarding the structural and functional result of a reconstructive procedure prior to chest closure provides additional security to the surgeon (when the result is good) or an opportunity to revise the repair (when it is suboptimal) [2–6]. Revision was necessary in 10 (7%) of the 143 patients who underwent mitral valve repair at the Mayo clinic [3]. Significant mitral regurgitation may still be present due to systolic anterior motion of the repaired mitral valve, usually in the setting of hypovolemia and/or hyperdynamic left ventricle (LV). Systolic anterior motion and mitral regurgitation usually resolve when LV volume is repleted. It should also be emphasized that mitral regurgitation severity after the repair be assessed under physiologic hemodynamic milieu.

Intraoperative echocardiography occasionally (< 3%) detects clinically unsuspected abnormalities that alter or add operative procedures [3]. Examples include patent foramen ovale (Fig. 17-7), atrial septal defect, cardiac mass (thrombus or tumor), unsuspected valvular regurgitation, and vascular abnormalities. Other surgical procedures that routinely employ intraoperative echocardiography are myectomy (for hypertrophic obstructive cardiomyopathy), tricuspid valve repair, shunt or congenital defect repair, and repair of aortic dissection (Figs. 17-8 and 17-9).

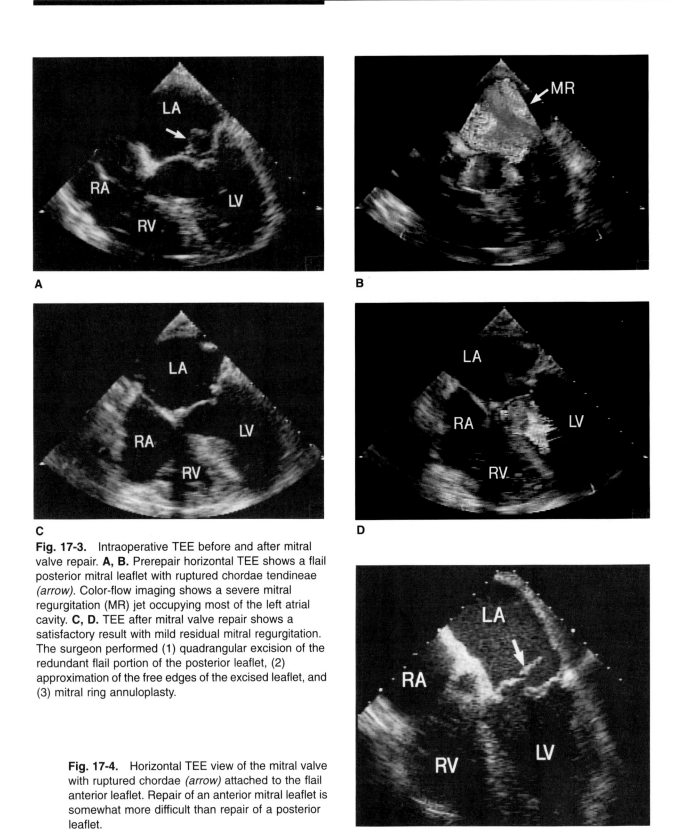

A

B

C

D

Fig. 17-3.   Intraoperative TEE before and after mitral valve repair. **A, B.** Prerepair horizontal TEE shows a flail posterior mitral leaflet with ruptured chordae tendineae *(arrow)*. Color-flow imaging shows a severe mitral regurgitation (MR) jet occupying most of the left atrial cavity. **C, D.** TEE after mitral valve repair shows a satisfactory result with mild residual mitral regurgitation. The surgeon performed (1) quadrangular excision of the redundant flail portion of the posterior leaflet, (2) approximation of the free edges of the excised leaflet, and (3) mitral ring annuloplasty.

Fig. 17-4.   Horizontal TEE view of the mitral valve with ruptured chordae *(arrow)* attached to the flail anterior leaflet. Repair of an anterior mitral leaflet is somewhat more difficult than repair of a posterior leaflet.

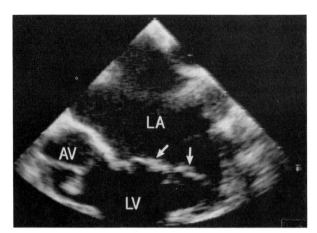

Fig. 17-5. Horizontal TEE view of bileaflet mitral valve prolapse *(arrows).*

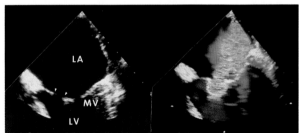

Fig. 17-6. Intraoperative horizontal TEE view of the mitral valve in a young patient with progressive dyspnea. He was stabbed in the chest several years earlier. Prerepair 2D imaging (left) shows a large perforation *(arrowheads)* of the anterior mitral leaflet (presumably due to previous stabbing). Color-flow imaging (right) shows a severe mitral regurgitation jet via the defect. The perforation was repaired with a patch closure with no residual mitral regurgitation.

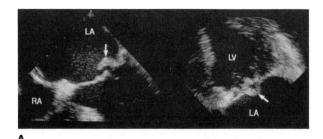

A

B

Fig. 17-7. **A.** Horizontal (left) and longitudinal (right) TEE imaging of a flail myxomatous mitral leaflet *(arrow)* obtained by intraoperative TEE. **B.** Comprehensive intraoperative TEE examination showed severe mitral regurgitation (MR) and patent foramen ovale *(double arrows)* with left-to-right shunt. This was best shown in a longitudinal atrial septum–superior vena cava (SVC) view. The mitral valve was successfully repaired and the patent foramen ovale closed with sutures.

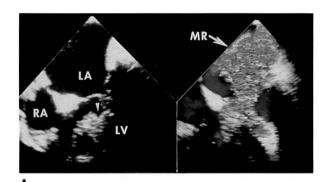
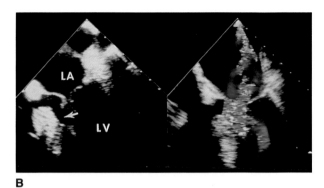

A   **B**

Fig. 17-8.   After the initial myectomy (*arrowhead,* **A**), there was still systolic anterior motion (SAM) of the mitral valve and severe mitral regurgitation (MR). Since the systolic anterior motion contact was distal to the myectomy site, myectomy was extended further distally *(arrow,* **B**). Color-flow imaging after additional myectomy shows only a mild degree of residual mitral regurgitation.

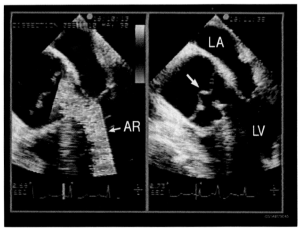
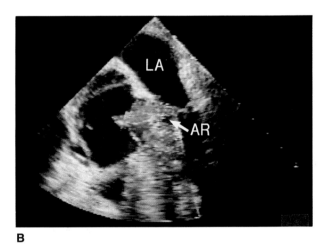

A   **B**

Fig. 17-9.   An elderly man with history of hypertension presented to the emergency room with severe back pain, pulse deficit, hypotension, and pulmonary edema. Aortic dissection was suspected, and he was urgently taken to the operating room. **A.** Intraoperative TEE shows proximal aortic dissection with an intimal flap *(arrow)* in the ascending aorta and severe aortic regurgitation on color-flow imaging. **B.** TEE after repair of aortic dissection demonstrates mild residual aortic regurgitation *(arrow).*

Intraoperative Monitoring

Intraoperative echocardiography is also useful for monitoring [10–12] such as for air embolism during neurosurgical procedure, fat embolism during hip arthroplasty, and regional wall motion abnormalities (as a marker of ischemia) in patients with severe coronary artery disease undergoing noncardiac surgery. Intraoperative TEE for monitoring is best performed by the anesthesiologist trained in echocardiography. Although there was an initial enthusiasm for routine monitoring of regional wall motion abnormalities in patients with suspected or known coronary artery disease during noncardiac surgery to detect intraoperative ischemia, the positive predictive value is very low and the correlation between transient wall motion abnormalities and intraoperative infarct is not strong [10]. The additive clinical value of intraoperative TEE in noncardiac surgery requires further study and there are no compelling data to support routine TEE monitoring of LV regional myocardial function during noncardiac surgical procedures.

In unstable patients another important use of intraoperative echocardiography is to evaluate unsuspected structural or hemodynamic problems perioperatively [3, 5]. The problems range from the totally unrelated to the planned surgical procedure to the complication of the surgical procedure—for example, unsuspected cardiac tumor during mitral valve surgery, aortic dissection during coronary artery bypass surgery, and rupture of a cardiac structure after routine valve replacement or bypass surgery (Figs. 17-10 and 17-11). Therefore, intraoperative echocardiography is valuable in troubleshooting unstable hemodynamic conditions after any type of surgical procedure.

Fig. 17-10. Persistent hypotension after a repeat mitral valve replacement. Intraoperative TEE was performed to evaluate the patient's unstable hemodynamic condition after the third mitral valve replacement. The study shows a pseudoaneurysm *(arrow)* in the left atrioventricular groove. Surgical inspection confirmed the pseudoaneurysm and it was closed.

Fig. 17-11. Emergency intraoperative echocardiography was requested to evaluate an unstable hemodynamic condition after routine coronary bypass surgery. The patient had a transmural inferior wall myocardial infarction, and coronary angiography showed 80% left main coronary artery stenosis and 100% right coronary occlusion. Until the time of operation, he was stable with no audible murmur. After bypass surgery, he could not come off the bypass pump. Transgastric TEE short-axis view of the LV demonstrates a large inferoseptal ventricular septal defect (VSD), with left-to-right shunt shown by color-flow imaging (orange-red flow indicates flow from the LV to the right ventricle).

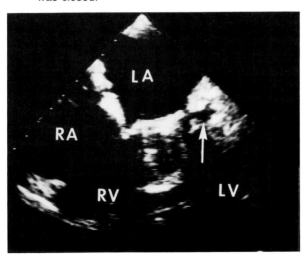

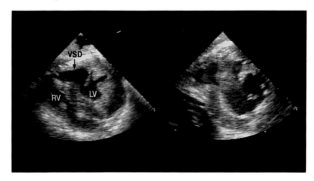

References

1. Johnson ML, et al. Usefulness of echocardiography in patients undergoing mitral valve surgery. *J Thorac Cardiovasc Surg* 1972;64:922–933.

2. Stewart WJ, et al. Intraoperative Doppler color flow mapping for decision-making in valve repair for mitral regurgitation: technique and results in 100 patients. *Circulation* 1990;81:556–566.

3. Freeman WK, et al. Intraoperative evaluation of mitral valve regurgitation and repair by transesophageal echocardiography: incidence and significance of systolic anterior motion. *J Am Coll Cardiol* 1992;3:599–609.

4. Goldman ME, et al. Mitral valvuloplasty is superior to valve replacement for preservation of left ventricular function: an intraoperative two-dimensional study. *J Am Coll Cardiol* 1987;10:568–575.

5. Sheikh KH, et al. The utility of transesophageal echocardiography and Doppler color flow imaging in patients undergoing cardiac valve surgery. *J Am Coll Cardiol* 1990;15:363–372.

6. Reichert SLA, et al. Intraoperative transesophageal color-coded Doppler echocardiography for evaluation of residual regurgitation after mitral valve repair. *J Thorac Cardiovasc Surg* 1990;100:756–761.

7. Orszulak TA, et al. Mitral regurgitation due to ruptured chordae tendineae: early and late results of valve repair. *J Thorac Cardiovasc Surg* 1985;89:491–498.

8. Sand ME, et al. A comparison of repair and replacement for mitral valve incompetence. *J Thorac Cardiovasc Surg* 1987;94:208–219.

9. Cosgrove DM, et al. Results of mitral valve reconstruction. *Circulation* 1986;74(suppl I):82–87.

10. Eisenberg MJ, et al. Monitoring for myocardial ischemia during noncardiac surgery. *JAMA* 1992;268:210–216.

11. Ereth MH, et al. Cemented versus noncemented total hip arthroplasty—embolism, hemodynamics, and intrapulmonary shunting. *Mayo Clin Proc* 1992;67:1066–1074.

12. Black S, et al. Preoperative and intraoperative echocardiography to detect right to left shunt in patients undergoing neurosurgical procedures in the sitting position. *Anesthesiology* 1990;72:436–438.

18

Echocardiography in Conjunction with Other Procedures or Techniques

Since entire cardiovascular structures can be visualized by comprehensive echocardiographic examination (using both the transthoracic and the transesophageal windows), echocardiography has been coupled with diagnostic or interventional cardiovascular procedures to improve diagnostic accuracy or to perform the procedures more efficiently and more safely.

Stress Echocardiography

Myocardial ischemia is manifested as new or worsening of regional wall motion abnormalities. Therefore, to diagnose myocardial ischemia, baseline wall motion of the left ventricle (LV) is compared to wall motion at peak or immediately after stress. Stress can be applied in the form of exercise, medication (dobutamine, dipyridamole, adenosine), or atrial pacing [1–7]. The baseline and (peak or post) stress images are stored in a digital format using a cine loop for a side-by-side comparison. In patients who cannot perform exercise for various reasons, pharmacologic stress can be performed. If the transthoracic approach yields inadequate imaging quality, transesophageal echocardiography (TEE) can be combined with pharmacologic stress. See Chapter 6 for additional information.

Pericardiocentesis

Pericardiocentesis (see also Chap. 12) can be carried out safely under 2D echocardiographic guidance [8–10]. The echocardiogram identifies the optimal puncture site (where the largest amount of pericardial effusion can be reached from the shortest distance), and the result of pericardiocentesis can be monitored easily by repeated examinations. The characteristic appearance of pericardial effusion on echocardiography can occasionally be useful in determining the etiology of pericardial effusion (such as hemopericardium versus infectious pericardial effusion). Doppler examination is useful in assessing the hemodynamic significance of residual pericardial effusion and in detecting effusive-constrictive pericarditis [11–12].

Intraoperative Echocardiography

The results of cardiac valve repair and other corrective surgeries can be assessed intraoperatively by echocardiography [13–15] (see also Chap. 17). This can be done by the epicardial or transesophageal approach. TEE has the advantages of not interfering with the surgical field and visualizing almost all cardiovascular structures. In addition to assessment of the surgical repair, intraoperative echocardiography can aid in identifying the underlying cardiovascular pathologies, which may be useful for surgeons to formulate operative procedures. Another important role of intraoperative echocardiography is to troubleshoot unexpected clinical deterioration perioperatively. For example, a patient with normal LV function and normal hemodynamic conditions before mitral valve repair becomes hypotensive and hemodynamically quite unstable after successful mitral valve repair. The patient may have hypovolemia, hemopericardium, LV outflow tract obstruction secondary to systolic anterior motion of the mitral valve which was just repaired, severe myocardial ischemia due to inadequate cardioplegia, or other mechanical complications associated with surgical procedures. This can be promptly evaluated by TEE which should help to identify the exact etiology of a patient's condition. The patient may be undergoing noncardiac surgery and become hemodynamically unstable. Intraoperative

echocardiography again is quite useful for prompt patient evaluation in the operating room. TEE has been utilized routinely at the Mayo Clinic to monitor air embolism in patients undergoing neurosurgical procedures and also to monitor regional wall motion abnormalities in selected high-risk patients undergoing noncardiac surgery [16–17].

Mitral Balloon Valvuloplasty

Balloon valvuloplasty is the procedure of choice for symptomatic mitral valve stenosis unless there is significant calcification of the mitral valve, subvalvular abnormalities, or severe mitral regurgitation. The procedure involves the transseptal passage of a balloon catheter and enlargement of the stenotic mitral valve orifice by inflation of the balloon. The procedure is usually performed under fluoroscopic guidance. TEE may be more useful in guiding the transseptal catheter to the fossa ovalis region, positioning the balloon in the mitral valve orifice area, and assessing results or complications of the procedure [18] (Fig. 18-1). Continuous-wave Doppler (Fig. 18-2) and color-flow imaging accurately provide the transmitral gradient and the amount of mitral regurgitation after each inflation. At the end of the procedure, the amount of left-to-right shunt secondary to the transseptal procedure can be measured by color-flow Doppler echocardiographic examination.

Closure of Atrial Septal Defect or Patent Foramen Ovale

Since the entire atrial septum can be visualized by TEE, closure of an atrial septal defect or patent foramen ovale can be guided or monitored [19]. A clamshell device has been utilized for this purpose; Figure 18-3 demonstrates the TEE imaging of closure by the device. A right-to-left shunt may result in significant hypoxemia, usually due to elevation of the right atrial pressure. In acute right-to-left shunt via the

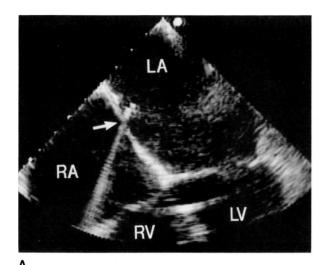

A

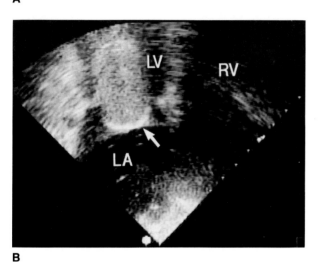

B

Fig. 18-1. TEE guidance and monitoring of mitral balloon valvuloplasty for mitral stenosis.
A. Horizontal four-chamber view showing the puncture of the atrial septum *(arrow)* by a catheter during the initial transseptal procedure.
B. Longitudinal view showing the position of the balloon *(arrow)* at the level of the mitral valve during inflation.

patent foramen ovale, it may be necessary to temporize the clinical situation by occluding the patent foramen ovale by balloon inflation. Figure 18-4 demonstrates such a case using a Rashkind balloon catheter in a critically ill patient with hypoxemia after right ventricular infarction. Oxygen saturation improved significantly after the procedure.

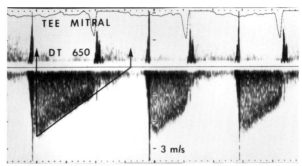

Fig. 18-2. Continuous-wave Doppler recording of a stenotic mitral valve using the transesophageal window. Since the mitral inflow is away from the esophagus, the velocities are recorded below the baseline. The peak velocity is 2.5 m/sec, corresponding to a 25 mm Hg gradient, and the pressure half-time is 190 msec ($= 0.29 \times 650$ msec) since the deceleration time (DT) is 650 msec. The velocity profile can be converted to above the baseline electronically.

Catheter Placement

TEE has been used to guide a catheter to a desired location during radiofrequency ablation and to assess any potential complication of the procedure. Initially, all radiofrequency ablations at the Mayo Clinic were carried out under the guidance of TEE monitoring. No significant structural complication was noted. Although not routinely utilized, TEE is potentially useful in positioning a bioptome for endomyocardial biopsy.

Contrast Echocardiography for Detection of Shunt

Although color-flow imaging is highly sensitive for detecting left-to-right shunt, right-to-left shunt is more difficult to detect by color-flow Doppler since it occurs with a relatively low pressure gradient (or low flow velocity). Therefore, contrast study is more sensitive in detecting right-to-left shunt, especially via the patent foramen ovale [20]. It is also useful in the detection of arteriovenous fistula in the lung. In patients with right-to-left shunt via the patent foramen ovale, the contrast agent

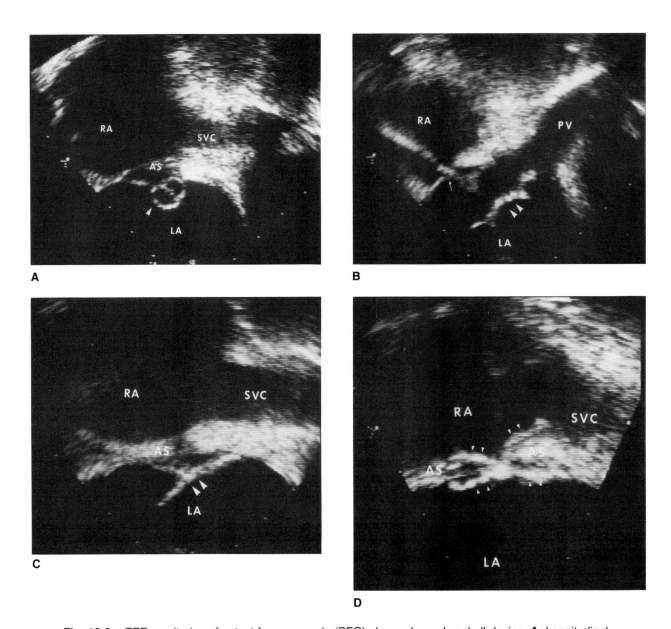

Fig. 18-3.   TEE monitoring of patent foramen ovale (PFO) closure by a clamshell device. **A.** Longitudinal view showing a balloon catheter *(arrowhead)* across the patent foramen ovale to size the defect. **B.** The clamshell device *(arrowheads)* is seen in the left atrium (LA) near the left upper pulmonary vein (PV). **C.** The device is pulled gently toward the atrial septum (AS) to close the patent foramen ovale. **D.** The arms *(arrowheads)* of the clamshell device are anchored onto the superior and inferior limbi of the atrial septum (AS).

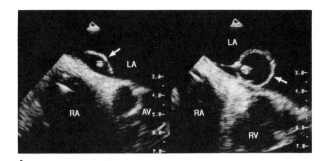

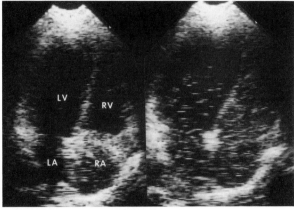

Fig. 18-5. Apical four-chamber contrast echocardiography in a patient with pulmonary arteriovenous (A-V) fistula. A contrast agent (indocyanine green) is injected into the right atrium (RA; left) and there is *no* immediate appearance of the agent in the left atrium. After four cardiac cycles (right), the left cardiac chambers are opacified by the contrast agent.

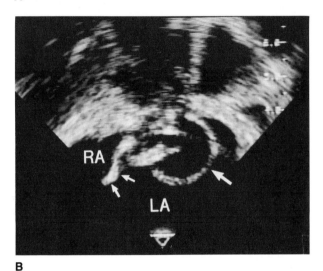

Fig. 18-4. TEE guidance and monitoring of occlusion of the patent foramen ovale by a balloon catheter in a patient with severe hypoxemia due to severe right-to-left shunt via the patent foramen ovale. **A.** Horizontal view showing a bulged atrial septum (*arrow* in left) toward the left atrium due to increased right atrial pressure. A Rashkind balloon (*arrow* in right) is inflated in the left atrium and pulled toward the atrial septum to occlude the patent foramen ovale. **B.** Longitudinal view of the same procedure as in **A.** The balloon (*large arrow*) is pulled tight toward the atrial septum (*small arrows*).

appears immediately in the left atrium after appearing in right atrium, whereas it takes longer than three cardiac cycles in arteriovenous fistula [21] (Fig. 18-5).

The most optimal contrast agent is indocyanine green followed by saline flush usually via a right-arm vein. Similar opacification can be achieved by injection of agitated saline solution. The study is performed at rest and after a provocative maneuver such as Valsalva or coughs. When a contrast agent is used to identify or verify the persistent left superior vena cava, contrast injection should be made via a left-arm vein. When cor atriatum Dexter is suspected as an explanation of right-to-left shunt and cyanosis, contrast injection may be necessary via a leg vein since only the flow from the inferior vena cava may shunt across the patent foramen ovale or atrial septal defect. Left-to-right shunt is seen as a negative contrast effect, shown in Figure 18-6, which is mostly replaced by color-flow imaging.

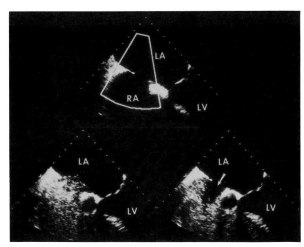

Fig. 18-6. Horizontal TEE view of atrial septal defect, demonstrating a negative contrast effect due to left-to-right shunt. A large atrial septal defect is shown in the upper panel. At onset of the QRS complex, few contrast bubbles cross the defect to the left atrium (left lower panel), but the most significant shunt is left to right, creating a beautiful negative contrast effect (*arrow* in right lower panel).

TEE is more sensitive in detecting atrial shunt and also is helpful in detecting intrapulmonary vascular shunt, since all four pulmonary veins are well visualized by TEE. By detecting contrast material in specific pulmonary veins, arteriovenous fistula not only can be diagnosed but also can be localized [22]. Intrapulmonary shunt may be aggravated by a standing position (orthodeoxia), especially in patients with liver disease or after pneumonectomy [23]. Hence, contrast echocardiography may be necessary with the patient in different positions (supine and upright). Contrast echocardiography also enhances weak continuous-wave Doppler spectral signals to allow better measurement of transvalvular flow velocities [24].

References

1. Sawada SG, et al. Exercise echocardiography detection of coronary artery disease in women. *J Am Coll Cardiol* 1989;14:140–147.

2. Sawada SG, et al. Prognostic value of a normal exercise echocardiogram. *Am Heart J* 1990; 120:49.

3. Crouse LJ, Harbrecht JJ, Vacek JL. Exercise echocardiography as a screening test for coronary artery disease and correlation with coronary angiography. *Am J Cardiol* 1991; 67:1213–1218.

4. Quinones MA, et al. Exercise echocardiography versus 201-Tl single-photon emission computed tomography in evaluation of coronary artery disease: analysis of 292 patients. *Circulation* 1992;85:1026–1031.

5. Picano E, Lattanzi F, L'Abbate A. Present application, practical aspects, and future issues on dipyridamole echocardiography. *Circulation* 1991;83(suppl III):111–115.

6. Berthe C, Pierard LA, Hiernaux M. Predicting the extent and location of coronary artery disease in acute myocardial infarction by echocardiography during dobutamine infusion. *Am J Cardiol* 1986;58:1167–1172.

7. Sawada SG, Segar DS, Ryan T. Echocardiographic detection of coronary artery disease during dobutamine infusion. *Circulation* 1991;83:1605–1614.

8. Callahan JA, et al. Pericardiocentesis assisted by two-dimensional echocardiography. *J Thorac Cardiovasc Surg* 1983;85:877–879.

9. Callahan JA, et al. Two-dimensional echocardiography guided pericardiocentesis: experience in 117 consecutive patients. *Am J Cardiol* 1985;55:476–479.

10. Kopecky SL, et al. Percutaneous pericardial catheter drainage: report of 42 consecutive cases. *Am J Cardiol* 1986;58:633–635.

11. Appleton CP, Hatle LK, Popp RL. Cardiac tamponade and pericardial effusion: respiratory variation in transvalvular flow velocities studied by Doppler echocardiography. *J Am Coll Cardiol* 1988;11:1020.

12. Burstow DJ, et al. Cardiac tamponade: characteristic Doppler observations. *Mayo Clin Proc* 1989;64:312–324.

13. Freeman WK, et al. Intraoperative evaluation of mitral valve regurgitation and repair by transesophageal echocardiography: incidence and significance of systolic anterior motion. *J Am Coll Cardiol* 1992;3:599–609.

14. Stewart WJ, et al. Intraoperative Doppler color flow mapping for decision-making in valve repair for mitral regurgitation: technique and results in 100 patients. *Circulation* 1990; 81:556–566.

15. Sheikh KH, et al. The utility of transesophageal echocardiography and Doppler color flow imaging in patients undergoing cardiac valve surgery. *J Am Coll Cardiol* 1990;15:363–372.

16. Ereth MH, et al. Cemented versus noncemented total hip arthroplasty—embolism, hemodynamics, and intrapulmonary shunting. *Mayo Clin Proc* 1992;67:1066–1074.

17. Black S, et al. Preoperative and intraoperative echocardiography to detect right to left shunt in patients undergoing neurosurgical procedures in the sitting position. *Anesthesiology* 1990;72:436–438.

18. Ballal RS, et al. Utility of transesophageal echocardiography in interatrial septal puncture during percutaneous mitral balloon commissurotomy. *Am J Cardiol* 1990;66:230–232.

19. Hellenbrand WE, et al. Transesophageal echocardiographic guidance of transcatheter closure of atrial septal defect. *Am J Cardiol* 1990;66:207–213.

20. Seward JB, et al. Peripheral venous contrast echocardiography. *Am J Cardiol* 1977; 39:202–212.

21. Shub C, et al. Detecting intrapulmonary right-to-left shunt with contrast echocardiography. Observations in a patient with diffuse pulmonary arteriovenous fistulas. *Mayo Clin Proc* 1976;51:81–84.

22. Nemec JJ, et al. Detection and evaluation of intrapulmonary vascular shunt with "contrast Doppler" transesophageal echocardiography. *J Am Soc Echocardiogr* 1991;4:79–83.

23. Mills TJ, et al. Platypnea-orthodeoxia: assessment with a unique cardiac catheterization procedure. *Cathet Cardiovasc Diagn* 1986; 12:100–102.

24. Hagler DJ, et al. Echocardiographic contrast enhancement of poor or weak continuous-wave Doppler signals. *Echocardiography* 1987; 4:63–67.

19

Comprehensive Examination According to the Referral Diagnosis

Echocardiography has become an extension of the physical examination in cardiovascular practice. Frequently, it is used to confirm clinical diagnostic suspicion and provide more detailed structural, functional, and hemodynamic information. Another important role of echocardiography is to detect the underlying cardiovascular pathology to explain the patient's symptom complex or laboratory abnormalities (chest x-ray, electrocardiography [ECG], or cardiac enzymes). Many patients are referred to the echocardiography laboratory because of their symptoms or nonspecific laboratory abnormalities and echocardiographers are expected to come up with a definite diagnosis or a clue to explain the patient's symptoms. In this last chapter, the comprehensive diagnostic approach is described according to the referral diagnosis.

Evaluation of Ventricular Function

Knowledge of left ventricular (LV) function is the basic step in all cardiology practice. General status of LV function is usually evident from history and examination. However, quantitation of LV function may be important to explain a patient's symptoms, to select the optimal therapeutic options, to select the optimal surgical timing, or to monitor the efficacy of a therapy. When a patient is referred for evaluation of ventricular function, the following systolic and diastolic function information should be provided:

1. LV cavity and wall dimensions, LV mass index

2. LV ejection fraction, fractional shortening
3. Description of regional wall motion abnormalities
4. The wall motion score index (especially in patients with ischemic heart disease)
5. Right ventricular (RV) cavity and wall dimensions
6. Description of RV function
7. Stroke volume and cardiac output
8. Diastolic filling parameters (mitral and tricuspid inflow velocities, pulmonary and hepatic vein flow velocity profile)

Evaluation of Dyspnea or Heart Failure

Dyspnea is a clinical manifestation of various cardiac or noncardiac disorders. This referral diagnosis requires a complete evaluation of the following:

1. Ventricular systolic and diastolic function as described above
2. Valvular anatomy and function
3. Exclude cardiac shunt
4. Respiratory variation in transvalvular and central venous flow (? constrictive pericarditis)
5. Evidence of cardiomyopathy?
6. Pulmonary artery pressure
7. Other cardiac or pericardial structural abnormalities of the heart

Stress echocardiography should be considered if the dyspnea is thought to be angina-equivalent.

Murmur or Mitral Valve Prolapse

Although various bedside maneuvers are helpful in determining the etiology of murmur by auscultation, it is often necessary to confirm clinical suspicion or to characterize further morphologic and hemodynamic detail. Another frequent reason for referral to echocardiography is mitral valve prolapse. It is still the most common cause for severe mitral regurgi-

tation and mitral valve repair (or replacement), but the majority of patients with mitral valve prolapse enjoy a relatively symptom-free life-style. Because of the medical, financial, and psychological impact of the diagnosis of mitral valve prolapse, strict diagnostic criteria should be utilized: (1) thickened or myxomatous mitral leaflets, (2) systolic displacement of the mitral leaflet into left atrium of at least 3 mm or more beyond the mitral annulus in the parasternal or apical long-axis view, and (3) mitral regurgitation.

2D echocardiography should be able to detect abnormal cardiac valve morphology such as bicuspid valve or pulmonic stenosis. Once the abnormal valve is identified, its hemodynamic severity should be established by Doppler and color-flow imaging. If 2D echocardiography does not identify a source of cardiac murmur, continuous-wave Doppler interrogation of all four valves and the septa (atrial and ventricular) should be performed. Occasionally, color-flow imaging can provide the first clue for an abnormal valve: trivial to mild aortic regurgitation from the bicuspid aortic valve or turbulent pulmonary artery flow from the pulmonic stenosis. Dynamic ventricular outflow obstruction is a frequent finding, especially in the elderly patient with a thickened basal septum with or without hypertension. Congenital heart lesions in adults, such as atrial septal defect, tiny ventricular septal defect, or patent ductus arteriosus, should be looked for when the usual causes of heart murmur are absent.

Nonspecific ECG Abnormalities

Although ECG is very useful when it is diagnostic for certain cardiac pathologies (i.e., ST-segment elevation for myocardial transmural infarct, diffuse ST-segment elevation for pericarditis), many ECG abnormalities are not specific or diagnostic. T-wave inversion may be a result of myocardial ischemia, electrolyte abnormalities, apical hypertrophic cardiomyopathy, or subarachnoid hemorrhage, or may even be a normal variation. Since an ECG abnormality can indicate a serious underlying cardiovascular condition, it therefore raises concern in preoperative assessment and, similarly, a nonspecific ECG abnormality may develop after a surgical or interventional procedure and creates a concern for procedure-related myocardial ischemia or infarction.

Echocardiography is a logical next diagnostic step since it can clarify the significance of ECG abnormalities by assessing the following:

1. Regional wall motion abnormalities for ischemia/infarction
2. Cardiomyopathy
3. Pericardial effusion
4. Intracardiac mass
5. Pulmonary embolism
6. LV hypertrophy
7. Valvular heart disease

Transient myocardial dysfunction has been noted after electroconvulsive therapy (ECT) or subarachnoid hemorrhage, along with ECG repolarization changes [1]. It is most likely related to a catecholamine surge, and gradual resolution of wall motion abnormalities has been documented by serial echocardiographic examination.

Chest Pain

Echocardiography is very helpful in the evaluation of chest pain syndrome, especially when the chest pain is not accompanied by diagnostic ECG changes. In a significant portion of patients with acute myocardial infarction, the initial ECG is nondiagnostic for myocardial ischemia. The diagnostic value is greatest if the study is performed while the patient is having chest pain. If the pain is of ischemic etiology, the regional wall motion abnormalities are usually present, even before typical ECG changes occur. The presence of regional wall motion abnormalities is not, however, specific for acute ischemia, but their absence strongly suggests a nonischemic etiology. Other cardiac reasons for chest pain can be readily detected by echocardiography. The following diagnoses should be considered when one evaluates patients with nonspecific chest pain:

1. Ischemia or infarction
2. Aortic dissection
3. Pericarditis
4. Valvular heart disease, especially aortic stenosis
5. Cardiomyopathies, especially hypertrophic cardiomyopathy
6. Pulmonary embolism
7. Intracardiac or extracardiac mass

Cardiac Source of Emboli

The cardiac sources of systemic or cerebral embolism include intracardiac thrombus, mass, vegetation, atrial septal aneurysm, paradoxical embolism via the patent foramen ovale, and ulcerated plaques in the aorta [2, 3]. Transthoracic echocardiography alone is inadequate to evaluate all the above pathologies. The left atrial appendage is not well visualized by transthoracic echocardiography and patent foramen ovale is not recognized in almost half of patients on transthoracic examination. Therefore, for comprehensive evaluation of the cardiac source of emboli, transesophageal echocardiography (TEE) should be performed.

Evaluation by transthoracic echocardiography should include the following:

1. Evaluate LV function.
2. Evaluate the anatomic substrate for thrombi formation such as aneurysm, dyskinetic segments, left atrial enlargement, mitral valve disease, hypereosinophilic syndrome, and atrial septal aneurysm.
3. Identify vegetations.
4. Detect cardiac tumors.

Evaluation by TEE should include the following:

1. Search for intracardiac mass or thrombi.
2. Visualize the left atrial appendage.
3. Look for spontaneous echo contrast in the left atrium, in multiple planes.

4. Scan the atrial septum for patent foramen ovale or atrial aneurysm.

5. Contrast echocardiography for detection of right-to-left shunt by injection of agitated saline solution via an arm vein at rest and with the release of Valsalva maneuver.

Hypotension or Cardiogenic Shock

Echocardiography is the most valuable bedside diagnostic tool to evaluate the patient with hypotension and/or shock syndrome. If a patient's symptoms are of cardiac origin, echocardiography should be able to identify the responsible etiology in these patients. The following should be evaluated by echocardiography:

1. LV and RV function
2. Valvular abnormalities (severe aortic stenosis, mitral regurgitation, aortic regurgitation, endocarditis, etc.)
3. Cardiac tamponade (search for localized, regional tamponade in postoperative patients)
4. Dynamic LV outflow tract obstruction
5. Hypovolemia (small LV cavity size with hypercontractile walls)
6. Pulmonary embolism (acute RV dilatation with generalized RV hypokinesis)
7. Cardiac shunt (e.g., infarct ventricular septal defect)
8. Aortic dissection
9. Cardiac rupture

Patients in the intensive care unit who are critically ill have multiple monitoring and life-saving devices. It may not be possible to perform echocardiography from the transthoracic window. TEE can be performed safely and provide diagnostic-quality images in this patient population [4]. For TEE in the critically ill patient:

1. Sedate the patient well (midazolam, meperidine hydrochloride [Demerol], and/or pancuronium for severely agitated patients on a ventilator).

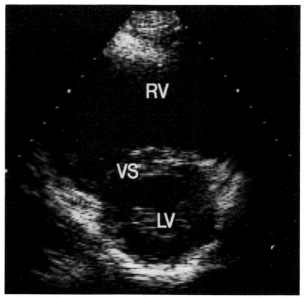

Fig. 19-1. Parasternal short-axis view showing a dilated right ventricle (RV) due to cardiac contusion. A similar finding is seen in right ventricular infarction, right ventricular cardiomyopathy, right ventricular volume overload as in atrial septal defect, and severe tricuspid regurgitation.

2. Administer glycopyrrolate (0.2 mg intravenously) for secretion control.
3. Monitor oxygen saturation and blood pressure during the examination.
4. Perform a comprehensive examination expeditiously.

In addition, there is no need to remove the nasogastric tube.

Cardiac Contusion and Donor Heart Evaluation

Cardiovascular pathologies due to chest trauma are potentially fatal complications, but frequently unrecognized since they occur in the setting of injury to multiple organ systems. Clinical examination, cardiac enzyme measurements, chest x-ray, and ECG may not be sensitive or specific for cardiac contusion or

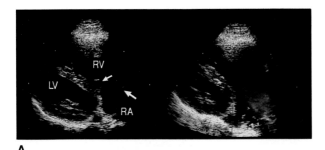

A

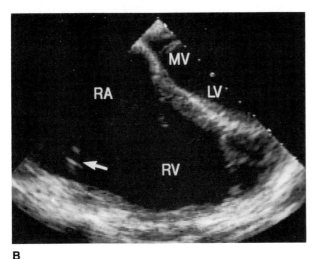

B

Fig. 19-2. A. Right ventricular inflow view shows a dilated right chamber and flail anterior tricuspid leaflet (*arrow* in right atrium), allowing severe tricuspid regurgitation. The tricuspid regurgitant color jet has laminar flow (without turbulence) due to a wide-open tricuspid regurgitation with no significant pressure gradient between the right ventricle and atrium. **B.** Horizontal TEE of the same patient shows a dilated and akinetic right ventricle (in real time) due to cardiac contusion. The tricuspid anterior leaflet is flail (*arrow*).

other cardiovascular structural abnormalities. Potential cardiac complications of chest trauma include ventricular dysfunction (especially contusion of the right ventricle since it is close to the sternum), cardiac tamponade, cardiac rupture, valvular rupture (especially the tricuspid valve), aortic rupture (see Fig. 15-10), and intracardiac thrombus. These cardiovascular pathologies can be promptly detected at the patient's bedside by 2D/Doppler echocardiography using both the transthoracic and the transesophageal approach. TEE is especially helpful in the evaluation of aortic pathology, cardiac or valvular rupture, and in patients with a suboptimal transthoracic window due to chest injury or motor vehicle accident [5–7].

Detection or exclusion of cardiac contusion is crucial when victims of motor vehicle accidents are evaluated as potential cardiac donors, to minimize the donor heart failure rate.

Examples of transthoracic and transesophageal echocardiographic findings of cardiac contusion are shown in Figures 19-1 and 19-2.

Systemic Hypertension

Hypertension is a common condition that contributes significantly to cardiovascular morbidity and mortality. LV hypertrophy is a characteristic response to systemic hypertension and is an independent prognostic indicator. 2D/M-mode echocardiography can measure LV wall thickness and estimate LV mass, both of which are indices of LV hypertrophy.

LV mass is derived from 2D-guided M-mode echocardiography of the LV from a parasternal short-axis view, as described in Chapter 4. When measuring LV mass by M-mode echocardiography, it is important to take into account patient age, body surface area, and sex. The values for the upper-normal LV mass index, as determined from M-mode echocardiography, is shown in Figure 4-4.

Not uncommonly, global systolic LV function is hyperdynamic due to hyperadrenergic state and intravascular volume contraction, resulting from diuretic therapy. Hypercontractile systolic function in the setting of LV hypertrophy may result in dynamic LV outflow tract obstruction, which produces a characteristic systolic late-peaking, dagger-shaped, continuous-wave Doppler signal.

Diastolic function is another important parameter that can be measured by 2D Doppler echocardiography in patients with systemic hypertension. The prominent diastolic abnormality in hypertension is a relaxation abnormality, and Doppler shows prolonged LV isovo-lumic relaxation time, reduced mitral inflow E velocity, increased mitral inflow A velocity, reduced E/A ratio, and prolonged mitral inflow deceleration time. However, the diastolic fill-ing pattern becomes pseudonormalized or re-strictive when a patient develops congestive heart failure during an end-stage hypertensive state.

In patients with hypertension and chronic renal failure, myocardial texture may become abnormal, simulating the appearance of car-diac amyloid, but is usually accompanied by a marked increase in QRS voltage on an elec-trocardiogram, compared to low voltage in cardiac amyloid. Therefore, the following in-formation needs to be assessed and evaluated in patients with systemic hypertension:

1. LV cavity and wall dimensions
2. LV mass index
3. LV systolic and diastolic function
4. Dynamic LV outflow tract obstruction

References

1. Zhu WX, et al. Myocardial stunning after elec-troconvulsive therapy. *Ann Intern Med* 1992;117:914–915.

2. DeRook FA, et al. Transesophageal echocardi-ography in the evaluation of stroke. *Ann Intern Med* 1992;117:922–932.

3. Amarenco P, et al. The prevalence of ulcerated plaques in the aortic arch in patients with stroke. *N Engl J Med* 1992;326:221–225.

4. Oh JK, et al. Transesophageal echocardiogra-phy in critically ill patients. *Am J Cardiol* 1990;66:1492–1495.

5. Miller FA Jr, et al. Two-dimensional echocardi-ographic findings in cardiac trauma. *Am J Cardiol* 1982;50:1022–1027.

6. Locke TJ, et al. Diagnosis of traumatic aortic rupture by transesophageal echocardiography. *J Thorac Cardiovasc Surg* 1991;101:555–556.

7. Galvin EF, et al. Transesophageal echocardiog-raphy in acute aortic transection. *Ann Thorac Surg* 1991;51:310–311.

Index

Note: Page numbers followed by f indicate figures; those followed by t indicate tables.

Abscess, aortic, 195
Acquired immunodeficiency syndrome (AIDS), heart involvement in, 162
Adenosine, 70–71
Alcohol, myocardial toxicity of, 162
Aliasing, 16, 18f
American College of Cardiology, echocardiography performance guidelines, 2
American College of Physicians, echocardiography performance guidelines, 2
American Heart Association, echocardiography performance guidelines, 2
American Society of Echocardiography
  congenital heart disease recommendations of, 205
  quantitation method recommendations of, 39
Amyloidosis
  cardiac, 156
  diastolic abnormalities of, 156
  echocardiographic features of, 154–157
  survival curve for, 157f
  ventricular wall thickness in, 153
Anatomic correlations, transesophageal echocardiographic, 22–34
Anatomic features, transthoracic echocardiography and, 7–13
Aneurysm
  aortic, 195, 196f, 201–203
  atrial septal, 210f

  mitral-aortic intervalvular fibrosa, 133–135
  ventricular, 79–80
Aneurysmal descending thoracic aorta, 197
Angiosarcoma, 187
Angiotensin-converting enzyme (ACE), 161
Anticoagulation therapy, 80
Aorta
  abscess of, 195
  anatomic relationships of, 34f
  aneurysm of, 195, 196f, 200–201
  ascending, in Marfan's syndrome, 196f
  biplane imaging planes of, 34
  coarctation of, 195, 203
    echocardiographic examination in, 217
  diseases of, 195–203
  long-axis view of, 196f
  M-mode echocardiography of, 53f
  overriding, 217
  pseudoaneurysm of, 201, 202f
  rupture of, 195, 200
  thoracic, 34, 35f, 195, 197
  views of, 34, 35f
  visualization of, 195
Aortic aneurysm, 201–203
Aortic annulus, 196f
Aortic debris, 200–201
Aortic disk prosthesis, 127
Aortic dissection, 196, 226f
  echocardiography of
    transesophageal, 198–200
    transthoracic, 196–197
  type I, 198f
  type II, 197f

  type III, 199f
Aortic plaque, 200
Aortic prosthesis
  dehisced, 118f, 126f
  obstruction of, 122–123
  pressure gradients of, 118–119f
Aortic regurgitation, 104
Aortic root abscess, 134f, 202f
Aortic stenosis, severe, 90–91
Aortic valve
  basal short-axis view of, 25f
  bicuspid, 87, 90f, 212f
  endocarditis of, 134f
  fibroelastoma of, 191f
  M-mode echocardiography of, 53f
  overriding, 217f
  prosthetic, Doppler hemodynamic profiles of, 120t
  regurgitation of, 88
    Doppler/color-flow imaging of, 101–104
    severity of, 60
    mild, 104
    severe, 103–104
    two-dimensional and M-mode echocardiography of, 101
    velocity of, 61
  in secondary long-axis view, 30f
  stenosis of
    differential diagnosis of, 95f
    Doppler echocardiography in, 89–96
    planimetry for, 112
    severe, 90–91
    subvalvular, 210
    supravalvular, 213f
    symptomatic, 209–210

Aortic valve, stenosis of—
Continued
two-dimensional and M-
mode echocardiography
in, 88–89
unicuspid and quadricuspid,
212f
Aortic valve area, 89
calculation of, 93
catheter-derived, 94f
continuity equation, 90
Apical hypertrophic cardiomyopathy
differential diagnosis of,
148–149
2D/M-mode echocardiography
of, 140, 142f
Arrhythmogenic right ventricular dysplasia, 139–140
Atherosclerotic plaques/debris,
195, 200
Atrial fibrillation
blood flow in, 64
cardioversion after TEE,
191
nonrheumatic, echocardiography in, 191
stroke prevention in, 191
Atrial filling phase (AFP), 46
Atrial myxoma, 185
transesophageal echocardiogram of, 187f
transthoracic echocardiogram
of, 186f
Atrial septum
aneurysmal, 210f
defect of
echocardiographic examination of, 208–209
echocardiography with closure of, 230–231
primum, 209f
secundum, 210f
sinus venosus, 211f, 219f
types of, 209f
lipomatous hypertrophy of,
192f
Atrioventricular septum, 210
Atrioventricular valve defect,
215f
Autocorrelation, 18
Automated edge detection system, 50

Bacterial endocarditis
prophylaxis for, 22, 23t
transesophageal echocardiography in, 133
transthoracic echocardiography in, 130
Bernoulli equation, 52, 54f
modified, 88
Bicuspid aortic valve, 87f, 90f,
212f
Bjork-Shiley aortic prosthesis obstruction, 121f
Bleeding disorder, with transesophageal echocardiog-
raphy, 35
Blood flow
in color-flow imaging, 18–19
pulmonary, 58f
through narrowed orifice, 54f
velocities of
acceleration of, 52
Doppler measurement of,
52
in normal, constriction, and
restriction, 171f
transvalvular gradients of,
55–58
in valvular stenosis, 88
Branciocephalic vessels, 195

Carcinoid heart disease, 157–159
Carcinoid plaque, 158–159
Cardiac amyloidosis. *See* Amyloidosis
Cardiac catheterization, 93, 127
Cardiac contusion, 240–241
Cardiac dimensions
measuring methods for, 14–15
normal values for, 15t
quantitative measurement of,
7
Cardiac disease. *See* Heart disease;
specific disorders
Cardiac hemodynamics, 51–64
Cardiac output, measurement of,
52–55
Cardiac prosthesis, infective endocarditis with, 129
Cardiac rupture, 74
Cardiac structures
detailed motion recordings of,
14–15
first ultrasound recording of, 1

Cardiac tamponade
detection of, 76–77
Doppler pattern of, 168f, 169f
echocardiography in, 165–166,
167f
Cardiac tumors
metastatic, 188–189
primary, 185–187, 188t
Cardiac valves. *See* specific valves
Cardiogenic shock
evaluation of, 238
post-myocardial infarction,
168f
transesophageal echocardiography in, 240
Cardiologist, role in interpreting
stress echocardiograms,
72
Cardiomyopathies
classification of, 137
dilated, 137–140
hypertrophic, 140–149
infiltrative, 150
primary, 138f
restrictive, 149–150
secondary, 153, 162
Cardiopulmonary resuscitation,
capabilities for, 22
Catecholamine crisis, 162
Catheter placement, 231
Caval–right atrial–atrial septal
view, 29f
Chest pain
evaluation of, 239
syndromes of, 72–73
Chondrosarcoma, 185
Chordal rupture, 147
Chronic obstructive pulmonary
disease, 69
Coanda effect, 104
Color-flow imaging
in comprehensive examina-
tion, 238
development of, 2
in hypertrophic cardiomyopathy, 143–146
instrumentation for, 5
in mitral regurgitation, 76, 106
in mitral stenosis assessment,
96–100
in prosthetic regurgitation,
123
in shunt detection, 231–234

in transthoracic echocardiography, 18–19
in valvular regurgitation, 101–110, 112
Congenital heart disease, 205
adult, 207–217
fetal, 217
infective endocarditis with, 129
intraoperative echocardiography in, 219
pediatric, 217
in pregnancy, 218
systematic tomographic approach in, 205–206
transesophageal echocardiography in, 218, 219f
two-dimensional examination in, 206–207
wide-field and three-dimensional imaging in, 218–219
Continuity equation, 58–59, 88
in determining aortic and mitral valve area, 90, 97
in determining prosthetic orifice area, 121–122
Continuous-wave Doppler echocardiography. *See* Doppler echocardiography, continuous-wave
Contrast agents, 233
Contrast echocardiography
in atrioventricular fistula, 233f
in evaluation of systemic embolism, 239
in myocardial viability and collateral circulation, 81
negative-contrast, 234
in shunt detection, 231–234
COPD. *See* Chronic obstructive pulmonary disease
Cor atriatum Dexter, 233
Cor pulmonale
transesophageal echocardiography in, 183–184
transthoracic echocardiography in, 182–183
Cor triatriatum, 219f
Coronary artery disease, 67–84
clinical impact of echocardiography in, 83–84
coronary artery visualization in, 82–83
diastolic function in, 82

digital echocardiography in, 69–70
intravascular ultrasound in, 84
morbidity and mortality of, 67
regional wall motion analysis in, 67–69
reperfusion therapy evaluation for, 80–81
risk stratification in, 81–82
stress echocardiography in, 70–72
viability, 81
wall motion score index, 46
Coronary artery visualization, 82–83
Coronary bypass surgery, intraoperative echocardiography after, 227f
Coronary flow reserve evaluation, 83
Coronary sinus aneurysm, 195
CPR. *See* Cardiopulmonary resuscitation
Cyanotic heart disease, 208

Deceleration time (DT), 46, 82
with myocardial infarction, 82f
pressure half-time and, 59–60
prolonged, 47
shortened, 47–49
Diagnosis, referral, 237–241
Diagnostic ultrasound, 4
Diastasis, 46
Diastole, definition of, 46–47
Diastolic filling
abnormalities of, 46–49
assessment of, 62
pattern of, 46–49
in post-myocardial infarction risk stratification, 82
relaxation abnormality, 47
respirometer recording, 171f
restrictive, 47–49, 64
venous flow pattern in, 49
Diastolic function assessment, 61–64, 82
Digital echocardiography
concept of, 69f
in coronary artery disease, 69–70
Dilated cardiomyopathy
Doppler echocardiography of, 139

familial, 139–140
two-dimensional echocardiography in, 137–139
Dipyridamole, 70–71
Dobutamine
in aortic stenosis with low output, 91
in stress echocardiography, 70–71
for stunned myocardium and myocardial viability, 81
Donor heart evaluation, 240–241
Doppler, Christian, 15
Doppler-derived pressure gradients, 2
Doppler echocardiography
accuracy of, 1–2
in aortic disease, 201–203
in cardiac disease due to systemic illness, 153, 156
in comprehensive examination, 240
in congenital heart disease, 208–209, 216
in constrictive pericarditis, 171
continuous-wave, 4–5, 16–17, 61–63, 110–112, 139, 230, 231f
in detecting complications of myocardial infarction, 73, 76
development of, 1
in dilated cardiomyopathy, 139
in hemodynamic assessment, 51–52, 55–59
in hypertrophic cardiomyopathy, 143–146
in infective endocarditis, 130
limitations and pitfalls of, 93–95
in mitral regurgitation evaluation, 76
in mitral stenosis assessment, 96–100
in pericardial effusion, 166
in prosthetic valve evaluation, 118–127
for pulmonary hypertension, 178–181
pulsed wave, 16–17, 139
transmitral, 82
transthoracic, 15–17

Doppler echocardiography—
Continued
in valvular heart disease evaluation, 87–113
in valvular regurgitation evaluation, 101–110
in valvular stenosis evaluation, 88, 89–100
Doppler effect, 15
demonstration of, 16f
Doppler equation, 16
Doppler measurements, normal maximal velocities in, 18t
Doppler shift, 15–16
Doppler spectra, 18f
Doxorubicin, myocardial toxicity of, 162
dP/dt, 61–62
Duchenne's dystrophy, heart involvement in, 162
Dyspnea evaluation, 238

Ebstein's anomaly, 214f
Echo-free space, 165
Echocardiography. *See also* Doppler echocardiography; M-mode echocardiography; Transesophageal echocardiography; Transthoracic echocardiography
for aortic diseases, 195–203
in cardiac disease due to systemic illness, 153–162
in cardiomyopathies, 137–150
clinical impact of
in coronary artery disease, 84
in pericardial disease, 175
in prosthetic valve dysfunction, 124–127
in valvular heart disease, 113
cognitive skills needed for, 3t
in comprehensive examination, 237–241
in congenital heart disease, 205–219
contrast, 231–234
in coronary artery disease, 67–84
development of, 1–2
in emergency room, 73
in endocarditis, 129–136
examination for, 2–5

in hemodynamic assessment, 51–64
instrumentation in, 3–5
intraoperative, 221–227, 230
in congenital heart disease, 219
introduction into clinical practice, 1
in myocardial infarction, 72–82
in nonrheumatic atrial fibrillation, 191
operator in, 2–3
with other procedures or techniques, 229–234
in pericardial diseases, 165–175
in prosthetic valve evaluation, 117–127
in pulmonary hypertension, 177–184
in regional wall motion analysis, 67–69
technical skills needed for, 3t
training for, 2–3
transesophageal, 21–37, 173–175, 198–200
transthoracic, 2, 7–19, 196–197
for tumors and masses, 185–193
in valvular heart disease, 87–113
in valvular regurgitation evaluation, 100–110
Effective regurgitant orifice (ERO), 107–109
Ejection fraction, 43
Elderly, dynamic left ventricular outflow tract obstruction in, 145–146
Electrocardiographic abnormalities, nonspecific, 238–239
Electroconvulsive therapy, 239
Embolism
air, 227
pulmonary, 182–184
with ventricular aneurysm, 80
Embolization, systemic, 200
Embolus, cardiac source of, 239–240
Emergency room, echocardiography in, 73
End-diastolic left ventricular volume, 43

Endocarditis
infective, 129
complications of, 132–133
diagnosis of, 129–132
echocardiographic-pathologic correlation in, 135–136
transesophageal echocardiography of, 133–135
Libman-Sacks, 161–162
Epicardial echocardiography, intraoperative, 222
Examination, comprehensive, 237–241
Exercise echocardiography, 70, 229
Exercise hemodynamics, in mitral stenosis, 100

Fetus, congenital heart disease in, 217
Fibroelastoma, aortic valve, 191f
Fibroma, left ventricle, 187f, 188f
Fibrosarcoma, 187
Field depth, 4
Filters, setting of, 4–5
Four-chamber view
in heart disease, 206
in two-dimensional examination, 207
Fractional shortening, 43–44
Frequency shift. *See* Doppler shift
Friedreich's ataxia, heart involvement in, 162

Gain setting, 5
Gorlin formula, 88
Gray scales, 4

Heart
anatomic section of, 9f, 11f, 12f
contusion, 240–241
first ultrasound examination of, 1
four-chamber view of, 26f
left ventricle-left atrial two-chamber view of, 28f
long- and short-axis views of, 7
longitudinal views from transthoracic transducer positions, 9f
parasternal short-axis views of, 10f

primary longitudinal TEE
views of, 27f
suprasternal notch long-axis
view of, 13f
tumors and masses of, 185–193
Heart failure
evaluation of, 238
with restrictive filling pattern,
82
Heart murmur, 238
Heart muscle disease, classification of, 138f
Hemangiosarcoma, 187
Hemochromatosis, heart disease
with, 159–160
Hemodynamics
abnormalities of, 52t
signs of, 52t
assessment of, 51–65
time constant of LV relaxation (TAU), 64–65
in constrictive pericarditis,
170–171
in mitral stenosis, 100
restrictive, 149–150
of stenotic valves, 111–112
in valve prostheses, 120t
Hepatic vein
Doppler velocities from, 171f
flow velocities of, 48f, 49, 64
pulsed-wave Doppler of, 110f
Hibernating myocardium, 81–82
Holodiastolic flow reversal,
103f
Horizontal plane
transesophageal, 23–24
transgastric, 28f
Hydraulic orifice formula, 55f
Hypereosinophilic syndrome,
160
Hypertension
aortic pathology in, 200f
echocardiographic evaluation
of, 241
pulmonary, 149, 177–184
systemic, 241–242
Hypertrophic cardiomyopathy
diastolic function, 144
Doppler/color-flow imaging in,
143–146
hypertensive, 146
isovolumic relaxation flow,
145, 146f

limitations and pitfalls of echocardiography in, 147–149
transesophageal echocardiography in, 146–147
two-dimensional and M-mode
echocardiography in,
140–143
Hypotension
evaluation of, 240
Hypothyroidism, heart involvement in, 162

Indocyanine green, 233
Infarct ventricular septal defect,
73, 74–76
Innominate artery stenosis, 95f
Instantaneous gradients, 55
maximum (MIG), 55–58, 59f
Instrumentation, 3–5
for transesophageal echocardiography, 21–22
Internal cardiac crux, 210–214
Intracardiac flow, 51t
Intracardiac pressures
echocardiographic determina-
tion of, 51t
measurement of, 60–61
Intracavitary flow, abnormal, 19
Intramural hematoma, 195
Intraoperative echocardiography,
221–227, 230
implementation of, 222
indications of, 222–223
mode of, 222
in monitoring, 227
purposes of, 221–222
Intrapulmonary shunt, 234
Intravascular ultrasound, 84
Intravenous drug users, infective
endocarditis in, 129
Ipecac syrup (Emetin), myocardial toxicity of, 162
Iron, myocardial deposit of, 159
Isovolumic contraction period,
61
Isovolumic relaxation flow, 62
apical obstruction with, 147f
with hypertrophic cardiomyopathy, 145
Isovolumic relaxation time
(IVRT), 46
prolonged, 46–47
shortened, 47, 49

Left atrial pressure, 64
Left ventricle
basal contractile function measurement, 42f
cavity size of, 81
concentric hypertrophy of, 162
dimensions of, 50
filling pressure of in pericardial
effusion, 166
linear dimensions and areas
from base of, 40t, 41
mass of, 41–43
quantitation of, 39–43
volumes of, 41, 42f
Left ventricular outflow tract,
52–55
diameter of, 93
dynamic obstruction of in
elderly, 146
obstruction of, 143
versus mitral regurgitation,
144
in stroke volume calculation,
56f
velocity of, 93, 95, 96f
Left ventricular outflow
tract–aortic valve time velocity integral ratio, 89,
90–93, 94f
Libman-Sacks endocarditis, cardiac lesions in, 161–162
Lipomatous atrial septal hypertrophy, 192f
Long-axis view
in heart disease, 206
of upper abdomen, 207
Longitudinal plane
transesophageal, 24–30
transgastric, 28f, 30f
Lung tumor, malignant, 35

M-mode echocardiography, 1,
14f
in aortic stenosis assessment,
88–89
in congenital heart disease,
208f
in constrictive pericarditis,
166–170
in hemodynamic assessment,
51–52, 53–54f
in hypertrophic cardiomyopathy, 140–143

M-mode echocardiography—
  Continued
  in infective endocarditis,
    129–130
  limitations of, 1
  in measuring cardiac dimen-
    sions, 14–15
  in pericardial effusion, 166
  in pulmonary hypertension,
    177–178
  transthoracic, 7–15
  in valvular regurgitation evalu-
    ation, 100, 101, 104,
    109
Mahan's equation, 180
Marfan's syndrome, 195
  ascending aorta in, 196f
Masses
  apical, 190f
  hiatal hernia, 193f
  intracardiac, 185, 192
  left atrial, 187f
  metastatic, 188–189
  transesophageal echocardiogra-
    phy for, 189–191
Mean gradient, 58
Mechanical valve, 117
  Doppler tracing of, 122
Melanoma, 185
Membranous subaortic stenosis,
  discrete, 213f
Metastatic cardiac tumors,
  188–189
Millar catheter, 62–63f
Mitral annulus area, 105
Mitral-aortic intervalvular fibrosa
  aneurysm, 133–135
Mitral balloon valvuloplasty,
  111–112
  echocardiography with, 230
  predicted outcome of, 98t
Mitral commissurotomy, open,
  221
Mitral flow. *See also* Diastolic fil-
    ling
  assessment of, 62, 64
  pattern of relaxation abnor-
    mality, 82
  pattern of restriction, 47–49,
    64
  velocities of, 47f
Mitral leaflet
  myxomatous flail of, 136f

reconstruction of, 223
Mitral regurgitant fraction,
  107f
Mitral regurgitant volume, 107f
Mitral valve
  flail myxomatous, 225f
  murmur of, 238
  myxomatous degeneration of,
    222–223
  progressive dyspnea and, 225f
  prolapse of, 225f, 238
  prosthetic
    degenerative, 125f
    Doppler hemodynamic pro-
      files of, 120t
    flow through, 126f
    intermittent failure to close,
      125f
    regurgitation of, 122f
  regurgitation of
    assessment of, 76
    blood flow in, 64
    Doppler/color-flow imaging
      of, 104–106
    in estimating regurgitant
      volume and fraction, 57f
    with hypertrophic cardiomy-
      opathy, 143–144
    with mitral stenosis, 99
    new quantitative approaches
      to, 106–109
    peak flow rate of, 108f
    severity of, 105–106
    two-dimensional and M-
      mode echocardiography
      of, 104–105
    velocity of, 61
  repair of
    indications for, 222–223
    intraoperative echocardiogra-
      phy in, 224f
    replacement of, 222–223
      persistent hypotension after,
        227f
    with ruptured chordae, 224f
  stenosis of, 231f
    Doppler and color-flow im-
      aging of, 96–100
    exercise hemodynamics in,
      100
    severity of, 96–97, 99
    two-dimensional echocardi-
      ography of, 96, 97f

Mitral valve area, 96, 97, 99
Multigated ultrasound beams,
  18
Multiplane probe, 31–33
Myectomy, 226f
Myocardial fibrosis, with sarcoidosis, 160–161
Myocardial infarction, acute
  chest pain with, 72–73, 239
  complications of, 67, 74t
    detection, 73–80
  diagnosis of, 84
  echocardiography for, 72–82,
    84
  post-infarction risk stratifica-
    tion in, 82
  prognostic risk stratification
    for, 67
  reperfusion therapy evaluation
    in, 80–81
Myocardial relaxation
  abnormal, 47
  with aging, 62, 64
Myocarditis, 162
Myocardium
  akinetic to dyskinetic, 189
  excessive iron deposit in, 159
  hibernating, 81–82
  ischemic, 67
    stress echocardiography in,
      229
  mass in, 41–43
  metastasis in, 158f
  salvage of, 67
  in sarcoidosis, 160–161
  stunned, 81–82
  toxins in, 162
  transient dysfunction of, 239
Myxoma, 185
  transesophageal echocardio-
    gram of, 187f
  transthoracic echocardiogram
    of, 186f

Neuromuscular disease, heart
  involvement in, 162
Nyquist frequency, 16
  limit of, 4, 19
Nyquist phenomenon, 17

Orthogonal longitudinal plane,
  23
Osteogenic sarcoma, 185

Outflow tract obstruction, 209–210

Papillary muscle rupture, 76, 77f
Parasternal short-axis views, 10f
Patent ductus arteriosus, 216
Patent foramen ovale, 78–79, 192f
  echocardiography with closure of, 230–231
  monitoring of, 232f, 233f
Peak aortic valve velocity, 89–90
Peak-to-peak gradient, 58
Pediatric congenital heart disease, 217
Percutaneous transluminar coronary angioplasty, 83
Pericardial cavity, 165–166
Pericardial effusion, 193f
  compromising loculated, 173–174
  detection of, 76–77, 165
  echocardiography of, 165–166, 167f
  first ultrasound detection of, 1
  versus pleural effusion, 173
  TEE four-chamber view of, 175f
Pericardiocentesis
  echo-guided, 166, 169f
  echocardiography with, 229–230
  site for, 175
Pericarditis, constrictive, 166–171
  data from patients with, 173t
  Doppler pattern of, 172f
  evaluation of, 174
  transient, 176
  versus restrictive cardiomyopathy, 150
Pericardium
  congenitally absent, 172, 173f
  cyst of, 173, 174f
  diseases of, 165–175
Pharmacologic stress echocardiography, 70–71
Pheochromocytoma, heart involvement in, 162
PHT. *See* Pressure half-time
PISAs, 106–108
Planimetry, 111

Pleural effusion
  versus pericardial effusion, 173
  two-dimensional imaging of, 175f
Pneumopericardium, 166
Precordial examination, 207
Pregnancy, heart disease in, 218
Pressure gradients
  of aortic prosthesis, 118–119f
  Doppler-derived, 88
    versus catheter-derived, 127
  equation for, 52
  mean, 89, 90
  in mitral valve stenosis, 96
Pressure half-time, 59–60
  from continuous-wave Doppler spectrum, 98f
  in mitral stenosis, 99
  in obstructed prosthetic valve, 121–122
  in regurgitant prosthetic valve, 123–124
  in valvular stenosis, 88
Pressure recovery phenomenon, 118
Prosthetic orifice area, effective, 123
Prosthetic valve
  classification of, 117; *See also* specific valves
  dysfunction of, 117–119
  echo reflectance with, 21
  evaluation of, 117–127
  obstruction of, 120–123
  regurgitation of, 123–124
Pseudoaneurysm, 80
  aortic, 201, 202f
Pseudonormalization, 49
Pseudotumor, 191–192
PTCA. *See* Percutaneous transluminar coronary angioplasty
Pulmonary arteries
  left, short-axis view of, 24f
  main, short-axis view of, 24f
  right, short-axis view of, 24f
  thromboembolism of, 177
Pulmonary arteriovenous fistula, 233f
Pulmonary artery pressure
  determination of, 97, 177
  end-diastolic, 61

  in mitral valve stenosis, 100
Pulmonary atresia, 214
  with ventricular septal defect, 217
Pulmonary embolism
  transesophageal echocardiography in, 183–184
  transthoracic echocardiography in, 182–183
Pulmonary flow
  calculation of, 55
  estimation of, 58f
Pulmonary hypertension, 177
  with cor pulmonale and pulmonary embolism, 182–184
  Doppler echocardiography in, 178–181
  pulmonary regurgitation with, 181
  with restrictive cardiomyopathy, 149
  two-dimensional echocardiography in, 177–178
Pulmonary-systemic flow ratio (Qp/Qs), 55
Pulmonary valve
  in carcinoid, 158f
  M-mode echocardiography of, 53f
  regurgitation of
    end-diastolic velocity of, 180–181
    velocity of, 61
Pulmonary vein
  flow velocities of, 48f, 49, 64
  systolic flow reversals of, 112
  TEE images of connections of, 37f
Pulmonary venous connections
  anomalous, 207–208
  partial anomalous (PAVC), 208
Pulse repetition frequency (PRF), 16

Q-tip appearance, 192, 193f

Rapid filling phase (RFP), 46
Reconstructive cardiac surgery, 222–223
Regional expansion selection (RES) function, 4

Regurgitant fraction, 55, 106
  estimation of, 57f, 106, 107f
  of regurgitant prosthetic valve,
    123–124
Regurgitant valve velocity, 60
Regurgitant volume, 55, 106
  estimation of, 57f, 103
Regurgitation, prosthetic valve,
  123–124
Relaxation abnormality, 46–47,
  62
  mitral flow pattern of, 82
Reperfusion therapy, 67
  evaluation of, 80–81
Restrictive cardiomyopathy
  primary, 149
  secondary, 150
Restrictive filling pattern, 82
Restrictive physiology, 47, 49, 62
Rhabdomyoma, 185
Rhabdomyosarcoma, 187
Right atrial thrombus, mobile,
  183, 188
Right ventricle
  end-diastolic pressure of, 61
  infarct of, 78–79, 184f
  M-mode echocardiography of,
    54f
  outflow of, 29f
Right ventricular outflow tract,
  55, 60–61
  flow acceleration time for, 180
  flow velocity acceleration time
    for, 181f
  in pulmonary flow estimation,
    58f
Risk stratification, post-myocardial infarction, 82

St. Jude prosthesis, 118
Sarcoidosis, 160–161
Septal hypertrophy, asymmetric,
  140–142, 162
Short-axis view
  in heart disease, 206
  of upper abdomen, 207
Shunt detection, 231–234
Simpson's method, modified, 41,
  43
Sonographer, role of in transesophageal echocardiog-
  raphy, 35–36

Spontaneous echo contrast, 189
Square root sign, 149
Straddling, 214
Streptokinase, 183
Stress echocardiography, 229
  caveats for technical and inter-
    pretation of, 72
  for coronary artery disease,
    70–71
Stroke volume
  across aortic valve, 92f
  calculation of, 56f
  measurement of, 52
Stunned myocardium, 81–82
Subclavian artery stenosis,
  95f
Suprasternal notch long-axis
  view, 13f
Systemic hypertension, 241–242
Systemic illness, heart disease
  due to, 153–162
Systemic lupus erythematosus
  (SLE), 161–162
Systolic function
  assessment of, 61–64
  global, 43–44
    decreased, 137
  regional, 44–46

Tamponade. *See* Cardiac Tamponade
Technical skills, 3, 72
TEE. *See* Transesophageal echocardiography
Tetralogy of Fallot, 214, 217
Three-dimensional imaging,
  218–219
Thromboembolism
  prediction of, 191
  pulmonary artery, 177
Thrombolytic therapy, 183
Thrombus
  left atrial, 190f
  mobile, 182–183
  pulmonary, 182–184
  versus tumors, 188–189
  ventricular, 80
Time constant of left ventricular
  relaxation (TAV), 64–65
Time velocity integral ratio,
  90–93, 94f, 122–123
Time velocity integral (TVI), 52,

55f
  measurement of, 56f
Tissue characterization, 2
Tissue valve, 117
Tomographic imaging planes,
  long and short, 7
Tomography, 205–206
Training
  guidelines and levels of, 2–3
  for transesophageal echocardi-
    ographer, 35–36
Transducers, 4
  aortic stenosis evaluation posi-
    tions of, 91f
  optimal position of, 72
  precordial position of, 207
  rotating multiplane, 31
  standard transthoracic posi-
    tions of, 7, 8–9f
  for transesophageal echocardi-
    ography, 21
Transesophageal
  echocardiographic probes,
    4f
Transesophageal echocardiography, 2, 21
  anatomic correlations in,
    22–34
  in aortic disease, 196–202
  in aortic dissection, 198–200
  in aortic regurgitation, 101
  in atrial septal defect, 234
  in carcinoid, 158
  clinical applications of, 35
  complications with, 35
  in comprehensive examina-
    tion, 238–241
  in congenital heart disease,
    210–215, 218–219
  in coronary artery visualiza-
    tion, 83
  of degenerative mitral prosthe-
    sis, 125f
  of dehisced aortic prosthesis,
    126f
  in detecting myocardial in-
    farction complications,
    73–74, 77f
  in endocarditis, 130–132,
    133–135
  future development of, 36–
    37

in hypertrophic cardiomyopathy, 146–147
indications for, 35t
instrumentation for, 21–22
intraoperative, 221–227
in mitral balloon valvuloplasty, 230, 231f
in patent foramen ovale monitoring, 232f, 233f
patient preparation for, 22
in pericardial disease, 173–175
of prosthetic valve, 122f, 124
in pulmonary embolism and cor pulmonale, 183–184
in pulmonary hypertension, 177
training for and sonographer in, 35–36
in tumors and masses, 189–191
in valvular heart disease assessment, 110–112
Transesophageal probe, 21
Transgastric views
long-axis, 32–33f
longitudinal, 30f
multiplane, 32–33f
short-axis, 26–27f, 32–33f
Transmitral pressure change, 46
Transposition of great arteries, corrected, 215f
Transthoracic echocardiography
in aortic dissection, 196–197
color-flow imaging, 18–19
Doppler, 15–17
M-mode and two-dimensional, 7–15
Transvalvular gradients, 55–58
Treadmill exercise, with echo images, 70
Tricuspid flow assessment, 62–64
Tricuspid inflow velocities, 171f
Tricuspid valve
abnormalities of in carcinoid, 157–159
atresia of, 215f
prosthetic, Doppler hemodynamic profiles of, 120t
regurgitation of
blood flow in, 64
Doppler/color-flow imaging of, 109–110

two-dimensional and M-mode echocardiography of, 109
velocity of, 60, 178–180
Truncus arteriosus, 217
Tumors
metastatic, 188–189
primary cardiac, 185–188
transesophageal echocardiography for, 189–191
Turbulence, detection of, 19
Two-dimensional echocardiography
of anatomic sections, 9f, 11f, 12f
in aortic stenosis assessment, 88–89
in cardiac disease due to systemic illness, 153–162
in chest pain syndrome evaluation, 72–73
in comprehensive examination, 238, 240
in congenital heart disease, 206–207, 208, 209
in constrictive pericarditis, 166–170
in detecting myocardial infarction complications, 73–76, 79
in dilated cardiomyopathy, 137–139
in emergency room, 73
heart chamber measurements of, 40t
in hemodynamic assessment, 51–52, 54f
in hypertrophic cardiomyopathy, 140–143
in mitral stenosis assessment, 96, 97f
in pericardial effusion, 166
with pericardiocentesis, 229–230
in pulmonary hypertension, 177–178
of stenotic aortic valve, 93f
in valvular regurgitation evaluation, 100, 101, 104, 109
in valvular stenosis evaluation, 87–88

Uhl's anomaly, 139–140
Ulcer, aortic, 195
Ultrasonography
high-frequency, 1
intravascular, 84
Ultrasound units, equipment for, 3–5

V waves, 110
Valve area
continuity equation for, 58–59
pressure half-time and, 59–60
Valvular heart disease, 87–113
infective endocarditis and, 129
integrated approach to, 113
tricuspid regurgitation in, 110
Valvular regurgitation
evaluation of, 100–110
integrated approach to assessing, 101
in normal subjects, 110
PISA and, 106–109
transesophageal echocardiography for, 112
Valvular stenosis, 87–100
Valvular vegetation
complications from, 132–133
limitations to detection of, 135
Variance, turbulence, 19
Vegetations
complications from, 132–133
limitations to detection of, 135
as mobile masses, 130, 131f
Venous flow, 49
Ventricles. *See also* Left ventricle; Right ventricle
aneurysms of, 79–80
assessment of function of, 39–50
evaluation of function of, 237–238
systolic function of in cardiomyopathies, 137
thrombus of
detection of, 80
versus tumors, 188–189
Ventricular septum
defect of
detection of, 73–76
echocardiographic examination of, 214–216

Ventricular septum, defect of—
  Continued
    membranous, 216f
    diffuse hypertrophy of, 142
    hypertrophic, 140–142
Ventricular wall thickness
    abnormal, 67–68
    with amyloidosis, 154, 156
    increased, 153

Venturi effect, 140

Wall motion
    abnormalities of exercise-in-
      duced regional, 70
    regional, 46
    analysis of
      interpretation of stress echo-
        cardiography by, 71t

    regional, 44–46, 67–69
Wall motion score index, 46,
    68–69, 238
    with myocardial infarction, 83f
    in post-myocardial infarction
      risk stratification, 82
Wide-field imaging, 218–219
WMSI. *See* Wall motion score
    index